*Skill Checklists for*

# Taylor's Clinical Nursing Skills

## A NURSING PROCESS APPROACH

**THIRD EDITION**

**Pamela Lynn, MSN, RN**
Instructor
School of Nursing
Gwynedd-Mercy College
Gwynedd Valley, Pennsylvania

**Marilee LeBon, BA**
Editor
Brigantine, New Jersey

. Wolters Kluwer | Lippincott Williams & Wilkins
Health
Philadelphia · Baltimore · New York · London
Buenos Aires · Hong Kong · Sydney · Tokyo

*Executive Acquisitions Editor:* Carrie Brandon
*Product Manager:* Helene T. Caprari
*Design Coordinator:* Holly McLaughlin
*Manufacturing Coordinator:* Karin Duffield
*Prepress Vendor:* Aptara, Inc.

3rd edition

9 8 7 6 5 4 3 2

Printed in the United States of America.

ISBN: 978-0-7817-9518-0

LWW.com

# Introduction

Developing clinical competency is a major challenge for each fundamentals student. To facilitate the mastery of nursing skills, we are happy to provide Skill Checklists for each skill in *Taylor Clinical Nursing Skills: A Nursing Process Approach,* 3rd edition. The skill checklists follow each step of the skill to provide a complete evaluative tool. Students can use the checklists to facilitate self-evaluation, and faculty will find them useful in measuring and recording student performance. Three-hole punched and perforated, these checklists can be easily reproduced and brought to the simulation laboratory or clinical area. The checklists are designed to record an evaluation of each step of the skill.

- Checkmark in the "Excellent" column denotes mastering the procedure.
- Checkmark in the "Satisfactory" column indicates use of the recommended technique.
- Checkmark in the "Needs Practice" column indicates use of some but not all of each recommended technique.

The Comments section allows you to highlight suggestions that will improve skills. Space is available at the top of each checklist to record a final pass/fail evaluation, date, and the signature of the student and evaluating faculty member.

# List of Skills by Chapter

**Chapter 1    Vital Signs**
**Skill 1-1:**    Assessing Body Temperature    1
**Skill 1-2:**    Monitoring Temperature Using an Overhead Radiant Warmer    5
**Skill 1-3:**    Using a Cooling Blanket    6
**Skill 1-4:**    Assessing a Peripheral Pulse by Palpation    8
**Skill 1-5:**    Assessing the Apical Pulse by Auscultation    9
**Skill 1-6:**    Assessing Respiration    10
**Skill 1-7:**    Assessing Brachial Artery Blood Pressure    11

**Chapter 2    Health Assessment**
**Skill 2-1:**    Performing a General Survey    14
**Skill 2-2:**    Using a Bed Scale    16
**Skill 2-3:**    Assessing the Skin, Hair, and Nails    18
**Skill 2-4:**    Assessing the Head and Neck    20
**Skill 2-5:**    Assessing the Thorax and Lungs    23
**Skill 2-6:**    Assessing the Cardiovascular System    25
**Skill 2-7:**    Assessing the Abdomen    27
**Skill 2-8:**    Assessing the Neurologic, Musculoskeletal, and Peripheral Vascular Systems    29

**Chapter 3    Safety**
**Skill 3-1:**    Fall Prevention    32
**Skill 3-2:**    Implementing Alternatives to the Use of Restraints    34
**Skill 3-3:**    Applying an Extremity Restraint    36
**Skill 3-4:**    Applying a Waist Restraint    38
**Skill 3-5:**    Applying an Elbow Restraint    40
**Skill 3-6:**    Applying a Mummy Restraint    42

**Chapter 4    Asepsis and Infection Control**
**Skill 4-1:**    Performing Hand Hygiene Using Soap and Water (Handwashing)    43
**Skill 4-2:**    Performing Hand Hygiene Using an Alcohol-Based Hand Rub    44
**Skill 4-3:**    Preparing a Sterile Field Using a Packaged Sterile Drape    45
**Skill 4-4:**    Preparing a Sterile Field Using a Commercially Prepared Sterile Kit or Tray    46
**Skill 4-5:**    Adding Sterile Items to a Sterile Field    48
**Skill 4-6:**    Putting on Sterile Gloves and Removing Soiled Gloves    50
**Skill 4-7:**    Using Personal Protective Equipment    52

**Chapter 5    Medications**
**Skill 5-1:**    Administering Oral Medications    54
**Skill 5-2:**    Administering Medications via a Gastric Tube    57
**Skill 5-3:**    Removing Medication from an Ampule    60
**Skill 5-4:**    Removing Medication from a Vial    62
**Skill 5-5:**    Mixing Medications From Two Vials in One Syringe    64
**Skill 5-6:**    Administering an Intradermal Injection    66
**Skill 5-7:**    Administering a Subcutaneous Injection    69
**Skill 5-8:**    Administering an Intramuscular Injection    72
**Skill 5-9:**    Administering Continuous Subcutaneous Infusion: Applying an Insulin Pump    75
**Skill 5-10:**    Administering Medications by Intravenous Bolus or Push Through an Intravenous Infusion    78
**Skill 5-11:**    Administering a Piggyback Intermittent Intravenous Infusion of Medication    81

**Skill 5-12:**   Administering an Intermittent Intravenous Infusion of Medication via a Mini-infusion Pump   84
**Skill 5-13:**   Administering an Intermittent Intravenous Infusion of Medication via a Volume-Control Administration Set   87
**Skill 5-14:**   Introducing Drugs Through a Medication or Drug-Infusion Lock Using the Saline Flush (Intermittent Peripheral Venous Access Device)   90
**Skill 5-15:**   Applying a Transdermal Patch   93
**Skill 5-16:**   Instilling Eye Drops   95
**Skill 5-17:**   Administering an Eye Irrigation   98
**Skill 5-18:**   Instilling Ear Drops   100
**Skill 5-19:**   Administering an Ear Irrigation   102
**Skill 5-20:**   Instilling Nose Drops   104
**Skill 5-21:**   Administering a Vaginal Cream   106
**Skill 5-22:**   Administering a Rectal Suppository   109
**Skill 5-23:**   Administering Medication via a Metered-Dose Inhaler (MDI)   111
**Skill 5-24:**   Administering Medication via a Small-Volume Nebulizer   113
**Skill 5-25:**   Administering Medication via a Dry Powder Inhaler   115

**Chapter 6**   **Perioperative Nursing**
**Skill 6-1:**   Providing Preoperative Patient Care: Hospitalized Patient   117
**Skill 6-2:**   Deep Breathing Exercises, Coughing, and Splinting   120
**Skill 6-3:**   Leg Exercises   122
**Skill 6-4:**   Providing Preoperative Patient Care: Hospitalized Patient (Day of Surgery)   123
**Skill 6-5:**   Providing Postoperative Care When Patient Returns to Room   125
**Skill 6-6:**   Applying a Forced-Air Warming Device   128

**Chapter 7**   **Hygiene**
**Skill 7-1:**   Giving a Bed Bath   129
**Skill 7-2:**   Assisting the Patient With Oral Care   132
**Skill 7-3:**   Providing Oral Care for the Dependent Patient   134
**Skill 7-4:**   Providing Denture Care   135
**Skill 7-5:**   Removing Contact Lenses   136
**Skill 7-6:**   Shampooing a Patient's Hair in Bed   137
**Skill 7-7:**   Assisting the Patient to Shave   139
**Skill 7-8:**   Making an Unoccupied Bed   140
**Skill 7-9:**   Making an Occupied Bed   142

**Chapter 8**   **Skin Integrity and Wound Care**
**Skill 8-1:**   Cleaning a Wound and Applying a Dry, Sterile Dressing   144
**Skill 8-2:**   Applying a Saline-Moistened Dressing   147
**Skill 8-3:**   Applying a Hydrocolloid Dressing   149
**Skill 8-4:**   Performing Irrigation of a Wound   151
**Skill 8-5:**   Collecting a Wound Culture   153
**Skill 8-6:**   Applying Montgomery Straps   155
**Skill 8-7:**   Caring for a Penrose Drain   157
**Skill 8-8:**   Caring for a T-Tube Drain   159
**Skill 8-9:**   Caring for a Jackson-Pratt Drain   162
**Skill 8-10:**   Caring for a Hemovac Drain   164
**Skill 8-11:**   Applying Negative Pressure Wound Therapy   166
**Skill 8-12:**   Removing Sutures   169
**Skill 8-13:**   Removing Surgical Staples   171
**Skill 8-14:**   Applying an External Heating Pad   173
**Skill 8-15:**   Applying a Warm Compress   175
**Skill 8-16:**   Assisting With a Sitz Bath   177
**Skill 8-17:**   Applying Cold Therapy   178

**Chapter 9**   **Activity**
**Skill 9-1:**   Assisting a Patient With Turning in Bed   180
**Skill 9-2:**   Moving a Patient Up in Bed With the Assistance of Another Nurse   182
**Skill 9-3:**   Transferring a Patient From the Bed to a Stretcher   184

Skill 9-4:     Transferring a Patient From the Bed to a Chair  186
Skill 9-5:     Transferring a Patient Using a Powered Full-Body Sling Lift  188
Skill 9-6:     Providing Range-of-Motion Exercises  190
Skill 9-7:     Assisting a Patient With Ambulation  192
Skill 9-8:     Assisting a Patient With Ambulation Using a Walker  194
Skill 9-9:     Assisting a Patient With Ambulation Using Crutches  196
Skill 9-10:    Assisting a Patient With Ambulation Using a Cane  198
Skill 9-11:    Applying and Removing Antiembolism Stockings  199
Skill 9-12:    Applying Pneumatic Compression Devices  201
Skill 9-13:    Applying a Continuous Passive Motion Device  203
Skill 9-14:    Applying a Sling  205
Skill 9-15:    Applying a Figure-Eight Bandage  206
Skill 9-16:    Assisting With Cast Application  208
Skill 9-17:    Caring for a Cast  210
Skill 9-18:    Applying Skin Traction and Caring for a Patient in Skin Traction  212
Skill 9-19:    Caring for a Patient in Skeletal Traction  214
Skill 9-20:    Caring for a Patient With an External Fixation Device  216

Chapter 10    Comfort
Skill 10-1:    Promoting Patient Comfort  218
Skill 10-2:    Giving a Back Massage  222
Skill 10-3:    Applying and Caring for a Patient Using a TENS Unit  224
Skill 10-4:    Caring for a Patient Receiving Patient-Controlled Analgesia  226
Skill 10-5:    Caring for a Patient Receiving Epidural Analgesia  228
Skill 10-6:    Caring for a Patient Receiving Continuous Wound Perfusion Pain Management  230

Chapter 11    Nutrition
Skill 11-1:    Assisting a Patient With Eating  232
Skill 11-2:    Inserting a Nasogastric (NG) Tube  234
Skill 11-3:    Administering a Tube Feeding  237
Skill 11-4:    Removing a Nasogastric Tube  240
Skill 11-5:    Caring for a Gastrostomy Tube  241

Chapter 12    Urinary Elimination
Skill 12-1:    Assisting With the Use of a Bedpan  243
Skill 12-2:    Assisting With the Use of a Urinal  245
Skill 12-3:    Assisting With the Use of a Bedside Commode  247
Skill 12-4:    Assessing Bladder Volume Using an Ultrasound Bladder Scanner  249
Skill 12-5:    Applying an External Condom Catheter  251
Skill 12-6:    Catheterizing the Female Urinary Bladder  253
Skill 12-7:    Catheterizing the Male Urinary Bladder  256
Skill 12-8:    Removing an Indwelling Catheter  259
Skill 12-9:    Performing Intermittent Closed Catheter Irrigation  260
Skill 12-10:   Administering a Continuous Closed Bladder Irrigation  262
Skill 12-11:   Emptying and Changing a Stoma Appliance on an Ileal Conduit  264
Skill 12-12:   Caring for a Suprapubic Urinary Catheter  266
Skill 12-13:   Caring for a Peritoneal Dialysis Catheter  268
Skill 12-14:   Caring for a Hemodialysis Access (Arteriovenous Fistula or Graft)  270

Chapter 13    Bowel Elimination
Skill 13-1:    Administering a Large-Volume Cleansing Enema  271
Skill 13-2:    Administering a Small-Volume Cleansing Enema  273
Skill 13-3:    Administering a Retention Enema  275
Skill 13-4:    Digital Removal of Stool  277
Skill 13-5:    Applying a Fecal Incontinence Pouch  279
Skill 13-6:    Changing and Emptying an Ostomy Appliance  280
Skill 13-7:    Irrigating a Colostomy  282
Skill 13-8:    Irrigating a Nasogastric Tube Connected to Suction  284

**Chapter 14   Oxygenation**
**Skill 14-1:**    Using a Pulse Oximeter   286
**Skill 14-2:**    Teaching Patient to Use an Incentive Spirometer   288
**Skill 14-3:**    Administering Oxygen by Nasal Cannula   290
**Skill 14-4:**    Administering Oxygen by Mask   291
**Skill 14-5:**    Using an Oxygen Tent   292
**Skill 14-6:**    Suctioning the Nasopharyngeal and Oropharyngeal Airways   293
**Skill 14-7:**    Inserting an Oropharyngeal Airway   296
**Skill 14-8:**    Suctioning an Endotracheal Tube: Open System   298
**Skill 14-9:**    Suctioning an Endotracheal Tube: Closed System   301
**Skill 14-10:**   Securing an Endotracheal Tube   304
**Skill 14-11:**   Suctioning the Tracheostomy: Open System   307
**Skill 14-12:**   Providing Tracheostomy Care   310
**Skill 14-13:**   Providing Care of a Chest Drainage System   313
**Skill 14-14:**   Assisting With Removal of a Chest Tube   315
**Skill 14-15:**   Using a Handheld Resuscitation Bag and Mask   316

**Chapter 15   Fluid, Electrolyte, and Acid–Base Balance**
**Skill 15-1:**    Initiating a Peripheral Venous Access IV Infusion   318
**Skill 15-2:**    Changing an IV Solution Container and Administration Set   322
**Skill 15-3:**    Monitoring an IV Site and Infusion   325
**Skill 15-4:**    Changing a Peripheral Venous Access Dressing   327
**Skill 15-5:**    Capping for Intermittent Use and Flushing a Peripheral Venous Access Device   329
**Skill 15-6:**    Administering a Blood Transfusion   330
**Skill 15-7:**    Changing the Dressing and Flushing Central Venous Access Devices   333
**Skill 15-8:**    Accessing an Implanted Port   335
**Skill 15-9:**    Deaccessing an Implanted Port   337
**Skill 15-10:**   Removing a Peripherally Inserted Central Catheter (PICC)   339

**Chapter 16   Cardiovascular Care**
**Skill 16-1:**    Obtaining an Electrocardiogram (ECG)   340
**Skill 16-2:**    Applying a Cardiac Monitor   343
**Skill 16-3:**    Obtaining an Arterial Blood Sample From an Arterial Line–Stopcock System   345
**Skill 16-4:**    Removing Arterial and Femoral Lines   347
**Skill 16-5:**    Performing Cardiopulmonary Resuscitation (CPR)   349
**Skill 16-6:**    Performing Emergency Automated External Defibrillation   351
**Skill 16-7:**    Performing Emergency Manual External Defibrillation (Asynchronous)   353
**Skill 16-8:**    Using an External (Transcutaneous) Pacemaker   355

**Chapter 17   Neurologic Care**
**Skill 17-1:**    Logrolling a Patient   358
**Skill 17-2:**    Applying a Two-Piece Cervical Collar   360
**Skill 17-3:**    Employing Seizure Precautions and Seizure Management   362
**Skill 17-4:**    Caring for a Patient in Halo Traction   364
**Skill 17-5:**    Caring for a Patient with an External Ventriculostomy (Intraventricular Catheter–Closed Fluid-Filled System)   366
**Skill 17-6:**    Caring for a Patient With a Fiber Optic Intracranial Catheter   368

**Chapter 18   Laboratory Specimen Collection**
**Skill 18-1:**    Testing Stool for Occult Blood   369
**Skill 18-2:**    Collecting a Stool Specimen for Culture   371
**Skill 18-3:**    Obtaining a Capillary Blood Sample for Glucose Testing   372
**Skill 18-4:**    Obtaining a Nasal Swab   374
**Skill 18-5:**    Obtaining a Nasopharyngeal Swab   376
**Skill 18-6:**    Collecting a Sputum Specimen for Culture   378
**Skill 18-7:**    Collecting a Urine Specimen (Clean Catch, Midstream) for Urinalysis and Culture   380
**Skill 18-8:**    Obtaining a Urine Specimen From an Indwelling Urinary Catheter   382
**Skill 18-9:**    Using Venipuncture to Collect a Venous Blood Sample for Routine Testing   384
**Skill 18-10:**   Obtaining a Venous Blood Specimen for Culture and Sensitivity   387
**Skill 18-11:**   Obtaining an Arterial Blood Specimen for Blood Gas Analysis   390

# List of Skills in Alphabetical Order

**Skill 2-7:** Abdomen, Assessing the 27
**Skill 9-7:** Ambulation, Assisting a Patient With 192
**Skill 9-10:** Ambulation Using a Cane, Assisting a Patient With 198
**Skill 9-9:** Ambulation Using Crutches, Assisting a Patient With 212
**Skill 9-8:** Ambulation Using a Walker, Assisting a Patient With 194
**Skill 9-11:** Antiembolism Stockings, Applying and Removing 199
**Skill 16-4:** Arterial and Femoral Lines, Removing 347
**Skill 10-2:** Back Massage, Giving a 222
**Skill 9-1:** Bed, Assisting a Patient With Turning in 000
**Skill 7-9:** Bed, Making an Occupied 142
**Skill 7-8:** Bed, Making an Unoccupied 140
**Skill 12-1:** Bedpan, Assisting With the Use of a 243
**Skill 12-3:** Bedside Commode, Assisting With the Use of a 247
**Skill 7-1:** Bed Bath, Giving a 129
**Skill 2-2:** Bed Scale, Using a 16
**Skill 12-10:** Bladder Irrigation, Administering a Continuous Closed 262
**Skill 12-4:** Bladder Volume Using an Ultrasound Bladder Scanner, Assessing 249
**Skill 1-7:** Blood Pressure, Assessing Brachial Artery 11
**Skill 18-9:** Blood Sample for Routine Testing, Using Venipuncture to Collect a Venous 384
**Skill 16-3:** Blood Sample From an Arterial Line–Stopcock System, Obtaining an Arterial 345
**Skill 18-11:** Blood Specimen for Blood Gas Analysis, Obtaining an Arterial 390
**Skill 18-10:** Blood Specimen for Culture and Sensitivity, Obtaining a Venous 387
**Skill 15-6:** Blood Transfusion, Administering a 330
**Skill 6-2:** Breathing Exercises, Deep: Coughing, and Splinting 120
**Skill 16-2:** Cardiac Monitor, Applying a 343
**Skill 16-5:** Cardiopulmonary Resuscitation (CPR), Performing 349
**Skill 2-6:** Cardiovascular System, Assessing the 25
**Skill 9-17:** Cast, Caring for a 210
**Skill 9-16:** Cast Application, Assisting With 208
**Skill 12-5:** Catheter, Applying an External Condom 251
**Skill 17-6:** Catheter, Caring for a Patient With a Fiber Optic Intracranial 368
**Skill 12-13:** Catheter, Caring for a Peritoneal Dialysis 247
**Skill 12-12:** Catheter, Caring for a Suprapubic Urinary 266
**Skill 18-8:** Catheter, Obtaining a Urine Specimen From an Indwelling Urinary 382
**Skill 12-8:** Catheter, Removing an Indwelling 259
**Skill 12-9:** Catheter Irrigation, Performing Intermittent Closed 260
**Skill 15-10:** Catheter (PICC), Removing a Peripherally Inserted Central 339
**Skill 12-6:** Catheterizing the Female Urinary Bladder 253
**Skill 12-7:** Catheterizing the Male Urinary Bladder 256
**Skill 15-7:** Central Venous Access Devices, Changing the Dressing and Flushing 333
**Skill 17-2:** Cervical Collar, Applying a Two-Piece 360
**Skill 14-13:** Chest Drainage System, Providing Care of a 290
**Skill 14-14:** Chest Tube, Assisting With Removal of a 315
**Skill 8-17:** Cold Therapy, Applying 178
**Skill 13-7:** Colostomy, Irrigating a 282
**Skill 10-1:** Comfort, Promoting Patient 218
**Skill 8-15:** Compress, Applying a Warm 175
**Skill 7-5:** Contact Lenses, Removing 136
**Skill 1-3:** Cooling Blanket, Using a 6

x **Contents**

**Skill 16-6:** Defibrillation, Performing Emergency Automated External  351
**Skill 16-7:** Defibrillation (Asynchronous), Performing Emergency Manual External  353
**Skill 7-4:** Denture Care, Providing  135
**Skill 8-10:** Drain, Caring for a Hemovac  164
**Skill 8-9:** Drain, Caring for a Jackson-Pratt  162
**Skill 8-7:** Drain, Caring for a Penrose  157
**Skill 8-8:** Drain, Caring for a T-Tube  159
**Skill 8-3:** Dressing, Applying a Hydrocolloid  149
**Skill 8-2:** Dressing, Applying a Saline-Moistened  147
**Skill 5-14:** Drug-Infusion Lock (Intermittent Peripheral Venous Access Device) Using the Saline Flush, Introducing Drugs Through a Medication or  90
**Skill 5-25:** Dry Powder Inhaler, Administering Medication via a  115
**Skill 5-18:** Ear Drops, Instilling  100
**Skill 5-19:** Ear Irrigation, Administering an  102
**Skill 11-1:** Eating, Assisting a Patient With  232
**Skill 16-1:** Electrocardiogram (ECG), Obtaining an  340
**Skill 14-8:** Endotracheal Tube: Open System, Suctioning an  298
**Skill 14-9:** Endotracheal Tube: Closed System, Suctioning an  301
**Skill 14-10:** Endotracheal Tube, Securing an  304
**Skill 13-1:** Enema, Administering a Large-Volume Cleansing  271
**Skill 13-3:** Enema, Administering a Retention  275
**Skill 13-2:** Enema, Administering a Small-Volume Cleansing  273
**Skill 10-5:** Epidural Analgesia, Caring for a Patient Receiving  228
**Skill 6-3:** Exercises, Leg  122
**Skill 9-6:** Exercises, Providing Range-of-Motion  190
**Skill 9-20:** External Fixation Device, Caring for a Patient With an  216
**Skill 5-16:** Eye Drops, Instilling  95
**Skill 5-17:** Eye Irrigation, Administering an  98
**Skill 3-1:** Fall Prevention  32
**Skill 13-5:** Fecal Incontinence Pouch, Applying a  279
**Skill 9-15:** Figure-Eight Bandage, Applying a  206
**Skill 6-6:** Forced-Air Warming Device, Applying a  128
**Skill 5-2:** Gastric Tube, Administering Medications via a  57
**Skill 11-5:** Gastrostomy Tube, Caring for a  241
**Skill 2-1:** General Survey, Performing a  14
**Skill 4-6:** Gloves, Putting on Sterile Gloves and Removing Soiled  50
**Skill 18-3:** Glucose Testing, Obtaining a Capillary Blood Sample for  372
**Skill 4-2:** Hand Hygiene, Performing: Using an Alcohol-Based Hand Rub  44
**Skill 4-1:** Hand Hygiene, Performing: Using Soap and Water (Handwashing)  43
**Skill 2-4:** Head and Neck, Assessing the  20
**Skill 8-14:** Heating Pad, Applying an External  173
**Skill 12-14:** Hemodialysis Access (Arteriovenous Fistula or Graft), Caring for a  270
**Skill 14-2:** Incentive Spirometer, Teaching Patient to Use an  288
**Skill 5-7:** Injection, Administering a Subcutaneous  69
**Skill 5-6:** Injection, Administering an Intradermal  66
**Skill 5-8:** Injection, Administering an Intramuscular  72
**Skill 5-10:** Intravenous Infusion, Administering Medications by Intravenous Bolus or Push Through an  75
**Skill 5-11:** Intravenous Infusion of Medication, Administering a Piggyback Intermittent  81
**Skill 5-12:** Intravenous Infusion of Medication via a Mini-Infusion Pump, Administering an Intermittent  84
**Skill 5-13:** Intravenous Infusion of Medication via a Volume-Control Administration Set, Administering an Intermittent  87
**Skill 5-9:** Insulin Pump, Applying an: Administering Continuous Subcutaneous Infusion  75
**Skill 15-1:** IV Infusion, Initiating a Peripheral Venous Access  318
**Skill 15-3:** IV Site and Infusion, Monitoring an  325
**Skill 15-2:** IV Solution Container and Administration Set, Changing an  322
**Skill 17-1:** Logrolling a Patient  358
**Skill 5-3:** Medication, Removing From an Ampule  60
**Skill 5-4:** Medication, Removing From a Vial  62
**Skill 5-1:** Medications, Administering Oral  54

**Skill 5-5:**    Medications, Mixing From Two Vials in One Syringe   64
**Skill 5-23:**   Metered-Dose Inhaler (MDI), Administering Medication via a   111
**Skill 8-6:**    Montgomery Straps, Applying   155
**Skill 9-2:**    Moving a Patient Up in Bed With the Assistance of Another Nurse   182
**Skill 18-4:**   Nasal Swab, Obtaining a   374
**Skill 11-2:**   Nasogastric (NG) Tube, Inserting a   234
**Skill 13-8:**   Nasogastric Tube Connected to Suction, Irrigating a   284
**Skill 11-4:**   Nasogastric Tube, Removing a   240
**Skill 14-6:**   Nasopharyngeal and Oropharyngeal Airways, Suctioning the   293
**Skill 18-5:**   Nasopharyngeal Swab, Obtaining a   376
**Skill 5-24:**   Nebulizer, Administering Medication via a Small-Volume   113
**Skill 2-8:**    Neurologic, Musculoskeletal, and Peripheral Vascular Systems, Assessing the   29
**Skill 5-20:**   Nose Drops, Instilling   104
**Skill 18-1:**   Occult Blood, Testing Stool for   369
**Skill 7-2:**    Oral Care, Assisting the Patient With   132
**Skill 7-3:**    Oral Care for the Dependent Patient, Providing   134
**Skill 14-7:**   Oropharyngeal Airway, Inserting an   296
**Skill 13-6:**   Ostomy Appliance, Changing and Emptying an   280
**Skill 14-4:**   Oxygen by Mask, Administering   291
**Skill 14-3:**   Oxygen by Nasal Cannula, Administering   290
**Skill 14-5:**   Oxygen Tent, Using an   292
**Skill 16-8:**   Pacemaker, Using an External (Transcutaneous)   355
**Skill 9-13:**   Passive Motion Device, Applying a Continuous   203
**Skill 10-4:**   Patient-Controlled Analgesia, Caring for a Patient Receiving   226
**Skill 15-5:**   Peripheral Venous Access Device, Capping for Intermittent Use and Flushing a   329
**Skill 15-4:**   Peripheral Venous Access Dressing, Changing a   327
**Skill 4-7:**    Personal Protective Equipment, Using   52
**Skill 9-12:**   Pneumatic Compression Devices, Applying   201
**Skill 15-8:**   Port, Accessing an Implanted   335
**Skill 15-9:**   Port, Deaccessing an Implanted   337
**Skill 6-5:**    Postoperative Care When Patient Returns to Room, Providing   125
**Skill 6-4:**    Preoperative Patient Care: Hospitalized Patient (Day of Surgery), Providing   123
**Skill 6-1:**    Preoperative Patient Care: Hospitalized Patient, Providing   117
**Skill 1-5:**    Pulse by Auscultation, Assessing the Apical   9
**Skill 1-4:**    Pulse by Palpation, Assessing a Peripheral   8
**Skill 14-1:**   Pulse Oximeter, Using a   286
**Skill 5-22:**   Rectal Suppository, Administering a   109
**Skill 1-6:**    Respiration, Assessing   10
**Skill 3-5:**    Restraint, Applying an Elbow   40
**Skill 3-3:**    Restraint, Applying an Extremity   36
**Skill 3-6:**    Restraint, Applying a Mummy   42
**Skill 3-4:**    Restraint, Applying a Wrist   42
**Skill 3-2:**    Restraints, Implementing Alternatives to the Use of   34
**Skill 14-15:**  Resuscitation Bag and Mask, Using a Handheld   316
**Skill 17-3:**   Seizure Precautions and Seizure Management, Employing   362
**Skill 7-6:**    Shampooing a Patient's Hair in Bed   137
**Skill 7-7:**    Shave, Assisting the Patient to   139
**Skill 8-16:**   Sitz Bath, Assisting With a   177
**Skill 2-3:**    Skin, Hair, and Nails; Assessing the   18
**Skill 9-14:**   Sling, Applying a   205
**Skill 18-6:**   Sputum Specimen for Culture, Collecting a   378
**Skill 4-5:**    Sterile Field, Adding Sterile Items to a   48
**Skill 4-4:**    Sterile Field Using a Commercially Prepared Sterile Kit or Tray, Preparing a   46
**Skill 4-3:**    Sterile Field Using a Packaged Sterile Drape, Preparing a   45
**Skill 12-11:**  Stoma Appliance on an Ileal Conduit, Emptying and Changing a   243
**Skill 13-4:**   Stool, Digital Removal of   277
**Skill 18-2:**   Stool Specimen for Culture, Collecting a   371
**Skill 8-13:**   Surgical Staples, Removing   171
**Skill 8-12:**   Sutures, Removing   169

xii   **Contents**

**Skill 1-1:**   Temperature, Assessing Body   1
**Skill 1-2:**   Temperature, Monitoring Using an Overhead Radiant Warmer,   5
**Skill 10-3:**   TENS Unit, Applying and Caring for a Patient Using a   224
**Skill 2-5:**   Thorax and Lungs, Assessing the   23
**Skill 14-12:**   Tracheostomy Care, Providing   310
**Skill 14-11:**   Tracheostomy: Open System, Suctioning the   307
**Skill 9-18:**   Traction, Applying Skin Traction and Caring for a Patient in Skin   212
**Skill 17-4:**   Traction, Caring for a Patient in Halo   364
**Skill 9-19:**   Traction, Caring for a Patient in Skeletal   214
**Skill 5-15:**   Transdermal Patch, Applying a   93
**Skill 9-4:**   Transferring a Patient From the Bed to a Chair   186
**Skill 9-3:**   Transferring a Patient From the Bed to a Stretcher   184
**Skill 9-5:**   Transferring a Patient Using a Powered Full-Body Sling Lift   188
**Skill 11-3:**   Tube Feeding, Administering a   237
**Skill 12-2:**   Urinal, Assisting With the Use of a   245
**Skill 18-7:**   Urine Specimen (Clean Catch, Midstream) for Urinalysis and Culture, Collecting a   382
**Skill 5-21:**   Vaginal Cream, Administering a   105
**Skill 17-5:**   Ventriculostomy (Intraventricular Catheter-Closed Fluid-Filled System), Caring for a Patient With an External   366
**Skill 8-1:**   Wound, Cleaning a, and Applying a Dry Sterile Dressing   144
**Skill 8-4:**   Wound, Performing Irrigation of a   151
**Skill 10-6:**   Wound Perfusion Pain Management, Caring for a Patient Receiving Continuous   230
**Skill 8-5:**   Wound Culture, Collecting a   153
**Skill 8-11:**   Wound Therapy, Applying Negative Pressure   166

*Skill Checklists for Taylor's Clinical Nursing Skills:*
*A Nursing Process Approach, 3rd edition*

Name _____   Date _____

Unit _____   Position _____

Instructor/Evaluator: _____   Position _____

| Excellent | Satisfactory | Needs Practice | SKILL 1-1<br><br>**Assessing Body Temperature** | |
|---|---|---|---|---|
| | | | **Goal:** The patient's temperature is assessed accurately without injury and the patient experiences only minimal discomfort. | **Comments** |
| ___ | ___ | ___ | 1. Check medical order or nursing care plan for frequency of measurement and route. More frequent temperature measurement may be appropriate based on nursing judgment. Bring necessary equipment to the bedside stand or overbed table. | |
| ___ | ___ | ___ | 2. Perform hand hygiene and put on PPE, if indicated. | |
| ___ | ___ | ___ | 3. Identify the patient. | |
| ___ | ___ | ___ | 4. Close curtains around bed and close the door to the room, if possible. Discuss the procedure with patient and assess the patient's ability to assist with the procedure. | |
| ___ | ___ | ___ | 5. Ensure the electronic or digital thermometer is in working condition. | |
| ___ | ___ | ___ | 6. Put on gloves, if appropriate or indicated. | |
| ___ | ___ | ___ | 7. Select the appropriate site based on previous assessment data. | |
| ___ | ___ | ___ | 8. Follow the steps as outlined below for the appropriate type of thermometer. | |
| ___ | ___ | ___ | 9. When measurement is completed, remove gloves, if worn. Remove additional PPE, if used. Perform hand hygiene. | |
| | | | **Measuring a Tympanic Membrane Temperature** | |
| ___ | ___ | ___ | 10. If necessary, push the "on" button and wait for the "ready" signal on the unit. | |
| ___ | ___ | ___ | 11. Slide disposable cover onto the tympanic probe. | |
| ___ | ___ | ___ | 12. *Insert the probe snugly into the external ear using gentle but firm pressure, angling the thermometer toward the patient's jaw line. Pull pinna up and back to straighten the ear canal in an adult.* | |
| ___ | ___ | ___ | 13. Activate the unit by pushing the trigger button. The reading is immediate (usually within 2 seconds). Note the reading. | |
| ___ | ___ | ___ | 14. Discard the probe cover in an appropriate receptacle by pushing the probe-release button or use rim of cover to remove from probe. Replace the thermometer in its charger, if necessary. | |

| Excellent | Satisfactory | Needs Practice | | Comments |
|---|---|---|---|---|

SKILL 1-1

**Assessing Body Temperature** *(Continued)*

**Assessing Oral Temperature**

‗ ‗ ‗    10. Remove the electronic unit from the charging unit, and remove the probe from within the recording unit.

‗ ‗ ‗    11. Cover thermometer probe with disposable probe cover and slide it on until it snaps into place.

‗ ‗ ‗    12. *Place the probe beneath the patient's tongue in the posterior sublingual pocket. Ask the patient to close his or her lips around the probe.*

‗ ‗ ‗    13. *Continue to hold the probe until you hear a beep. Note the temperature reading.*

‗ ‗ ‗    14. Remove the probe from the patient's mouth. Dispose of the probe cover by holding the probe over an appropriate receptacle and pressing the probe release button.

‗ ‗ ‗    15. Return the thermometer probe to the storage place within the unit. Return the electronic unit to the charging unit, if appropriate.

**Assessing Rectal Temperature**

‗ ‗ ‗    10. Adjust the bed to a comfortable working height, usually elbow height of the care giver (VISN 8 Patient Safety Center, 2009). Put on nonsterile gloves.

‗ ‗ ‗    11. Assist the patient to a side-lying position. Pull back the covers sufficiently to expose only the buttocks.

‗ ‗ ‗    12. Remove the rectal probe from within the recording unit of the electronic thermometer. Cover the probe with a disposable probe cover and slide it into place until it snaps in place.

‗ ‗ ‗    13. *Lubricate about 1 inch of the probe with a water-soluble lubricant.*

‗ ‗ ‗    14. Reassure the patient. Separate the buttocks until the anal sphincter is clearly visible.

‗ ‗ ‗    15. *Insert the thermometer probe into the anus about 1.5 inches in an adult or 1 inch in a child.*

‗ ‗ ‗    16. Hold the probe in place until you hear a beep, then carefully remove the probe. Note the temperature reading on the display.

‗ ‗ ‗    17. Dispose of the probe cover by holding the probe over an appropriate waste receptacle and pressing the release button.

‗ ‗ ‗    18. Using toilet tissue, wipe the anus of any feces or excess lubricant. Dispose of the toilet tissue. Remove gloves and discard them.

## SKILL 1-1

# Assessing Body Temperature *(Continued)*

| Excellent | Satisfactory | Needs Practice | | Comments |
|---|---|---|---|---|
| —— | —— | —— | 19. Cover the patient and help him or her to a position of comfort. | |
| —— | —— | —— | 20. Place the bed in the lowest position; elevate rails as needed. | |
| —— | —— | —— | 21. Return the thermometer to the charging unit. | |

**Assessing Axillary Temperature**

| Excellent | Satisfactory | Needs Practice | | Comments |
|---|---|---|---|---|
| —— | —— | —— | 10. Move the patient's clothing to expose only the axilla. | |
| —— | —— | —— | 11. Remove the probe from the recording unit of the electronic thermometer. Place a disposable probe cover on by sliding it on and snapping it securely. | |
| —— | —— | —— | 12. *Place the end of the probe in the center of the axilla. Have the patient bring the arm down and close to the body.* | |
| —— | —— | —— | 13. Hold the probe in place until you hear a beep, and then carefully remove the probe. Note the temperature reading. | |
| —— | —— | —— | 14. Cover the patient and help him or her to a position of comfort. | |
| —— | —— | —— | 15. Dispose of the probe cover by holding the probe over an appropriate waste receptacle and pushing the release button. | |
| —— | —— | —— | 16. Place the bed in the lowest position and elevate rails, as needed. Leave the patient clean and comfortable. | |
| —— | —— | —— | 17. Return the electronic thermometer to the charging unit. | |

**Assessing Temporal Artery Temperature**

| Excellent | Satisfactory | Needs Practice | | Comments |
|---|---|---|---|---|
| —— | —— | —— | 10. Brush the patient's hair aside if it is covering the temporal artery area. | |
| —— | —— | —— | 11. Apply a probe cover. | |
| —— | —— | —— | 12. Hold the thermometer like a remote control device, with your thumb on the red 'ON' button. Place the probe flush on the center of the forehead, with the body of the instrument sideways (not straight up and down), so it is not in the patient's face. | |
| —— | —— | —— | 13. Depress the ON button. Keep the button depressed throughout the measurement. | |
| —— | —— | —— | 14. Slowly slide the probe straight across the forehead, midline, to the hair line. The thermometer will click; fast clicking indicates a rise to a higher temperature, slow clicking indicates the instrument is still scanning, but not finding any higher temperature. | |

SKILL 1-1

## Assessing Body Temperature *(Continued)*

| Excellent | Satisfactory | Needs Practice | | Comments |
|---|---|---|---|---|
| —— | —— | —— | 15. Brush hair aside if it is covering the ear, exposing the area of the neck under the ear lobe. Lift the probe from the forehead and touch on the neck just behind the ear lobe, in the depression just below the mastoid. | |
| —— | —— | —— | 16. Release the button and read the thermometer measurement. | |
| —— | —— | —— | 17. Hold the thermometer over a waste receptacle. Gently push the probe cover with your thumb against the proximal edge to dispose of probe cover. | |
| —— | —— | —— | 18. Instrument will automatically turn off in 30 seconds, or press and release the power button. | |

*Skill Checklists for Taylor's Clinical Nursing Skills:*
*A Nursing Process Approach, 3rd edition*

Name _____    Date _____

Unit _____    Position _____

Instructor/Evaluator: _____    Position _____

| Excellent | Satisfactory | Needs Practice | SKILL 1-2<br><br>**Monitoring Temperature Using an Overhead Radiant Warmer** | |
|---|---|---|---|---|
| | | | **Goal:** The infant's temperature is maintained within normal limits without injury. | **Comments** |
| ___ | ___ | ___ | 1. Check medical order or nursing care plan for the use of a radiant warmer. | |
| ___ | ___ | ___ | 2. Perform hand hygiene and put on PPE, if indicated. | |
| ___ | ___ | ___ | 3. Identify the patient. | |
| ___ | ___ | ___ | 4. Close curtains around bed and close the door to the room, if possible. Discuss the procedure with the patient's family. | |
| ___ | ___ | ___ | 5. Plug in the warmer. Turn the warmer to the manual setting. Allow the blankets to warm before placing the infant under the warmer. | |
| ___ | ___ | ___ | 6. *Switch the warmer setting to automatic. Set the warmer to the desired abdominal skin temperature, usually 36.5°C.* | |
| ___ | ___ | ___ | 7. Place the infant under the warmer. Attach the probe to the infant's abdominal skin at mid-epigastrium, halfway between the xiphoid and the umbilicus. Cover with a foil patch. | |
| ___ | ___ | ___ | 8. When the abdominal skin temperature reaches the desired set point, check the patient's axillary or rectal temperature, based on facility policy, to be sure it is within the normal range. | |
| ___ | ___ | ___ | 9. Adjust the warmer's set point slightly, as needed, if the axillary or rectal temperature is abnormal. Do not change the set point if the axillary or rectal temperature is normal. | |
| ___ | ___ | ___ | 10. Remove additional PPE, if used. Perform hand hygiene. | |
| ___ | ___ | ___ | 11. Check frequently to be sure the probe maintains contact with the patient's skin. Continue to monitor temperature measurement and other vital signs. | |

*Skill Checklists for Taylor's Clinical Nursing Skills:*
*A Nursing Process Approach, 3rd edition*

Name _____   Date _____

Unit _____   Position _____

Instructor/Evaluator: _____   Position _____

## SKILL 1-3
# Using a Cooling Blanket

**Goal:** The patient maintains the desired body temperature.

| Excellent | Satisfactory | Needs Practice | | Comments |
|---|---|---|---|---|
| ___ | ___ | ___ | 1. Review the medical order for the application of the hypothermia blanket. Obtain consent for the therapy per facility policy. | |
| ___ | ___ | ___ | 2. Gather the necessary supplies and bring to the bedside stand or overbed table. | |
| ___ | ___ | ___ | 3. Perform hand hygiene and put on PPE, if indicated. | |
| ___ | ___ | ___ | 4. Identify the patient. Determine if the patient has had any previous adverse reaction to hypothermia therapy. | |
| ___ | ___ | ___ | 5. Close curtains around bed and close the door to the room, if possible. Explain what you are going to do and why you are going to do it to the patient. | |
| ___ | ___ | ___ | 6. Check that the water in the electronic unit is at the appropriate level. Fill the unit two thirds full with distilled water, or to the fill mark, if necessary. Check the temperature setting on the unit to ensure it is within the safe range. | |
| ___ | ___ | ___ | 7. Assess the patient's vital signs, neurologic status, peripheral circulation, and skin integrity. | |
| ___ | ___ | ___ | 8. Adjust bed to comfortable working height, usually elbow height of the care giver (VISN 8 Patient Safety Center, 2009). | |
| ___ | ___ | ___ | 9. Make sure the patient's gown has cloth ties, not snaps or pins. | |
| ___ | ___ | ___ | 10. Apply lanolin or a mixture of lanolin and cold cream to the patient's skin where it will be in contact with the blanket. | |
| ___ | ___ | ___ | 11. Turn on the blanket and make sure the cooling light is on. Verify that the temperature limits are set within the desired safety range. | |
| ___ | ___ | ___ | 12. Cover the hypothermia blanket with a thin sheet or bath blanket. | |
| ___ | ___ | ___ | 13. Position the blanket under the patient so that the top edge of the pad is aligned with the patient's neck. | |

SKILL 1-3
## Using a Cooling Blanket *(Continued)*

| Excellent | Satisfactory | Needs Practice | | Comments |
|---|---|---|---|---|
| —— | —— | —— | 14. Put on gloves. Lubricate the rectal probe and insert it into the patient's rectum unless contraindicated. Or tuck the skin probe deep into the patient's axilla and tape it in place. For patients who are comatose or anesthetized, use an esophageal probe. Remove gloves. Attach the probe to the control panel for the blanket. | |
| —— | —— | —— | 15. Wrap the patient's hands and feet in gauze if ordered, or if the patient desires. For male patients, elevate the scrotum off the cooling blanket with towels. | |
| —— | —— | —— | 16. Place the patient in a comfortable position. Lower the bed. Dispose of any other supplies appropriately. | |
| —— | —— | —— | 17. Recheck the thermometer and settings on the control panel. | |
| —— | —— | —— | 18. Remove any additional PPE, if used. Perform hand hygiene. | |
| —— | —— | —— | 19. *Turn and position the patient regularly (every 30 minutes to 1 hour).* Keep linens free from condensation. Reapply cream, as needed. Observe the patient's skin for change in color, changes in lips and nail beds, edema, pain, and sensory impairment. | |
| —— | —— | —— | 20. *Monitor vital signs and perform a neurologic assessment, per facility policy, usually every 15 minutes, until the body temperature is stable.* In addition, monitor the patient's fluid and electrolyte status. | |
| —— | —— | —— | 21. Observe for signs of shivering, including verbalized sensations, facial muscle twitching, hyperventilation, or twitching of extremities. | |
| —— | —— | —— | 22. Assess the patient's level of comfort. | |
| —— | —— | —— | 23. Turn off blanket according to facility policy, usually when the patient's body temperature reaches 1 degree above the desired temperature. Continue to monitor the patient's temperature until it stabilizes. | |

*Skill Checklists for Taylor's Clinical Nursing Skills:*
*A Nursing Process Approach, 3rd edition*

Name _____  Date _____

Unit _____  Position _____

Instructor/Evaluator: _____  Position _____

SKILL 1-4

# Assessing a Peripheral Pulse by Palpation

**Goal:** The patient's pulse is assessed accurately without injury and the patient experiences only minimal discomfort.

| Excellent | Satisfactory | Needs Practice | | Comments |
|---|---|---|---|---|
| ⎯ | ⎯ | ⎯ | 1. Check medical order or nursing care plan for frequency of pulse assessment. More frequent pulse measurement may be appropriate based on nursing judgment. | |
| ⎯ | ⎯ | ⎯ | 2. Perform hand hygiene and put on PPE, if indicated. | |
| ⎯ | ⎯ | ⎯ | 3. Identify the patient. | |
| ⎯ | ⎯ | ⎯ | 4. Close curtains around bed and close the door to the room, if possible. Discuss the procedure with patient and assess the patient's ability to assist with the procedure. | |
| ⎯ | ⎯ | ⎯ | 5. Put on gloves, as appropriate. | |
| ⎯ | ⎯ | ⎯ | 6. Select the appropriate peripheral site based on assessment data. | |
| ⎯ | ⎯ | ⎯ | 7. Move the patient's clothing to expose only the site chosen. | |
| ⎯ | ⎯ | ⎯ | 8. Place your first, second, and third fingers over the artery. *Lightly compress the artery so pulsations can be felt and counted.* | |
| ⎯ | ⎯ | ⎯ | 9. Using a watch with a second hand, count the number of pulsations felt for 30 seconds. Multiply this number by 2 to calculate the rate for 1 minute. *If the rate, rhythm, or amplitude of the pulse is abnormal in any way, palpate and count the pulse for 1 minute.* | |
| ⎯ | ⎯ | ⎯ | 10. Note the rhythm and amplitude of the pulse. | |
| ⎯ | ⎯ | ⎯ | 11. When measurement is completed, remove gloves, if worn. Cover the patient and help him or her to a position of comfort. | |
| ⎯ | ⎯ | ⎯ | 12. Remove additional PPE, if used. Perform hand hygiene. | |

*Skill Checklists for Taylor's Clinical Nursing Skills:*
*A Nursing Process Approach, 3rd edition*

Name _____     Date _____

Unit _____     Position _____

Instructor/Evaluator: _____     Position _____

|  |  |  | SKILL 1-5<br>**Assessing the Apical Pulse by Auscultation** |  |
|---|---|---|---|---|
| **Excellent** | **Satisfactory** | **Needs Practice** | **Goal:** The patient's pulse is assessed accurately without injury and the patient experiences minimal discomfort. | **Comments** |
| ___ | ___ | ___ | 1. Check medical order or nursing care plan for frequency of pulse assessment. More frequent pulse measurement may be appropriate based on nursing judgment. Identify the need to obtain an apical pulse measurement. | |
| ___ | ___ | ___ | 2. Perform hand hygiene and put on PPE, if indicated. | |
| ___ | ___ | ___ | 3. Identify the patient. | |
| ___ | ___ | ___ | 4. Close curtains around bed and close the door to the room, if possible. Discuss procedure with patient and assess patient's ability to assist with the procedure. | |
| ___ | ___ | ___ | 5. Put on gloves, as appropriate. | |
| ___ | ___ | ___ | 6. Use alcohol swab to clean the diaphragm of the stethoscope. Use another swab to clean the earpieces, if necessary. | |
| ___ | ___ | ___ | 7. Assist patient to a sitting or reclining position and expose chest area. | |
| ___ | ___ | ___ | 8. Move the patient's clothing to expose only the apical site. | |
| ___ | ___ | ___ | 9. Hold the stethoscope diaphragm against the palm of your hand for a few seconds. | |
| ___ | ___ | ___ | 10. *Palpate the space between the fifth and sixth ribs (fifth intercostal space), and move to the left midclavicular line.* Place the diaphragm over the apex of the heart. | |
| ___ | ___ | ___ | 11. Listen for heart sounds ("lub-dub"). Each "lub-dub" counts as one beat. | |
| ___ | ___ | ___ | 12. Using a watch with a second hand, count the heartbeat for 1 minute. | |
| ___ | ___ | ___ | 13. When measurement is completed, remove gloves, if worn. Cover the patient and help him or her to a position of comfort. | |
| ___ | ___ | ___ | 14. Clean the diaphragm of the stethoscope with an alcohol swab. | |
| ___ | ___ | ___ | 15. Remove additional PPE, if used. Perform hand hygiene. | |

*Skill Checklists for Taylor's Clinical Nursing Skills:*
*A Nursing Process Approach, 3rd edition*

Name _____  Date _____

Unit _____  Position _____

Instructor/Evaluator: _____  Position _____

SKILL 1-6

# Assessing Respiration

**Goal:** The patient's respirations are assessed accurately without injury and the patient experiences only minimal discomfort.

| Excellent | Satisfactory | Needs Practice | | Comments |
|---|---|---|---|---|
| ____ | ____ | ____ | 1. *While your fingers are still in place for the pulse measurement, after counting the pulse rate, observe the patient's respirations.* | |
| ____ | ____ | ____ | 2. Note the rise and fall of the patient's chest. | |
| ____ | ____ | ____ | 3. Using a watch with a second hand, count the number of respirations for 30 seconds. Multiply this number by 2 to calculate the respiratory rate per minute. | |
| ____ | ____ | ____ | 4. *If respirations are abnormal in any way, count the respirations for at least 1 full minute.* | |
| ____ | ____ | ____ | 5. Note the depth and rhythm of the respirations. | |
| ____ | ____ | ____ | 6. When measurement is completed, remove gloves, if worn. Cover the patient and help him or her to a position of comfort. | |
| ____ | ____ | ____ | 7. Remove additional PPE, if used. Perform hand hygiene. | |

*Skill Checklists for Taylor's Clinical Nursing Skills:*
*A Nursing Process Approach, 3rd edition*

Name _____  Date _____

Unit _____  Position _____

Instructor/Evaluator: _____  Position _____

SKILL 1-7
# Assessing Brachial Artery Blood Pressure

**Goal:** The patient's blood pressure is measured accurately
with minimal discomfort to the patient.

| Excellent | Satisfactory | Needs Practice | | Comments |
|---|---|---|---|---|
| ___ | ___ | ___ | 1. Check physician's order or nursing care plan for frequency of blood pressure measurement. More frequent measurement may be appropriate based on nursing judgment. | |
| ___ | ___ | ___ | 2. Perform hand hygiene and put on PPE, if indicated. | |
| ___ | ___ | ___ | 3. Identify the patient. | |
| ___ | ___ | ___ | 4. Close curtains around bed and close the door to the room, if possible. Discuss procedure with patient and assess patient's ability to assist with the procedure. Validate that the patient has relaxed for several minutes. | |
| ___ | ___ | ___ | 5. Put on gloves, if appropriate or indicated. | |
| ___ | ___ | ___ | 6. Select the appropriate arm for application of the cuff. | |
| ___ | ___ | ___ | 7. Have the patient assume a comfortable lying or sitting position with the forearm supported at the level of the heart and the palm of the hand upward. If the measurement is taken in the supine position, support the arm with a pillow. In the sitting position, support the arm yourself or by using the bedside table. If the patient is sitting, have the patient sit back in the chair so that the chair supports his or her back. In addition, make sure the patient keeps the legs uncrossed. | |
| ___ | ___ | ___ | 8. Expose the brachial artery by removing garments, or move a sleeve, if it is not too tight, above the area where the cuff will be placed. | |
| ___ | ___ | ___ | 9. Palpate the location of the brachial artery. *Center the bladder of the cuff over the brachial artery, about midway on the arm, so that the lower edge of the cuff is about 2.5 to 5 cm (1 to 2 inches) above the inner aspect of the elbow. Line the artery marking on the cuff up with the patient's brachial artery.* The tubing should extend from the edge of the cuff nearer the patient's elbow. | |
| ___ | ___ | ___ | 10. Wrap the cuff around the arm smoothly and snugly, and fasten it. Do not allow any clothing to interfere with the proper placement of the cuff. | |

| Excellent | Satisfactory | Needs Practice | SKILL 1-7 **Assessing Brachial Artery Blood Pressure** *(Continued)* | Comments |
|---|---|---|---|---|

____ ____ ____  11. Check that the needle on the aneroid gauge is within the zero mark. If using a mercury manometer, check to see that the manometer is in the vertical position and that the mercury is within the zero level with the gauge at eye level.

**Estimating Systolic Pressure**

____ ____ ____  12. Palpate the pulse at the brachial or radial artery by pressing gently with the fingertips.

____ ____ ____  13. Tighten the screw valve on the air pump.

____ ____ ____  14. *Inflate the cuff while continuing to palpate the artery. Note the point on the gauge where the pulse disappears.*

____ ____ ____  15. Deflate the cuff and wait 1 minute.

**Obtaining Blood Pressure Measurement**

____ ____ ____  16. Assume a position that is no more than 3 feet away from the gauge.

____ ____ ____  17. Place the stethoscope earpieces in your ears. Direct the earpieces forward into the canal and not against the ear itself.

____ ____ ____  18. Place the bell or diaphragm of the stethoscope firmly but with as little pressure as possible over the brachial artery. Do not allow the stethoscope to touch clothing or the cuff.

____ ____ ____  19. Pump the pressure 30 mm Hg above the point at which the systolic pressure was palpated and estimated. Open the valve on the manometer and allow air to escape slowly (allowing the gauge to drop 2 to 3 mm per second).

____ ____ ____  20. *Note the point on the gauge at which the first faint, but clear, sound appears that slowly increases in intensity. Note this number as the systolic pressure. Read the pressure to the closest 2 mm Hg.*

____ ____ ____  21. Do not reinflate the cuff once the air is being released to recheck the systolic pressure reading.

____ ____ ____  22. *Note the point at which the sound completely disappears.*

____ ____ ____  23. Allow the remaining air to escape quickly. Repeat any suspicious reading, but wait at least 1 minute. Deflate the cuff completely between attempts to check the blood pressure.

# Assessing Brachial Artery Blood Pressure *(Continued)*

| Excellent | Satisfactory | Needs Practice | | Comments |
|---|---|---|---|---|
| —— | —— | —— | 24. When measurement is completed, remove the cuff. Remove gloves, if worn. Cover the patient and help him or her to a position of comfort. | |
| —— | —— | —— | 25. Remove additional PPE, if used. Perform hand hygiene. | |
| —— | —— | —— | 26. Clean the diaphragm of the stethoscope with the alcohol wipe. Clean and store the sphygmomanometer, according to facility policy. | |

*Skill Checklists for Taylor's Clinical Nursing Skills:*
*A Nursing Process Approach, 3rd edition*

Name _____  Date _____

Unit _____  Position _____

Instructor/Evaluator: _____  Position _____

---

SKILL 2-1

# Performing a General Survey

**Goal:** The assessment is completed without the patient experiencing anxiety or discomfort, an overall impression of the patient is formulated, the findings are documented, and the appropriate referral is made to other healthcare professionals, as needed for further evaluation.

| Excellent | Satisfactory | Needs Practice | | Comments |
|---|---|---|---|---|
| ___ | ___ | ___ | 1. Perform hand hygiene and put on PPE, if indicated. | |
| ___ | ___ | ___ | 2. Identify the patient. | |
| ___ | ___ | ___ | 3. Close curtains around bed and the door to the room, if possible. Explain the purpose of the health examination and what you are going to do. Answer any questions. | |
| ___ | ___ | ___ | 4. Assess the patient's physical appearance. Observe if the patient appears his or her stated age. Note the patient's mental status. Is the person alert and oriented, responsive to questions and responding appropriately? Are the facial features symmetric? Note any signs of acute distress, such as shortness of breath, pain, or anxiousness. | |
| ___ | ___ | ___ | 5. Assess the patient's body structure. Does the person's height appear within normal range for stated age and genetic heritage? Does the person's weight appear within normal range for height and body build? Note if body fat is evenly distributed. Do body parts appear equal bilaterally and relatively proportionate? Is the patient's posture erect and appropriate for age? | |
| ___ | ___ | ___ | 6. Assess the patient's mobility. Is the patient's gait smooth, even, well-balanced, and coordinated? Is joint mobility smooth and coordinated with a general full range of motion (ROM)? Are involuntary movements evident? | |
| ___ | ___ | ___ | 7. Assess the patient's behavior. Are facial expressions appropriate for the situation? Does the patient maintain eye contact, based on cultural norms? Does the person appear comfortable and relaxed with you? Is the patient's speech clear and understandable? Observe the person's hygiene and grooming. Is the clothing appropriate for climate, fit well, appear clean, and appropriate for the person's culture and age group? Does the person appear clean and well groomed, appropriate for age and culture? | |
| ___ | ___ | ___ | 8. Assess for pain. (Refer to Chapter 10, Comfort.) | |

| Excellent | Satisfactory | Needs Practice | | Comments |
|---|---|---|---|---|
| | | | SKILL 2-1<br>**Performing a General Survey** *(Continued)* | |

| Excellent | Satisfactory | Needs Practice | | Comments |
|---|---|---|---|---|
| ___ | ___ | ___ | 9. Have the patient remove shoes and heavy outer clothing. Weigh the patient using a scale. Compare the measurement with previous weight measurements and recommended range for height. | |
| ___ | ___ | ___ | 10. With shoes off, and standing erect, measure the patient's height using a wall-mounted measuring device or measuring pole. Compare height and weight with recommended average weights on a standardized chart. | |
| ___ | ___ | ___ | 11. Use the patient's weight and height measurements to calculate the patient's BMI.<br><br>$$\text{Body mass index} = \frac{\text{weight in kilograms}}{\text{height in meters}^2}$$ | |
| ___ | ___ | ___ | 12. Using the tape measure, measure the patient's waist circumference. Place the tape measure snugly around the patient's waist at the level of the umbilicus. | |
| ___ | ___ | ___ | 13. Measure the patient's temperature, pulse, respirations, blood pressure, and oxygen saturation. (Refer to Chapter 1, Vital Signs, and Chapter 14, Oxygenation, for specific techniques.) | |
| ___ | ___ | ___ | 14. Remove PPE, if used. Perform hand hygiene. Continue with assessments of specific body systems as appropriate or indicated. Initiate appropriate referral to other healthcare practitioners for further evaluation as indicated. | |

*Skill Checklists for Taylor's Clinical Nursing Skills:*
*A Nursing Process Approach, 3rd edition*

Name _____     Date _____

Unit _____     Position _____

Instructor/Evaluator: _____     Position _____

SKILL 2-2

# Using a Bed Scale

| Excellent | Satisfactory | Needs Practice | **Goal:** The patient's weight is assessed accurately, without injury, and the patient experiences minimal discomfort. | Comments |
|---|---|---|---|---|
| ―― | ―― | ―― | 1. Check medical order or nursing care plan for frequency of weight measurement. More frequent pulse measurement may be appropriate based on nursing judgment. Obtain the assistance of a second caregiver, based on patient's mobility and ability to cooperate with procedure. | |
| ―― | ―― | ―― | 2. Perform hand hygiene and put on PPE, if indicated. | |
| ―― | ―― | ―― | 3. Identify the patient. | |
| ―― | ―― | ―― | 4. Close curtains around bed and close door to room if possible. Discuss procedure with patient and assess patient's ability to assist with the procedure. | |
| ―― | ―― | ―― | 5. Place a cover over the sling of the bed scale. | |
| ―― | ―― | ―― | 6. Attach the sling to the bed scale. Lay the sheet or bath blanket in the sling. Turn the scale on. *Adjust the dial so that weight reads 0.0.* | |
| ―― | ―― | ―― | 7. Adjust bed to comfortable working position, usually elbow height of the caregiver (VISN 8, 2009). Position one caregiver on each side of the bed, if two caregivers are present. Raise side rail on the opposite side of the bed from where the scale is located, if not already in place. Cover the patient with the sheet or bath blanket. Remove other covers and any pillows. | |
| ―― | ―― | ―― | 8. Turn patient onto his or her side facing the side rail, keeping his or her body covered with the sheet or blanket. Remove the sling from the scale. Roll sling long ways. Place rolled sling under patient, making sure the patient is centered in the sling. | |
| ―― | ―― | ―― | 9. Roll patient back over sling and onto other side. Pull sling through, as if placing sheet under patient, unrolling sling as it is pulled through. | |
| ―― | ―― | ―― | 10. Roll scale over the bed so that arms of scale are directly over patient. *Spread the base of the scale.* Lower arms of the scale and place arm hooks into holes on the sling. | |

| Excellent | Satisfactory | Needs Practice | | Comments |
|---|---|---|---|---|

___  ___  ___    11. Once scale arms are hooked onto the sling, gradually elevate the sling so that the patient is lifted up off of the bed. *Assess all tubes and drains, making sure that none have tension placed on them as the scale is lifted. Once the sling is no longer touching the bed, ensure that nothing else is hanging onto the sling (e.g., ventilator tubing, IV tubing). If any tubing is connected to the patient, raise it up so that it is not adding any weight to the patient.*

___  ___  ___    12. Note weight reading on the scale. Slowly and gently, lower patient back onto the bed. Disconnect scale arms from sling. Close base of scale and pull it away from the bed.

___  ___  ___    13. Raise the side rail. Turn patient to the side rail. Roll the sling up against the patient's backside.

___  ___  ___    14. Raise the other side rail. Roll patient back over the sling and up facing the other side rail. Remove sling from bed. Remove gloves, if used. Raise remaining side rail.

___  ___  ___    15. Cover the patient and help him or her to a position of comfort. Place the bed in the lowest position.

___  ___  ___    16. Remove disposable cover from sling and discard in appropriate receptacle.

___  ___  ___    17. Remove additional PPE, if used. Perform hand hygiene.

___  ___  ___    18. Replace scale and sling in appropriate spot. Plug scale into electrical outlet.

*Skill Checklists for Taylor's Clinical Nursing Skills:*
*A Nursing Process Approach, 3rd edition*

Name _____  Date _____

Unit _____  Position _____

Instructor/Evaluator: _____  Position _____

SKILL 2-3

# Assessing the Skin, Hair, and Nails

**Goal:** The assessment is completed without the patient experiencing anxiety or discomfort, the findings are documented, and the appropriate referral is made to the other healthcare professionals, as needed, for further evaluation.

| Excellent | Satisfactory | Needs Practice | | Comments |
|---|---|---|---|---|
| —— | —— | —— | 1. Perform hand hygiene and put on PPE, if indicated. | |
| —— | —— | —— | 2. Identify the patient. | |
| —— | —— | —— | 3. Close curtains around bed and the door to room, if possible. Explain the purpose of the integumentary examination and what you are going to do. Answer any questions. | |
| —— | —— | —— | 4. Ask the patient to remove all clothing and put on an examination gown (if appropriate). The patient remains in the sitting position for most of the examination but will need to stand or lie on the side when the posterior part of the body is examined, exposing only the body part being examined. | |
| —— | —— | —— | 5. Use the bath blanket or drape to cover any exposed area other than the one being assessed. Inspect the overall skin coloration. | |
| —— | —— | —— | 6. Inspect skin for vascularity, bleeding, or bruising. | |
| —— | —— | —— | 7. Inspect the skin for lesions. Note bruises, scratches, cuts, insect bites, and wounds (Refer to Wound Assessment [Fundamentals Review 8-3] in Chapter 8, Skin Integrity and Wound Care). If present, note size, shape, color, exudates, and distribution/pattern. | |
| —— | —— | —— | 8. Palpate skin using the backs of your hands to assess temperature. Wear gloves when palpating any potentially open area of the skin. | |
| —— | —— | —— | 9. Palpate for texture and moisture. | |
| —— | —— | —— | 10. Assess for skin turgor by gently pinching the skin under the clavicle. | |
| —— | —— | —— | 11. Palpate for edema, which is characterized by swelling, with taut and shiny skin over the edematous area. | |
| —— | —— | —— | 12. If lesions are present, put on gloves and palpate the lesion. | |
| —— | —— | —— | 13. Inspect the nail condition, including the shape and color as well as the nail angle, noting if any clubbing is present. | |
| —— | —— | —— | 14. Palpate nails for texture and capillary refill. | |

SKILL 2-3

# Assessing the Skin, Hair, and Nails *(Continued)*

| Excellent | Satisfactory | Needs Practice | | Comments |
|---|---|---|---|---|
| —— | —— | —— | 15. Inspect the hair and scalp. Wear gloves for palpation if lesions or infestation is suspected or if hygiene is poor. | |
| —— | —— | —— | 16. Remove gloves and any additional PPE, if used. Perform hand hygiene. Continue with assessments of specific body systems, as appropriate or indicated. Initiate appropriate referral to other healthcare practitioners for further evaluation, as indicated. | |

*Skill Checklists for Taylor's Clinical Nursing Skills:*
*A Nursing Process Approach, 3rd edition*

Name _____  Date _____

Unit _____  Position _____

Instructor/Evaluator: _____  Position _____

## SKILL 2-4

# Assessing the Head and Neck

| Excellent | Satisfactory | Needs Practice | | Comments |
|:---:|:---:|:---:|---|---|
| | | | **Goal:** The assessment is completed without the patient experiencing anxiety or discomfort, the findings are documented, and the appropriate referral is made to the other healthcare professionals, as needed, for further evaluation. | |
| —— | —— | —— | 1. Perform hand hygiene and put on PPE, if indicated. | |
| —— | —— | —— | 2. Identify the patient. | |
| —— | —— | —— | 3. Close curtains around bed and close the door to the room, if possible. Explain the purpose of the head and neck examination and what you are going to do. Answer any questions. | |
| —— | —— | —— | 4. Inspect the head and then the face for color, symmetry, lesions, and distribution of facial hair. Note facial expression. Palpate the skull. | |
| —— | —— | —— | 5. Inspect the external eye structures (eyelids, eyelashes, eyeball, and eyebrows), cornea, conjunctiva, and sclera. Note color, edema, symmetry, and alignment. | |
| —— | —— | —— | 6. Examine the pupils for equality of size, shape, and reaction to light by darkening the room and using a penlight to shine the light on each pupil. | |
| —— | —— | —— | 7. To test for pupillary accommodation and convergence, ask the patient to focus on an object as you bring it closer to the nose. | |
| —— | —— | —— | 8. Using an ophthalmoscope, check the red reflex. | |
| —— | —— | —— | 9. Test the patient's visual acuity with a Snellen chart. Ask the patient to read the smallest possible line of letters, first with both eyes and then with one eye at a time. | |
| —— | —— | —— | 10. With the patient about 2 feet away, ask the patient to focus on your finger and move the patient's eyes through the six cardinal positions of gaze. | |
| —— | —— | —— | 11. Inspect the external ear bilaterally for shape, size, and lesions. Palpate the ear and mastoid process. | |
| —— | —— | —— | 12. Perform an otoscopic examination. For an adult, pull the auricle up and back; for a child, pull the auricle down and back. Note cerumen (wax), edema, discharge, or foreign bodies and condition of the tympanic membrane. | |
| —— | —— | —— | 13. Use a whispered voice to test hearing. Stand about 1 to 2 feet away from the patient out of the patient's line of vision. Ask the patient to cover the ear not being tested. Perform test on each ear. | |

| Excellent | Satisfactory | Needs Practice | SKILL 2-4 **Assessing the Head and Neck** *(Continued)* | Comments |
|---|---|---|---|---|
| —— | —— | —— | 14. Use a tuning fork to perform Weber's test and Rinne test if the patient reports diminished hearing in either ear. | |
| —— | —— | —— | 15. Put on gloves. Inspect and palpate the external nose. | |
| —— | —— | —— | 16. Palpate and lightly percuss over the frontal and maxillary sinuses. | |
| —— | —— | —— | 17. Occlude one nostril externally with a finger while patient breathes through the other; repeat for the other side. | |
| —— | —— | —— | 18. Inspect the internal nostrils using an otoscope with a nasal speculum attachment. | |
| —— | —— | —— | 19. Palpate the temporomandibular joint by placing your index finger over the front of each ear as you ask the patient to open and close the mouth. | |
| —— | —— | —— | 20. Inspect the lips, oral mucosa, hard and soft palates, gingivae, teeth, and salivary gland openings by asking the patient to open the mouth wide using a tongue blade and penlight. | |
| —— | —— | —— | 21. Inspect the tongue. Ask the patient to stick out the tongue. Place a tongue blade at the side of the tongue while patient pushes it to the left and right with the tongue. Inspect the uvula by asking the patient to say "ahh" while sticking out the tongue. Palpate the tongue for muscle tone and tenderness. Remove gloves. | |
| —— | —— | —— | 22. Palpate from the forehead to the posterior triangle of the neck for the posterior cervical lymph nodes using the finger pads in a slow, circular motion. | |
| —— | —— | —— | 23. Inspect and palpate in front of and behind the ears, under the chin, and in the anterior triangle for the anterior cervical lymph nodes. | |
| —— | —— | —— | 24. Inspect and palpate the left and then the right carotid arteries. *Only palpate one carotid artery at a time.* Use the bell of the stethoscope to auscultate the arteries. | |
| —— | —— | —— | 25. Inspect and palpate for the trachea. | |
| —— | —— | —— | 26. Palpate the thyroid gland (illustrate the two techniques). Then, if enlarged, auscultate the thyroid gland using the bell of the stethoscope. | |
| —— | —— | —— | 27. Inspect and palpate the supraclavicular area. | |

SKILL 2-4

# Assessing the Head and Neck *(Continued)*

| Excellent | Satisfactory | Needs Practice | | Comments |
|---|---|---|---|---|
| —— | —— | —— | 28. Inspect the ability of the patient to move the neck. Ask the patient to touch chin to chest and to each shoulder, each ear to the corresponding shoulder, and then tip the head back as far as possible. | |
| —— | —— | —— | 29. Remove any additional PPE, if used. Perform hand hygiene. Continue with assessments of specific body systems, as appropriate or indicated. Initiate appropriate referral to other healthcare practitioners for further evaluation, as indicated. | |

*Skill Checklists for Taylor's Clinical Nursing Skills:*
*A Nursing Process Approach, 3rd edition*

Name _____  Date _____

Unit _____  Position _____

Instructor/Evaluator: _____  Position _____

## SKILL 2-5
# Assessing the Thorax and Lungs

**Goal:** The assessment is completed without causing the patient to experience anxiety or discomfort, the findings are documented, and the appropriate referral is made to other healthcare professionals, as needed, for further evaluation.

| Excellent | Satisfactory | Needs Practice | | Comments |
|---|---|---|---|---|
| —— | —— | —— | 1. Perform hand hygiene and put on PPE, if indicated. | |
| —— | —— | —— | 2. Identify the patient. | |
| —— | —— | —— | 3. Close curtains around bed and close the door to the room, if possible. Explain the purpose of the thorax and lung examination and what you are going to do. Answer any questions. | |
| —— | —— | —— | 4. Help the patient undress, if needed, and provide a patient gown. Assist the patient to a sitting position and expose the posterior thorax. | |
| —— | —— | —— | 5. Use the bath blanket to cover any exposed area other than the one being assessed. Inspect the posterior thorax. Examine the skin, bones, and muscles of the spine, shoulder blades, and back as well as symmetry of expansion and accessory muscle use during respirations. | |
| —— | —— | —— | 6. Assess the anteroposterior (AP) and lateral diameters of the thorax. | 2 : 1 ratio |
| —— | —— | —— | 7. Palpate over the spine and posterior thorax. | |
| —— | —— | —— | a. Use the palmar surface of the hand to palpate for temperature, tenderness, muscle development, and masses. | |
| —— | —— | —— | b. Instruct patient to take a deep breath. Assess for tactile fremitus by using the ball of the hands to palpate over the posterior thorax and while the patient says "ninety-nine". | |
| —— | —— | —— | 8. Assess thoracic expansion by standing behind the patient, placing both thumbs on either side of the patient's spine at the level of T9 or T10. Ask the patient to take a deep breath and note movement of your hands. | |
| —— | —— | —— | 9. Percuss over the posterior and lateral lung fields for tone using a zigzag pattern, starting above the scapulae to the bases of the lungs. Note intensity, pitch, duration, and quality of sounds produced. Percuss for diaphragmatic excursion on each side of the posterior thorax. | |

| Excellent | Satisfactory | Needs Practice | SKILL 2-5<br>**Assessing the Thorax and Lungs** *(Continued)* | Comments |
|---|---|---|---|---|
| —— | —— | —— | 10. Auscultate the lungs across and down the posterior thorax to the bases of lungs as the patient breathes slowly and deeply through the mouth. | |
| —— | —— | —— | 11. Examine the anterior thorax. With the patient sitting, rearrange the gown so the anterior chest is exposed. Inspect the skin, bones, and muscles, as well as symmetry of lung expansion and accessory muscle use. | |
| —— | —— | —— | 12. Palpate the anterior thorax using the proper sequence. Palpate for tactile fremitus (as the patient repeats the word "ninety-nine"). | |
| —— | —— | —— | 13. Percuss over the anterior thorax using the proper sequence. | |
| —— | —— | —— | 14. Auscultate the lungs through the anterior thorax as the patient breathes slowly and deeply through the mouth. | |
| —— | —— | —— | 15. Inspect the breasts and axillae with the patient's hands resting on both sides of the body, placed on the hips, and then raised above the head. | |
| —— | —— | —— | 16. Palpate the axillae with the patient's arms resting against the side of the body. Assist the patient into a supine position. Place a small pillow or towel under the patient's back. Palpate the breasts and nipples. Wear gloves if there is any discharge from the nipples or if a lesion is present. | |
| —— | —— | —— | 17. Assist the patient in replacing the gown. Remove gloves and any additional PPE, if used. Perform hand hygiene. Continue with assessments of specific body systems, as appropriate or indicated. Initiate appropriate referral to other healthcare practitioners for further evaluation, as indicated. | |

*Skill Checklists for Taylor's Clinical Nursing Skills:*
*A Nursing Process Approach, 3rd edition*

Name _____ Date _____

Unit _____ Position _____

Instructor/Evaluator: _____ Position _____

SKILL 2-6
# Assessing the Cardiovascular System

**Goal:** The assessment is completed without causing the patient to experience anxiety or discomfort, the findings are documented, and the appropriate referral is made to other healthcare professionals, as needed, for further evaluation.

| Excellent | Satisfactory | Needs Practice | | Comments |
|---|---|---|---|---|
| ____ | ____ | ____ | 1. Perform hand hygiene and put on PPE, if indicated. | |
| ____ | ____ | ____ | 2. Identify the patient. | |
| ____ | ____ | ____ | 3. Close curtains around bed and close the door to the room, if possible. Explain the purpose of the cardiovascular examination and what you are going to do. Answer any questions. | |
| ____ | ____ | ____ | 4. Help the patient undress, if needed, and provide a patient gown. Assist the patient to a supine position with the head elevated about 30 to 45 degrees and expose the anterior chest. Use the bath blanket to cover any exposed area other than the one being assessed. | |
| ____ | ____ | ____ | 5. Inspect and palpate the left and then the right carotid arteries. *Only palpate one carotid artery at a time.* Use the bell of the stethoscope to auscultate the arteries. | |
| ____ | ____ | ____ | 6. Inspect the neck for jugular vein distention, observing for pulsations. | |
| ____ | ____ | ____ | 7. Inspect the **precordium** for contour, pulsations, and heaves. Observe for the apical impulse at the fourth to fifth intercostal spaces (ICS). | |
| ____ | ____ | ____ | 8. Use the palmar surface with the four fingers held together and palpate the precordium gently for pulsations. Remember that hands should be warm. Palpation proceeds in a systematic manner, with assessment of specific cardiac landmarks—the aortic, pulmonic, tricuspid, and mitral areas and Erb's point. Palpate the apical impulse in the mitral area. Note size, duration, force, and location in relationship to the midclavicular line. | |
| ____ | ____ | ____ | 9. Use systematic auscultation, beginning at the aortic area, moving to the pulmonic area, then to Erb's point, then to the tricuspid area, and finally to the mitral area. Ask the patient to breathe normally. The stethoscope diaphragm is first used to listen to high-pitched sounds, followed by use of the bell to listen to low-pitched sounds. Focus on the overall rate and rhythm of the heart and the normal heart sounds. | |

SKILL 2-6

# Assessing the Cardiovascular System *(Continued)*

| Excellent | Satisfactory | Needs Practice | | Comments |
|---|---|---|---|---|
| —— | —— | —— | 10. Assist the patient in replacing the gown. Remove PPE, if used. Perform hand hygiene. Continue with assessments of specific body systems as appropriate or indicated. Initiate appropriate referral to other healthcare practitioners for further evaluation, as indicated. | |

*Skill Checklists for Taylor's Clinical Nursing Skills:*
*A Nursing Process Approach, 3rd edition*

Name _____  Date _____

Unit _____  Position _____

Instructor/Evaluator: _____  Position _____

SKILL 2-7

## Assessing the Abdomen

**Goal:** The assessments are completed without causing the patient to experience anxiety or discomfort, the findings are documented, and the appropriate referral is made to other healthcare professionals, as needed, for further evaluation.

| Excellent | Satisfactory | Needs Practice | | Comments |
|---|---|---|---|---|
| —— | —— | —— | 1. Perform hand hygiene and put on PPE, if indicated. | |
| —— | —— | —— | 2. Identify the patient. | |
| —— | —— | —— | 3. Close curtains around bed and close the door to the room, if possible. Explain the purpose of the abdominal examination and what you are going to do. Answer any questions. | |
| —— | —— | —— | 4. Help the patient undress, if needed, and provide a patient gown. Assist the patient to a supine position and expose the abdomen. Use the bath blanket to cover any exposed area other than the one being assessed. | |
| —— | —— | —— | 5. Inspect the abdomen for skin color, contour, pulsations, the umbilicus, and other surface characteristics (rashes, lesions, masses, scars). | |
| —— | —— | —— | 6. Auscultate all four quadrants of the abdomen for bowel sounds by using the diaphragm of the stethoscope. Use a systematic method. | |
| —— | —— | —— | 7. Auscultate the abdomen for vascular sounds by using the bell of the stethoscope. | |
| —— | —— | —— | 8. Percuss the abdomen for tones. | |
| —— | —— | —— | 9. Palpate the abdomen lightly in all four quadrants and then palpate using deep palpation technique. *If the patient complains of pain or discomfort in a particular area of the abdomen, palpate that area last.* | |
| —— | —— | —— | 10. Palpate for the kidneys on each side of the abdomen. Palpate the liver at the right costal border. Palpate for the spleen at the left costal border. | |
| —— | —— | —— | 11. *Assess for rebound tenderness last if the patient reports pain by pressing deeply and gently into the abdomen with the hand and fingers downward and then withdrawing the hand rapidly.* | |
| —— | —— | —— | 12. Palpate and then auscultate the femoral pulses in the groin. | |

| Excellent | Satisfactory | Needs Practice | | SKILL 2-7 **Assessing the Abdomen** (Continued) | |
|:---:|:---:|:---:|---|---|---|
| | | | | | **Comments** |
| — | — | — | 13. | Assist the patient in replacing the gown. Remove PPE, if used. Perform hand hygiene. Continue with assessments of specific body systems, as appropriate, or indicated. Initiate appropriate referral to other healthcare practitioners for further evaluation, as indicated. | |

*Skill Checklists for Taylor's Clinical Nursing Skills:*
*A Nursing Process Approach, 3rd edition*

Name _____ Date _____

Unit _____ Position _____

Instructor/Evaluator: _____ Position _____

## SKILL 2-8

# Assessing the Neurologic, Musculoskeletal, and Peripheral Vascular Systems

| Excellent | Satisfactory | Needs Practice | **Goal:** The assessments are completed without causing the patient to experience anxiety or discomfort, the findings are documented, and the appropriate referral is made to other healthcare professionals, as needed, for further evaluation. | Comments |
|---|---|---|---|---|
| ___ | ___ | ___ | 1. Perform hand hygiene and put on PPE, if indicated. | |
| ___ | ___ | ___ | 2. Identify the patient. | |
| ___ | ___ | ___ | 3. Close curtains around bed and close the door to the room, if possible. Explain the purpose of the neurologic, musculoskeletal, and peripheral vascular examinations and what you are going to do. Answer any questions. | |
| ___ | ___ | ___ | 4. Help the patient undress, if needed, and provide a patient gown. Assist the patient to a supine position. Use the bath blanket to cover any exposed area other than the one being assessed. | |
| ___ | ___ | ___ | 5. Begin with a survey of the patient's overall hygiene and physical appearance. | |
| ___ | ___ | ___ | 6. Assess the patient's mental status. | |
| ___ | ___ | ___ |    a. Evaluate the patient's orientation to person, place, and time. | |
| ___ | ___ | ___ |    b. Evaluate level of consciousness. | |
| ___ | ___ | ___ |    c. Assess memory (immediate recall and past memory). | |
| ___ | ___ | ___ |    d. Assess abstract reasoning by asking the patient to explain a proverb, such as "The early bird catches the worm." | |
| ___ | ___ | ___ |    e. Evaluate the patient's ability to understand spoken and written word. | |
| ___ | ___ | ___ | 7. Test cranial nerve (CN) function. | |
| ___ | ___ | ___ |    a. Ask the patient to close the eyes, occlude one nostril, and then identify the smell of different substances, such as coffee, chocolate, or alcohol. Repeat with other nostril. | |
| ___ | ___ | ___ |    b. Test visual acuity and pupillary constriction. | |
| ___ | ___ | ___ |    c. Move the patient's eyes through the six cardinal positions of gaze. | |
| ___ | ___ | ___ |    d. Ask the patient to smile, frown, wrinkle forehead, and puff out cheeks. | |
| ___ | ___ | ___ |    e. Test hearing. | |
| ___ | ___ | ___ |    f. Test the gag reflex by touching the posterior pharynx with the tongue depressor. Explain to patient that this may be uncomfortable. | |

## SKILL 2-8

# Assessing the Neurologic, Musculoskeletal, and Peripheral Vascular Systems (Continued)

| Excellent | Satisfactory | Needs Practice | | Comments |
|---|---|---|---|---|
| —— | —— | —— | g. Place your hands on the patient's shoulders while he or she shrugs against resistance. Then place your hand on the patient's left cheek, then the right cheek, and have the patient push against it. | |
| —— | —— | —— | 8. Inspect the ability of the patient to move his or her neck. Ask the patient to touch his or her chin to chest and to each shoulder, each ear to the corresponding shoulder, and then tip head back as far as possible. | |
| —— | —— | —— | 9. Inspect the upper extremities. Observe for skin color, presence of lesions, rashes, and muscle mass. Palpate for skin temperature, texture, and presence of masses. | |
| —— | —— | —— | 10. Ask patient to extend arms forward and then rapidly turn palms up and down. | |
| —— | —— | —— | 11. Ask patient to flex upper arm and to resist examiner's opposing force. | |
| —— | —— | —— | 12. Inspect and palpate the hands, fingers, wrists, and elbow joints. | |
| —— | —— | —— | 13. Palpate the radial and brachial pulses. | |
| —— | —— | —— | 14. Have the patient squeeze two of your fingers. | |
| —— | —— | —— | 15. Ask the patient to close his or her eyes. Using your finger or applicator, trace a one-digit number on the patient's palm and ask him or her to identify the number. Repeat on the other hand with a different number. | |
| —— | —— | —— | 16. Ask the patient to close his or her eyes. Place a familiar object, such as a key, in the patient's hand and ask him or her to identify the object. Repeat using another object for the other hand. | |
| —— | —— | —— | 17. Assist the patient to a supine position. Examine the lower extremities. Inspect the legs and feet for color, lesions, varicosities, hair growth, nail growth, edema, and muscle mass. | |
| —— | —— | —— | 18. Test for pitting edema in the pretibial area by pressing fingers into the skin of the pretibial area. If an indentation remains in the skin after the fingers have been lifted, pitting edema is present. | |
| —— | —— | —— | 19. Palpate for pulses and skin temperature at the posterior tibial, dorsalis pedis, and popliteal areas. | |
| —— | —— | —— | 20. Have the patient perform the straight leg test with one leg at a time. | |
| —— | —— | —— | 21. Ask the patient to move one leg laterally with the knee straight to test abduction and medially to test adduction of the hips. | |

| Excellent | Satisfactory | Needs Practice | SKILL 2-8<br>**Assessing the Neurologic, Musculoskeletal, and<br>Peripheral Vascular Systems** *(Continued)* | Comments |
|---|---|---|---|---|
| — | — | — | 22. Ask the patient to raise the thigh against the resistance of your hand; next have the patient push outward against the resistance of your hand; then have the patient pull backward against the resistance of your hand. Repeat on the opposite side. | |
| — | — | — | 23. Assess the patient's deep tendon reflexes (DTR). | |
| — | — | — | a. Place your fingers above the patient's wrist and tap with a reflex hammer; repeat on the other arm. | |
| — | — | — | b. Place your fingers at the elbow area with the thumb over the antecubital area and tap with a reflex hammer; repeat on the other side. | |
| — | — | — | c. Place your fingers over the triceps tendon area and tap with a reflex hammer; repeat on the other side. | |
| — | — | — | d. Tap just below the patella with a reflex hammer; repeat on the other side. | |
| — | — | — | e. Tap over the Achilles' tendon area with reflex hammer; repeat on the other side. | |
| — | — | — | 24. Stroke the sole of the patient's foot with the end of a reflex hammer handle or other hard object such as a key; repeat on the other side. | |
| — | — | — | 25. Ask patient to dorsiflex and then plantarflex both feet against opposing resistance. | |
| — | — | — | 26. As needed, assist the patient to a standing position. Observe the patient as he or she walks with a regular gait, on the toes, on the heels, and then heel to toe. | |
| — | — | — | 27. Perform the Romberg's test; ask the patient to stand straight with feet together, both eyes closed with arms at side. Wait 20 seconds and observe for patient swaying and ability to maintain balance. Be alert to prevent patient fall or injury related to losing balance during this assessment. | |
| — | — | — | 28. Assist the patient to a comfortable position. | |
| — | — | — | 29. Remove PPE, if used. Perform hand hygiene. Continue with assessments of specific body systems, as appropriate, or indicated. Initiate appropriate referral to other health-care practitioners for further evaluation, as indicated. | |

*Skill Checklists for Taylor's Clinical Nursing Skills:*
*A Nursing Process Approach, 3rd edition*

Name _____ Date _____

Unit _____ Position _____

Instructor/Evaluator: _____ Position _____

SKILL 3-1

# Fall Prevention

**Goal:** The patient does not experience a fall and remains free of injury.

| Excellent | Satisfactory | Needs Practice | | Comments |
|---|---|---|---|---|
| —— | —— | —— | 1. Perform hand hygiene and put on PPE, if indicated. | |
| —— | —— | —— | 2. Identify the patient. | |
| —— | —— | —— | 3. Explain the rationale for fall prevention interventions to the patient and family/significant others. | |
| —— | —— | —— | 4. Include the patient's family and/or significant others in the plan of care. | |
| —— | —— | —— | 5. Provide adequate lighting. Use a night light during sleeping hours. | |
| —— | —— | —— | 6. Remove excess equipment, supplies, furniture, and other objects from rooms and walkways. Pay particular attention to high traffic areas and the route to the bathroom. | |
| —— | —— | —— | 7. Orient patient and significant others to new surroundings, including use of the telephone, call signal, patient bed, and room illumination. Indicate the location of the patient bathroom. | |
| —— | —— | —— | 8. Provide a 'low bed' to replace regular hospital bed. | |
| —— | —— | —— | 9. Use floor mats if patient is at risk for serious injury. | |
| —— | —— | —— | 10. Provide nonskid footwear and/or walking shoes. | |
| —— | —— | —— | 11. Institute a toileting regimen and/or continence program, if appropriate. | |
| —— | —— | —— | 12. Provide a bedside commode and/or urinal/bedpan, if appropriate. Ensure that it is near the bed at all times. | |
| —— | —— | —— | 13. Ensure that the call bell, bedside table, telephone, and other personal items are within the patient's reach at all times. | |
| —— | —— | —— | 14. Confer with primary care provider regarding appropriate exercise and physical therapy. | |
| —— | —— | —— | 15. Confer with primary care provider regarding appropriate mobility aids, such as a cane or walker. | |
| —— | —— | —— | 16. Confer with primary care provider regarding the use of bone-strengthening medications, such as calcium, vitamin D, and drugs to prevent/treat osteoporosis. | |
| —— | —— | —— | 17. Encourage the patient to rise or change position slowly and sit for several minutes before standing. | |

| | | | SKILL 3-1 |
|---|---|---|---|

## Fall Prevention *(Continued)*

| Excellent | Satisfactory | Needs Practice | | Comments |
|---|---|---|---|---|
| —— | —— | —— | 18. Evaluate the appropriateness of elastic stockings for lower extremities. | |
| —— | —— | —— | 19. Review medications for potential hazards. | |
| —— | —— | —— | 20. Keep the bed in the lowest position during use. If elevated to provide care (to reduce caregiver strain), ensure that it is lowered when care is completed. | |
| —— | —— | —— | 21. Make sure locks on the bed or wheelchair are secured at all times. | |
| —— | —— | —— | 22. Use bed rails according to facility policy, when appropriate. | |
| —— | —— | —— | 23. Anticipate patient needs and provide assistance with activities instead of waiting for the patient to ask. | |
| —— | —— | —— | 24. Consider the use of an electronic personal alarm or pressure sensor alarm for the bed or chair. | |
| —— | —— | —— | 25. Discuss the possibility of appropriate family member(s) staying with patient. | |
| —— | —— | —— | 26. Consider the use of patient attendant or sitter. | |
| —— | —— | —— | 27. Increase the frequency of patient observation and surveillance; 1- or 2-hour nursing rounds, including pain assessment, toileting assistance, patient comfort, personal items in reach, and patient needs. | |
| —— | —— | —— | 28. Remove PPE, if used. Perform hand hygiene. | |

34

*Skill Checklists for Taylor's Clinical Nursing Skills:*
*A Nursing Process Approach, 3rd edition*

Name _____ Date _____

Unit _____ Position _____

Instructor/Evaluator: _____ Position _____

| Excellent | Satisfactory | Needs Practice | SKILL 3-2<br><br>**Implementing Alternatives to the Use of Restraints**<br><br>**Goal:** The use of restraints is avoided and the patient and others remain free from harm. | Comments |
|---|---|---|---|---|
| —— | —— | —— | 1. Perform hand hygiene and put on PPE, if indicated. | |
| —— | —— | —— | 2. Identify the patient. | |
| —— | —— | —— | 3. Explain the rationale for interventions to the patient and family/significant others. | |
| —— | —— | —— | 4. Include the patient's family and/or significant others in the plan of care. | |
| —— | —— | —— | 5. Identify behavior(s) that place the patient at risk for restraint use. Assess the patient's status and environment, as outlined above. | |
| —— | —— | —— | 6. Identify triggers or contributing factors to patient behaviors. Evaluate medication usage for medications that can contribute to cognitive and movement dysfunction and contribute to increased risk for falls. | |
| —— | —— | —— | 7. Assess the patient's functional, mental, and psychological status and the environment, as outlined above. | |
| —— | —— | —— | 8. Provide adequate lighting. Use a nightlight during sleeping hours. | |
| —— | —— | —— | 9. Consult with primary care provider and other appropriate healthcare providers regarding the continued need for treatments/therapies and the use of the least invasive method to deliver care. | |
| —— | —— | —— | 10. Assess the patient for pain and discomfort. Provide appropriate pharmacologic and nonpharmacologic interventions. (Refer to Chapter 10, Comfort.) | |
| —— | —— | —— | 11. Ask a family member or significant other to stay with patient. | |
| —— | —— | —— | 12. Reduce unnecessary environmental stimulation and noise. | |
| —— | —— | —— | 13. Provide simple, clear, and direct explanations for treatments and care. Repeat to reinforce as needed. | |
| —— | —— | —— | 14. Distract and redirect using a calm voice. | |
| —— | —— | —— | 15. Increase the frequency of patient observation and surveillance; 1- or 2-hour nursing rounds, including pain assessment, toileting assistance, patient comfort, personal items in reach, and patient needs. | |

## SKILL 3-2

# Implementing Alternatives to the Use of Restraints *(Continued)*

| Excellent | Satisfactory | Needs Practice | | Comments |
|---|---|---|---|---|
| —— | —— | —— | 16. Implement fall precaution interventions. Refer to Skill 3-1. | |
| —— | —— | —— | 17. Camouflage tube and other treatment sites with clothing, elastic sleeves, or bandaging. | |
| —— | —— | —— | 18. Ensure the use of glasses and hearing aids, if necessary. | |
| —— | —— | —— | 19. Consider relocation to a room close to the nursing station. | |
| —— | —— | —— | 20. Encourage daily exercise/provide exercise and activities or relaxation techniques. | |
| —— | —— | —— | 21. Make the environment as homelike as possible; provide familiar objects. | |
| —— | —— | —— | 22. Allow restless patient to walk after ensuring that environment is safe. Use a large plant or piece of furniture as a barrier to limit wandering from designated area. | |
| —— | —— | —— | 23. Consider the use of patient attendant or sitter. | |
| —— | —— | —— | 24. Remove PPE, if used. Perform hand hygiene. | |

*Skill Checklists for Taylor's Clinical Nursing Skills:*
*A Nursing Process Approach, 3rd edition*

Name _____    Date _____

Unit _____    Position _____

Instructor/Evaluator: _____    Position _____

## SKILL 3-3
## Applying an Extremity Restraint

**Goal:** The patient is constrained by the restraint, remains free from injury, and the restraint does not interfere with therapeutic devices.

| Excellent | Satisfactory | Needs Practice | | Comments |
|---|---|---|---|---|
| —— | —— | —— | 1. Determine need for restraints. Assess patient's physical condition, behavior, and mental status. (Refer to Fundamentals Review 3-1, 3-2, 3-3, and 3-4 at the beginning of the chapter.) | |
| —— | —— | —— | 2. Confirm agency policy for application of restraints. *Secure an order from the primary care provider, or validate that the order has been obtained within the past 24 hours.* | |
| —— | —— | —— | 3. Perform hand hygiene and put on PPE, if indicated. | |
| —— | —— | —— | 4. Identify the patient. | |
| —— | —— | —— | 5. Explain reason for restraint use to patient and family. Clarify how care will be given and how needs will be met. Explain that restraint is a temporary measure. | |
| —— | —— | —— | 6. Include the patient's family and/or significant others in the plan of care. | |
| —— | —— | —— | 7. Apply restraint according to manufacturer's directions: | |
| —— | —— | —— | a. Choose the least restrictive type of device that allows the greatest possible degree of mobility. | |
| —— | —— | —— | b. Pad bony prominences. | |
| —— | —— | —— | c. Wrap the restraint around the extremity with the soft part in contact with the skin. If a hand mitt is being used, pull over the hand with cushion to the palmar aspect of hand. Secure in place with the Velcro straps. | |
| —— | —— | —— | 8. *Ensure that two fingers can be inserted between the restraint and patient's wrist or ankle.* | |
| —— | —— | —— | 9. Maintain restrained extremity in normal anatomic position. *Use a quick-release knot to tie the restraint to the bed frame, not side rail. The restraint may also be attached to a chair frame.* The site should not be readily accessible to patient. | |
| —— | —— | —— | 10. Remove PPE, if used. Perform hand hygiene. | |

SKILL 3-3

# Applying an Extremity Restraint *(Continued)*

| Excellent | Satisfactory | Needs Practice | | Comments |
|---|---|---|---|---|
| — | — | — | 11. Assess the patient at least every hour or according to facility policy. Assessment should include the placement of the restraint, neurovascular assessment of the affected extremity, and skin integrity. In addition, assess for signs of sensory deprivation, such as increased sleeping, daydreaming, anxiety, panic, and hallucinations. | |
| — | — | — | 12. *Remove restraint at least every 2 hours, or according to agency policy and patient need.* Perform range-of-motion exercises. | |
| — | — | — | 13. Evaluate patient for continued need of restraint. Reapply restraint only if continued need is evident and order is still valid. | |
| — | — | — | 14. Reassure patient at regular intervals. Provide continued explanation of rationale for interventions, reorientation if necessary, and plan of care. *Keep call bell within easy reach.* | |

*Skill Checklists for Taylor's Clinical Nursing Skills:*
*A Nursing Process Approach, 3rd edition*

Name _____  Date _____

Unit _____  Position _____

Instructor/Evaluator: _____  Position _____

## SKILL 3-4

# Applying a Waist Restraint

**Goal:** The patient is constrained by the restraint, remains free from injury, and the restraint does not interfere with therapeutic devices.

| Excellent | Satisfactory | Needs Practice | | Comments |
|---|---|---|---|---|
| —— | —— | —— | 1. Determine need for restraints. Assess patient's physical condition, behavior, and mental status. (Refer to Fundamentals Review 3-1, 3-2, 3-3, and 3-4 at the beginning of the chapter.) | |
| —— | —— | —— | 2. Confirm agency policy for application of restraints. *Secure an order from the primary care provider or validate that the order has been obtained within the past 24 hours.* | |
| —— | —— | —— | 3. Perform hand hygiene and put on PPE, if indicated. | |
| —— | —— | —— | 4. Identify the patient. | |
| —— | —— | —— | 5. Explain reason for use to patient and family. Clarify how care will be given and how needs will be met. Explain that restraint is a temporary measure. | |
| —— | —— | —— | 6. Include the patient's family and/or significant others in the plan of care. | |
| —— | —— | —— | 7. Apply restraint according to manufacturer's directions: | |
| —— | —— | —— | a. Choose the correct size of the least restrictive type of device that allows the greatest possible degree of mobility. | |
| —— | —— | —— | b. Pad bony prominences that may be affected by the waist restraint. | |
| —— | —— | —— | c. Assist patient to a sitting position, if not contraindicated. | |
| —— | —— | —— | d. *Place waist restraint on patient over gown. Bring ties through slots in restraint. Position slots at patient's back.* | |
| —— | —— | —— | e. Pull the ties secure. *Ensure that the restraint is not too tight and there are no wrinkles in it.* | |
| —— | —— | —— | f. *Insert fist between restraint and patient to ensure that breathing is not constricted. Assess respirations after restraint is applied.* | |
| —— | —— | —— | 8. *Use a quick-release knot to tie the restraint to the bed frame, not side rail.* If patient is in a wheelchair, lock the wheels and place the ties under the arm rests and tie behind the chair. Site should not be readily accessible to the patient. | |

SKILL 3-4

# Applying a Waist Restraint *(Continued)*

| Excellent | Satisfactory | Needs Practice | | Comments |
|---|---|---|---|---|
| ___ | ___ | ___ | 9. Remove PPE, if used. Perform hand hygiene. | |
| ___ | ___ | ___ | 10. Assess the patient at least every hour or according to facility policy. An assessment should include the placement of the restraint, respiratory assessment, and skin integrity. Assess for signs of sensory deprivation, such as increased sleeping, daydreaming, anxiety, panic, and hallucinations. | |
| ___ | ___ | ___ | 11. ***Remove restraint at least every 2 hours or according to agency policy and patient need.*** Perform ROM exercises. | |
| ___ | ___ | ___ | 12. Evaluate patient for continued need of restraint. Reapply restraint only if continued need is evident and order is still valid. | |
| ___ | ___ | ___ | 13. Reassure patient at regular intervals. Provide continued explanation of rationale for interventions, reorientation if necessary, and plan of care. ***Keep call bell within easy reach.*** | |
| ___ | ___ | ___ | 14. Perform hand hygiene. | |

*Skill Checklists for Taylor's Clinical Nursing Skills:*
*A Nursing Process Approach, 3rd edition*

Name _____     Date _____

Unit _____     Position _____

Instructor/Evaluator: _____     Position _____

| Excellent | Satisfactory | Needs Practice | SKILL 3-5<br>**Applying an Elbow Restraint**<br><br>**Goal:** The patient is constrained by the restraint, remains free from injury, and the restraint does not interfere with therapeutic devices. | Comments |
|---|---|---|---|---|
| ___ | ___ | ___ | 1. Determine need for restraints. Assess patient's physical condition, behavior, and mental status. Refer to review material in the chapter introduction. | |
| ___ | ___ | ___ | 2. Confirm agency policy for application of restraints. *Secure an order from the primary care provider or validate that the order has been obtained within the past 24 hours.* | |
| ___ | ___ | ___ | 3. Perform hand hygiene and put on PPE, if indicated. | |
| ___ | ___ | ___ | 4. Identify the patient. | |
| ___ | ___ | ___ | 5. Explain reason for use to patient and family. Clarify how care will be given and how needs will be met. Explain that restraint is a temporary measure. | |
| ___ | ___ | ___ | 6. Apply restraint according to manufacturer's directions: | |
| ___ | ___ | ___ | a. Choose the correct size of the least restrictive type of device that allows the greatest possible degree of mobility. | |
| ___ | ___ | ___ | b. Pad bony prominences that may be affected by the restraint. | |
| ___ | ___ | ___ | c. Spread elbow restraint out flat. Place middle of elbow restraint behind patient's elbow. *The restraint should not extend below the wrist or place pressure on the axilla.* | |
| ___ | ___ | ___ | d. *Wrap restraint snugly around patient's arm, but make sure that two fingers can easily fit under restraint.* | |
| ___ | ___ | ___ | e. Secure Velcro straps around restraint. | |
| ___ | ___ | ___ | f. Apply restraint to opposite arm if patient can move arm. | |
| ___ | ___ | ___ | g. Thread Velcro strap from one elbow restraint across the back and into the loop on the opposite elbow restraint. | |
| ___ | ___ | ___ | 7. *Assess circulation to fingers and hand.* | |
| ___ | ___ | ___ | 8. Remove PPE, if used. Perform hand hygiene. | |
| ___ | ___ | ___ | 9. Assess the patient at least every hour or according to facility policy. An assessment should include the placement of the restraint, neurovascular assessment, and skin integrity. Assess for signs of sensory deprivation, such as increased sleeping, daydreaming, anxiety, inconsolable crying, and panic. | |

# Applying an Elbow Restraint (Continued)

| Excellent | Satisfactory | Needs Practice | | Comments |
|---|---|---|---|---|
| —— | —— | —— | 10. *Remove restraint at least every 2 hours or according to agency policy and patient need. Remove restraint at least every 2 hours for children ages 9 to 17 years and at least every 1 hour for children under age 9, or according to agency policy and patient need.* Perform ROM exercises. | |
| —— | —— | —— | 11. Evaluate patient for continued need of restraint. Reapply restraint only if continued need is evident. | |
| —— | —— | —— | 12. Reassure patient at regular intervals. *Keep call bell within easy reach.* | |

*Skill Checklists for Taylor's Clinical Nursing Skills:*
*A Nursing Process Approach, 3rd edition*

Name _____  Date _____

Unit _____  Position _____

Instructor/Evaluator: _____  Position _____

| Excellent | Satisfactory | Needs Practice | SKILL 3-6<br>**Applying a Mummy Restraint**<br><br>**Goal:** The patient is constrained by the restraint, remains free from injury, and the restraint does not interfere with therapeutic devices. | Comments |
|---|---|---|---|---|
| —— | —— | —— | 1. Determine need for restraints. Assess patient's physical condition, behavior, and mental status. Refer to review material in the chapter introduction. | |
| —— | —— | —— | 2. Confirm agency policy for application of restraints. *Secure an order from the primary care provider or validate that the order has been obtained within the past 24 hours.* | |
| —— | —— | —— | 3. Perform hand hygiene and put on PPE, if indicated. | |
| —— | —— | —— | 4. Identify the patient. | |
| —— | —— | —— | 5. Explain reason for use to patient and family. Clarify how care will be given and how needs will be met. Explain that restraint is a temporary measure. | |
| —— | —— | —— | 6. Open the blanket or sheet. Place the child on the blanket, with edge of blanket at or above neck level. | |
| —— | —— | —— | 7. Position the child's right arm alongside the child's body. Left arm should not be constrained at this time. Pull the right side of the blanket tightly over the child's right shoulder and chest. Secure under the left side of the child's body. | |
| —— | —— | —— | 8. Position the left arm alongside the child's body. Pull the left side of the blanket tightly over the child's left shoulder and chest. Secure under the right side of the child's body. | |
| —— | —— | —— | 9. Fold the lower part of blanket up and pull over the child's body. Secure under the child's body on each side or with safety pins. | |
| —— | —— | —— | 10. Stay with child while mummy wrap is in place. Reassure child and parents at regular intervals. Once examination or treatment is completed, unwrap child. | |
| —— | —— | —— | 11. Remove PPE, if used. Perform hand hygiene. | |

*Skill Checklists for Taylor's Clinical Nursing Skills:*
*A Nursing Process Approach, 3rd edition*

Name _____ Date _____

Unit _____ Position _____

Instructor/Evaluator: _____ Position _____

| Excellent | Satisfactory | Needs Practice | SKILL 4-1<br><br>**Performing Hand Hygiene Using Soap and Water (Handwashing)** | |
|---|---|---|---|---|
| | | | **Goal:** The hands will be free of visible soiling and transient microorganisms will be eliminated. | **Comments** |
| ___ | ___ | ___ | 1. Gather the necessary supplies. Stand in front of the sink. Do not allow your clothing to touch the sink during the washing procedure. | |
| ___ | ___ | ___ | 2. Remove jewelry, if possible, and secure in a safe place. A plain wedding band may remain in place. | |
| ___ | ___ | ___ | 3. Turn on water and adjust force. Regulate the temperature until the water is warm. | |
| ___ | ___ | ___ | 4. Wet the hands and wrist area. Keep hands lower than elbows to allow water to flow toward fingertips. | |
| ___ | ___ | ___ | 5. Use about 1 teaspoon liquid soap from dispenser or rinse bar of soap and lather thoroughly. Cover all areas of hands with the soap product. Rinse soap bar again and return to soap rack. | |
| ___ | ___ | ___ | 6. With firm rubbing and circular motions, wash the palms and backs of the hands, each finger, the areas between the fingers, and the knuckles, wrists, and forearms. ***Wash at least 1 inch above area of contamination.*** If hands are not visibly soiled, wash to 1 inch above the wrists. | |
| ___ | ___ | ___ | 7. Continue this friction motion for at least 15 seconds. | |
| ___ | ___ | ___ | 8. Use fingernails of the opposite hand or a clean orangewood stick to clean under fingernails. | |
| ___ | ___ | ___ | 9. Rinse thoroughly with water flowing toward fingertips. | |
| ___ | ___ | ___ | 10. Pat hands dry with a paper towel, beginning with the fingers and moving upward toward forearms, and discard it immediately. Use another clean towel to turn off the faucet. Discard towel immediately without touching other clean hand. | |
| ___ | ___ | ___ | 11. Use oil-free lotion on hands if desired. | |

*Skill Checklists for Taylor's Clinical Nursing Skills:*
*A Nursing Process Approach, 3rd edition*

Name _____  Date _____

Unit _____  Position _____

Instructor/Evaluator: _____  Position _____

SKILL 4-2

# Performing Hand Hygiene Using an Alcohol-Based Hand Rub

**Goal:** Transient microorganisms are eliminated from the hands.

| Excellent | Satisfactory | Needs Practice | | Comments |
|---|---|---|---|---|
| —— | —— | —— | 1. Remove jewelry, if possible, and secure in a safe place. A plain wedding band may remain in place. | |
| —— | —— | —— | 2. Check the product labeling for correct amount of product needed. | |
| —— | —— | —— | 3. Apply the correct amount of product to the palm of one hand. Rub hands together, covering all surfaces of hands and fingers, and between fingers. Also clean the fingertips and the area beneath the fingernails. | |
| —— | —— | —— | 4. Rub hands together until they are dry (at least 15 seconds). | |
| —— | —— | —— | 5. Use oil-free lotion on hands if desired. | |

*Skill Checklists for Taylor's Clinical Nursing Skills:*
*A Nursing Process Approach, 3rd edition*

Name _____ Date _____

Unit _____ Position _____

Instructor/Evaluator: _____ Position _____

| Excellent | Satisfactory | Needs Practice | SKILL 4-3<br>**Preparing a Sterile Field Using a Packaged Sterile Drape**<br><br>**Goal:** The sterile field is created without contamination and the patient remains free of exposure to potential infection-causing microorganisms. | Comments |
|---|---|---|---|---|
| ___ | ___ | ___ | 1. Perform hand hygiene and put on PPE, if indicated. | |
| ___ | ___ | ___ | 2. Identify the patient. Explain the procedure to the patient. | |
| ___ | ___ | ___ | 3. Check that packaged sterile drape is dry and unopened. Also note expiration date, making sure that the date is still valid. | |
| ___ | ___ | ___ | 4. Select a work area that is waist level or higher. | |
| ___ | ___ | ___ | 5. Open the outer covering of the drape. Remove sterile drape, lifting it carefully by its corners. Hold away from body and above the waist and work surface. | |
| ___ | ___ | ___ | 6. Continue to hold only by the corners. Allow the drape to unfold, away from your body and any other surface. | |
| ___ | ___ | ___ | 7. Position the drape on the work surface with the moisture-proof side down. This would be the shiny or blue side. Avoid touching any other surface or object with the drape. If any portion of the drape hangs off the work surface, that part of the drape is considered contaminated. | |
| ___ | ___ | ___ | 8. Place additional sterile items on field as needed. Refer to Skill 4-5. Continue with the procedure as indicated. | |
| ___ | ___ | ___ | 9. When procedure is completed, remove PPE, if used. Perform hand hygiene. | |

46

Name _____   Date _____

Unit _____   Position _____

Instructor/Evaluator: _____   Position _____

### SKILL 4-4

# Preparing a Sterile Field Using a Commercially Prepared Sterile Kit or Tray

**Goal:** A sterile field is created without contamination, the contents of the package remain sterile, and the patient remains free of exposure to potential infection-causing microorganisms.

| Excellent | Satisfactory | Needs Practice | | Comments |
|---|---|---|---|---|
| ___ | ___ | ___ | 1. Perform hand hygiene and put on PPE, if indicated. | |
| ___ | ___ | ___ | 2. Identify the patient. Explain the procedure to the patient. | |
| ___ | ___ | ___ | 3. Check that the packaged kit or tray is dry and unopened. Also note expiration date, making sure that the date is still valid. | |
| ___ | ___ | ___ | 4. Select a work area that is waist level or higher. | |
| ___ | ___ | ___ | 5. Open the outside cover of the package and remove the kit or tray. Place in the center of the work surface, with the topmost flap positioned on the far side of the package. | |
| ___ | ___ | ___ | 6. Reach around the package and grasp the outer surface of the end of the topmost flap, holding no more than 1 inch from the border of the flap. Pull open away from the body, keeping the arm outstretched and away from the inside of the wrapper. Allow the wrapper to lie flat on the work surface. | |
| ___ | ___ | ___ | 7. Reach around the package and grasp the outer surface of the first side flap, holding no more than 1 inch from the border of the flap. Pull open to the side of the package, keeping the arm outstretched and away from the inside of the wrapper. Allow the wrapper to lie flat on the work surface. | |
| ___ | ___ | ___ | 8. Reach around the package and grasp the outer surface of the remaining side flap, holding no more than 1 inch from the border of the flap. Pull open to the side of the package, keeping the arm outstretched and away from the inside of the wrapper. Allow the wrapper to lie flat on the work surface. | |

## SKILL 4-4

# Preparing a Sterile Field Using a Commercially Prepared Sterile Kit or Tray *(Continued)*

| Excellent | Satisfactory | Needs Practice | | Comments |
|---|---|---|---|---|

| Excellent | Satisfactory | Needs Practice | | |
|---|---|---|---|---|
| — | — | — | 9. Stand away from the package and work surface. Grasp the outer surface of the remaining flap closest to the body, holding not more than 1 inch from the border of the flap. Pull the flap back toward the body, keeping arm outstretched and away from the inside of the wrapper. Keep this hand in place. Use other hand to grasp the wrapper on the underside (the side that is down to the work surface). Position the wrapper so that when flat, edges are on the work surface, and do not hang down over sides of work surface. Allow the wrapper to lie flat on the work surface. | |
| — | — | — | 10. The outer wrapper of the package has become a sterile field with the packaged supplies in the center. Do not touch or reach over the sterile field. Place additional sterile items on field as needed. Refer to Skill 4-5. Continue with the procedure as indicated. | |
| — | — | — | 11. When procedure is completed, remove PPE, if used. Perform hand hygiene. | |

*Skill Checklists for Taylor's Clinical Nursing Skills:*
*A Nursing Process Approach, 3rd edition*

Name _____  Date _____

Unit _____  Position _____

Instructor/Evaluator: _____  Position _____

SKILL 4-5

# Adding Sterile Items to a Sterile Field

**Goal**: The sterile field is created without contamination, the sterile supplies are not contaminated, and the patient remains free of exposure to potential infection-causing microorganisms.

| Excellent | Satisfactory | Needs Practice | | Comments |
|---|---|---|---|---|
| —— | —— | —— | 1. Perform hand hygiene and put on PPE, if indicated. | |
| —— | —— | —— | 2. Identify the patient. Explain the procedure to the patient. | |
| —— | —— | —— | 3. Check that the sterile, packaged drape and supplies are dry and unopened. Also note expiration date, making sure that the date is still valid. | |
| —— | —— | —— | 4. Select a work area that is waist level or higher. | |
| —— | —— | —— | 5. Prepare sterile field as described in Skill 4-3 or Skill 4-4. | |
| —— | —— | —— | 6. Add sterile item: | |
| | | | **To Add an Agency-Wrapped and Sterilized Item** | |
| —— | —— | —— | a. Hold agency-wrapped item in the dominant hand, with top flap opening away from the body. With other hand, reach around the package and unfold top flap and both sides. | |
| —— | —— | —— | b. Keep a secure hold on the item through the wrapper with the dominant hand. Grasp the remaining flap of the wrapper closest to the body, taking care not to touch the inner surface of the wrapper or the item. Pull the flap back toward the wrist, so the wrapper covers the hand and wrist. | |
| —— | —— | —— | c. Grasp all the corners of the wrapper together with the nondominant hand and pull back toward wrist, covering hand and wrist. Hold in place. | |
| —— | —— | —— | d. Hold the item 6 inches above the surface of the sterile field and drop onto the field. Be careful to avoid touching the surface or other items or dropping onto the 1-inch border. | |
| | | | **To Add a Commercially Wrapped and Sterilized Item** | |
| —— | —— | —— | a. Hold package in one hand. Pull back top cover with other hand. Alternately, carefully peel the edges apart using both hands. | |
| —— | —— | —— | b. After top cover or edges are partially separated, hold the item 6 inches above the surface of the sterile field. Continue opening the package and drop the item onto the field. Be careful to avoid touching the surface or other items or dropping onto the 1-inch border. | |
| —— | —— | —— | c. Discard wrapper. | |

SKILL 4-5

# Adding Sterile Items to a Sterile Field *(Continued)*

| Excellent | Satisfactory | Needs Practice | | Comments |
|---|---|---|---|---|

**To Add a Sterile Solution**

a. Obtain appropriate solution and check expiration date.

b. Open solution container according to directions and *place cap on table away from the field with edges up.*

c. Hold bottle outside the edge of the sterile field with the label side facing the palm of your hand and prepare to pour from a height of 4 to 6 inches (10 to 15 cm). The tip of the bottle should never touch a sterile container or field.

d. Pour required amount of solution steadily into sterile container previously added to the sterile field and positioned at side of sterile field or onto dressings. *Avoid splashing any liquid.*

e. Touch only the outside of the lid when recapping. Label solution with date and time of opening.

7. Continue with procedure as indicated.

8. When procedure is completed, remove PPE, if used. Perform hand hygiene.

*Skill Checklists for Taylor's Clinical Nursing Skills:*
*A Nursing Process Approach, 3rd edition*

Name _____ Date _____

Unit _____ Position _____

Instructor/Evaluator: _____ Position _____

| | | | |
|---|---|---|---|
| | | | **SKILL 4-6** |

### SKILL 4-6
# Putting on Sterile Gloves and Removing Soiled Gloves

**Goal:** The gloves are applied and removed without contamination.

| Excellent | Satisfactory | Needs Practice | | Comments |
|---|---|---|---|---|
| ___ | ___ | ___ | 1. Perform hand hygiene and put on PPE, if indicated. | |
| ___ | ___ | ___ | 2. Identify the patient. Explain the procedure to the patient. | |
| ___ | ___ | ___ | 3. Check that the sterile glove package is dry and unopened. Also note expiration date, making sure that the date is still valid. | |
| ___ | ___ | ___ | 4. Place sterile glove package on clean, dry surface at or above your waist. | |
| ___ | ___ | ___ | 5. Open the outside wrapper by carefully peeling the top layer back. Remove inner package, handling only the outside of it. | |
| ___ | ___ | ___ | 6. Place the inner package on the work surface with the side labeled 'cuff end' closest to the body. | |
| ___ | ___ | ___ | 7. Carefully open the inner package. Fold open the top flap, then the bottom and sides. Take care not to touch the inner surface of the package or the gloves. | |
| ___ | ___ | ___ | 8. With the thumb and forefinger of the nondominant hand, grasp the folded cuff of the glove for the dominant hand, touching only the exposed inside of the glove. | |
| ___ | ___ | ___ | 9. Keeping the hands above the waistline, lift and hold the glove up and off the inner package with fingers down. *Be careful it does not touch any unsterile object.* | |
| ___ | ___ | ___ | 10. Carefully insert dominant hand palm up into glove and pull glove on. Leave the cuff folded until the opposite hand is gloved. | |
| ___ | ___ | ___ | 11. Hold the thumb of the gloved hand outward. Place the fingers of the gloved hand inside the cuff of the remaining glove. Lift it from the wrapper, taking care not to touch anything with the gloves or hands. | |
| ___ | ___ | ___ | 12. Carefully insert nondominant hand into glove. Pull the glove on, taking care that the skin does not touch any of the outer surfaces of the gloves. | |
| ___ | ___ | ___ | 13. *Slide the fingers of one hand under the cuff of the other and fully extend the cuff down the arm, touching only the sterile outside of the glove. Repeat for the remaining hand.* | |

SKILL 4-6

# Putting on Sterile Gloves and Removing Soiled Gloves *(Continued)*

| Excellent | Satisfactory | Needs Practice | | Comments |
|---|---|---|---|---|
| —— | —— | —— | 14. *Adjust gloves on both hands if necessary, touching only sterile areas with other sterile areas.* | |
| —— | —— | —— | 15. Continue with procedure as indicated. | |
| | | | **Removing Soiled Gloves** | |
| —— | —— | —— | 16. Use dominant hand to grasp the opposite glove near cuff end on the outside exposed area. Remove it by pulling it off, inverting it as it is pulled, keeping the contaminated area on the inside. Hold the removed glove in the remaining gloved hand. | |
| —— | —— | —— | 17. Slide fingers of ungloved hand between the remaining glove and the wrist. *Take care to avoid touching the outside surface of the glove.* Remove it by pulling it off, inverting it as it is pulled, keeping the contaminated area on the inside, and securing the first glove inside the second. | |
| —— | —— | —— | 18. Discard gloves in appropriate container. Remove additional PPE, if used. Perform hand hygiene. | |

*Skill Checklists for Taylor's Clinical Nursing Skills:*
*A Nursing Process Approach, 3rd edition*

Name _____ Date _____

Unit _____ Position _____

Instructor/Evaluator: _____ Position _____

| Excellent | Satisfactory | Needs Practice | | Comments |
|---|---|---|---|---|
| | | | **SKILL 4-7**<br>**Using Personal Protective Equipment** | |
| | | | **Goal:** The transmission of microorganisms is prevented. | |
| | ✓ | | 1. Check medical record and nursing plan of care for type of precautions and review precautions in infection control manual. | |
| | ✓ | | 2. Plan nursing activities before entering patient's room. | |
| | ✓ | | 3. Perform hand hygiene. | |
| | ✓ | | 4. Provide instruction about precautions to patient, family members, and visitors. | |
| | ✓ | | 5. Put on gown, gloves, mask, and protective eyewear, based on the type of exposure anticipated and category of isolation precautions. | |
| | ✓ | | a. Put on the gown, with the opening in the back. Tie gown securely at neck and waist. | |
| | ✓ | | b. Put on the mask or respirator over your nose, mouth, and chin. Secure ties or elastic bands at the middle of the head and neck. If respirator is used, perform a fit check. Inhale; the respirator should collapse. Exhale; air should not leak out. | |
| | ✓ | | c. Put on goggles. Place over eyes and adjust to fit. Alternately, a face shield could be used to take the place of the mask and goggles. | |
| | ✓ | | d. Put on clean disposable gloves. Extend gloves to cover the cuffs of the gown. | |
| | ✓ | | 6. Identify the patient. Explain the procedure to the patient. Continue with patient care as appropriate. | |
| | ✓ | | **Remove PPE**<br>7. Remove PPE: Except for respirator, remove PPE at the doorway or in an anteroom. Remove respirator after leaving the patient room and closing door. | |
| | ✓ | | a. If impervious gown has been tied in front of the body at the waistline, untie waist strings before removing gloves. | |
| | ✓ | | b. Grasp the outside of one glove with the opposite gloved hand and peel off, turning the glove inside out as you pull it off. Hold the removed glove in the remaining gloved hand. | |

SKILL 4-7

# Using Personal Protective Equipment *(Continued)*

| Excellent | Satisfactory | Needs Practice | | Comments |
|---|---|---|---|---|
| — | ✓ | — | c. Slide fingers of ungloved hand under the remaining glove at the wrist, taking care not to touch the outer surface of the glove. | |
| — | ✓ | — | d. Peel off the glove over the first glove, containing the one glove inside the other. Discard in appropriate container. | |
| — | ✓ | — | e. To remove the goggles or face shield: Handle by the headband or ear pieces. Lift away from the face. Place in designated receptacle for reprocessing or in an appropriate waste container. | |
| — | ✓ | — | f. To remove gown: Unfasten ties, if at the neck and back. Allow the gown to fall away from shoulders. Touching only the inside of the gown, pull away from the torso. Keeping hands on the inner surface of the gown, pull from arms. Turn gown inside out. Fold or roll into a bundle and discard. | |
| — | ✓ | — | g. To remove mask or respirator: Grasp the neck ties or elastic, then top ties or elastic and remove. Take care to avoid touching front of mask or respirator. Discard in waste container. If using a respirator, save for future use in the designated area. | |
| — | ✓ | — | 8. Perform hand hygiene immediately after removing all PPE. | |

*Skill Checklists for Taylor's Clinical Nursing Skills:*
*A Nursing Process Approach, 3rd edition*

Name _____  Date _____

Unit _____  Position _____

Instructor/Evaluator: _____  Position _____

## SKILL 5-1
# Administering Oral Medications

**Goal:** The patient will swallow the prescribed medication at the proper time.

| Excellent | Satisfactory | Needs Practice | | Comments |
|---|---|---|---|---|
| — | — | — | 1. Gather equipment. Check each medication order against the original in the medical record, according to facility policy. Clarify any inconsistencies. Check the patient's chart for allergies. | |
| — | — | — | 2. Know the actions, special nursing considerations, safe dose ranges, purpose of administration, and adverse effects of the medications to be administered. Consider the appropriateness of the medication for this patient. | |
| — | — | — | 3. Perform hand hygiene. | |
| — | — | — | 4. Move the medication cart to the outside of the patient's room or prepare for administration in the medication area. | |
| — | — | — | 5. Unlock the medication cart or drawer. Enter pass code into the computer and scan employee identification, if required. | |
| — | — | — | 6. *Prepare medications for one patient at a time.* | |
| — | — | — | 7. Read the CMAR/MAR and select the proper medication from the patient's medication drawer or unit stock. | |
| — | — | — | 8. Compare the label with the CMAR/MAR. Check expiration dates and perform calculations, if necessary. Scan the bar code on the package, if required. | |
| — | — | — | 9. Prepare the required medications: | |
| — | — | — | a. *Unit dose packages:* Place unit dose-packaged medications in a disposable cup. *Do not open the wrapper until at the bedside.* Keep narcotics and medications that require special nursing assessments in a separate container. | |
| — | — | — | b. *Multidose containers:* When removing tablets or capsules from a multidose bottle, pour the necessary number into the bottle cap and then place the tablets or capsules in a medication cup. Break only scored tablets, if necessary, to obtain the proper dosage. Do not touch tablets or capsules with hands. | |

SKILL 5-1

# Administering Oral Medications *(Continued)*

| Excellent | Satisfactory | Needs Practice | | Comments |
|---|---|---|---|---|
| — | — | — | c. *Liquid medication in multidose bottle:* When pouring liquid medications out of a multidose bottle, hold the bottle so the label is against the palm. Use the appropriate measuring device when pouring liquids, and read the amount of medication at the bottom of the meniscus at eye level. Wipe the lip of the bottle with a paper towel. | |
| — | — | — | 10. **When all medications for one patient have been prepared, recheck the labels with the CMAR/MAR before taking the medications to the patient. Replace any multidose containers in the patient's drawer or unit stock. Lock the medication cart before leaving it.** | *4 types of insulin* *cannot mix long acting* |
| — | — | — | 11. Transport medications to the patient's bedside carefully, and keep the medications in sight at all times. | |
| — | — | — | 12. **Ensure that the patient receives the medications at the correct time.** | *Regular – clear* *NPH – cloudy* |
| — | — | — | 13. Perform hand hygiene and put on PPE, if indicated. | |
| — | — | — | 14. Identify the patient. Usually, the patient should be identified using two methods. Compare the information with the CMAR/MAR. | |
| — | — | — | a. Check the name and identification number on the patient's identification band. | |
| — | — | — | b. Ask the patient to state his or her name and birth date, based on facility policy. | |
| — | — | — | c. If the patient cannot identify him- or herself, verify the patient's identification with a staff member who knows the patient, for the second source. | |
| — | — | — | 15. **Scan the patient's bar code on the identification band, if required.** | |
| — | — | — | 16. **Complete necessary assessments before administering medications. Check the patient's allergy bracelet or ask the patient about allergies. Explain the purpose and action of each medication to the patient.** | *inhaler – wait 1 min between doses* *gargle after* |
| — | — | — | 17. Assist the patient to an upright or lateral position. | |
| — | — | — | 18. Administer medications: | |
| — | — | — | a. Offer water or other permitted fluids with pills, capsules, tablets, and some liquid medications. | |
| — | — | — | b. Ask whether the patient prefers to take the medications by hand or in a cup. | |

SKILL 5-1

# Administering Oral Medications *(Continued)*

| Excellent | Satisfactory | Needs Practice | | Comments |
|---|---|---|---|---|
| —— | —— | —— | 19. *Remain with the patient until each medication is swallowed. Never leave medication at the patient's bedside.* | |
| —— | —— | —— | 20. Assist the patient to a comfortable position. Remove PPE, if used. Perform hand hygiene. | |
| —— | —— | —— | 21. Document the administration of the medication immediately after administration. | |
| —— | —— | —— | 22. Evaluate the patient's response to medication within appropriate time frame. | |

*Skill Checklists for Taylor's Clinical Nursing Skills:*
*A Nursing Process Approach, 3rd edition*

Name _____ Date _____

Unit _____ Position _____

Instructor/Evaluator: _____ Position _____

SKILL 5-2

# Administering Medications via a Gastric Tube

**Goal:** The patient receives the medication via the tube and experiences the intended effect of the medication.

| Excellent | Satisfactory | Needs Practice | | Comments |
|---|---|---|---|---|
| ___ | ___ | ___ | 1. Gather equipment. Check each medication order against the original in the medical record, according to facility policy. Clarify any inconsistencies. Check the patient's chart for allergies. | |
| ___ | ___ | ___ | 2. Know the actions, special nursing considerations, safe dose ranges, purpose of administration, and adverse effects of the medications to be administered. Consider the appropriateness of the medication for this patient. | |
| ___ | ___ | ___ | 3. Perform hand hygiene. | |
| ___ | ___ | ___ | 4. Move the medication cart to the outside of the patient's room or prepare for administration in the medication area. | |
| ___ | ___ | ___ | 5. Unlock the medication cart or drawer. Enter pass code and scan employee identification, if required. | |
| ___ | ___ | ___ | 6. *Prepare medications for one patient at a time.* | |
| ___ | ___ | ___ | 7. Read the CMAR/MAR and select the proper medication from the patient's medication drawer or unit stock. | |
| ___ | ___ | ___ | 8. Compare the label with the CMAR/MAR. Check expiration dates and perform calculations, if necessary. Scan the bar code on the package, if required. | |
| ___ | ___ | ___ | 9. Check to see if medications to be administered come in a liquid form. *If pills or capsules are to be given, check with pharmacy or drug reference to verify the ability to crush or open capsules.* | |
| ___ | ___ | ___ | 10. Prepare medication. | |
| ___ | ___ | ___ | *Pills:* Using a pill crusher, crush each pill one at a time. Dissolve the powder with water or other recommended liquid in a liquid medication cup, keeping each medication separate from the others. Keep the package label with the medication cup, for future comparison of information. | |
| ___ | ___ | ___ | *Liquid:* When pouring liquid medications from a multidose bottle, hold the bottle with the label against the palm. Use the appropriate measuring device when pouring liquids, and read the amount of medication at the bottom of the meniscus at eye level. Wipe the lip of the bottle with a paper towel. | |

| Excellent | Satisfactory | Needs Practice | SKILL 5-2<br><br>**Administering Medications via a<br>Gastric Tube** *(Continued)* |
|---|---|---|---|
| | | | **Comments** |
| —— | —— | —— | 11. *When all medications for one patient have been prepared, recheck the label with the MAR before taking the medications to the patient.* |
| —— | —— | —— | 12. Lock the medication cart before leaving it. |
| —— | —— | —— | 13. Transport medications to the patient's bedside carefully, and keep the medications in sight at all times. |
| —— | —— | —— | 14. *Ensure that the patient receives the medications at the correct time.* |
| —— | —— | —— | 15. Perform hand hygiene and put on PPE, if indicated. |
| —— | —— | —— | 16. Identify the patient. Usually, the patient should be identified using two methods. Compare information with the CMAR/MAR. |
| —— | —— | —— | a. Check the name and identification number on the patient's identification band. |
| —— | —— | —— | b. Ask the patient to state his or her name and birth date, based on facility policy. |
| —— | —— | —— | c. If the patient cannot identify him- or herself, verify the patient's identification with a staff member who knows the patient for the second source. |
| —— | —— | —— | 17. Complete necessary assessments before administering medications. Check the patient's allergy bracelet or ask the patient about allergies. Explain what you are going to do, and the reason for doing it, to the patient. |
| —— | —— | —— | 18. Scan the patient's bar code on the identification band, if required. |
| —— | —— | —— | 19. Assist the patient to the high Fowler's position, unless contraindicated. |
| —— | —— | —— | 20. Put on gloves. |
| —— | —— | —— | 21. If patient is receiving continuous tube feedings, pause the tube-feeding pump. |
| —— | —— | —— | 22. Pour the water into the irrigation container. Measure 30 mL of water. Apply clamp on feeding tube, if present. Alternately, pinch gastric tube below port with fingers, or position stopcock to correct direction. Open port on gastric tube delegated to medication administration or disconnect tubing for feeding from gastric tube and place cap on end of feeding tubing. |
| —— | —— | —— | 23. *Check placement of tube, depending on type of tube and facility policy.* (Refer to Chapter 11, Nutrition.) |

SKILL 5-2

# Administering Medications via a Gastric Tube *(Continued)*

| Excellent | Satisfactory | Needs Practice | | Comments |
|---|---|---|---|---|
| ___ | ___ | ___ | 24. Note the amount of any residual. Refer to Chapter 11, Nutrition. Replace residual back into stomach, based on facility policy. | |
| ___ | ___ | ___ | 25. Apply clamp on feeding tube, if present. Alternately, pinch gastric tube below port with fingers, or position stopcock to correct direction. Remove 60-mL syringe gastric tube. Remove the plunger of the syringe. Reinsert the syringe in the gastric tube without the plunger. Pour 30 mL of water into the syringe. *Unclamp the tube and allow the water to enter the stomach via gravity infusion.* | |
| ___ | ___ | ___ | 26. Administer the first dose of medication by pouring into the syringe. Follow with a 5- to 10-mL water flush between medication doses. Follow the last dose of medication with 30 to 60 mL of water flush. | |
| ___ | ___ | ___ | 27. Clamp the tube, remove the syringe, and replace the feeding tubing. If stopcock is used, position stopcock to correct direction. If tube medication port was used, cap port. Unclamp gastric tube and restart tube feeding, if appropriate for medications administered. | |
| ___ | ___ | ___ | 28. Remove gloves. Assist the patient to a comfortable position. If receiving a tube feeding, the head of the bed must remain elevated at least 30 degrees. | |
| ___ | ___ | ___ | 29. Remove additional PPE, if used. Perform hand hygiene. | |
| ___ | ___ | ___ | 30. Document the administration of the medication immediately after administration. | |
| ___ | ___ | ___ | 31. Evaluate the patient's response to medication within appropriate time frame. | |

*Skill Checklists for Taylor's Clinical Nursing Skills:*
*A Nursing Process Approach, 3rd edition*

Name _____   Date _____

Unit _____   Position _____

Instructor/Evaluator: _____   Position _____

| Excellent | Satisfactory | Needs Practice | SKILL 5-3<br><br>**Removing Medication from an Ampule** | |
|---|---|---|---|---|
| | | | **Goal:** The proper dose of medication will be removed in a sterile manner, and will be free from glass shards. | **Comments** |
| —— | —— | —— | 1. Gather equipment. Check the medication order against the original order in the medical record, according to facility policy. Clarify any inconsistencies. Check the patient's chart for allergies. | |
| —— | —— | —— | 2. Know the actions, special nursing considerations, safe dose ranges, purpose of administration, and adverse effects of the medications to be administered. Consider the appropriateness of the medication for this patient. | |
| —— | —— | —— | 3. Perform hand hygiene. | |
| —— | —— | —— | 4. Move the medication cart to the outside of the patient's room or prepare for administration in the medication area. | |
| —— | —— | —— | 5. Unlock the medication cart or drawer. Enter pass code and scan employee identification, if required. | |
| —— | —— | —— | 6. *Prepare medications for one patient at a time.* | |
| —— | —— | —— | 7. Read the CMAR/MAR and select the proper medication from the patient's medication drawer or unit stock. | |
| —— | —— | —— | 8. Compare the label with the CMAR/MAR. Check expiration dates and perform calculations, if necessary. Scan the bar code on the package, if required. | |
| —— | —— | —— | 9. Tap the stem of the **ampule** or twist your wrist quickly while holding the ampule vertically. | |
| —— | —— | —— | 10. Wrap a small gauze pad around the neck of the ampule. | |
| —— | —— | —— | 11. Use a snapping motion to break off the top of the ampule along the scored line at its neck. *Always break away from your body.* | |
| —— | —— | —— | 12. Attach filter needle to syringe. Remove the cap from the filter needle by pulling it straight off. | |
| —— | —— | —— | 13. Withdraw medication in the amount ordered plus a small amount more (approximately 30% more). *Do not inject air into the solution.* Use either of the following methods. *While inserting the filter needle into the ampule, be careful not to touch the rim.* | |
| —— | —— | —— | a. Insert the tip of the needle into the ampule, which is upright on a flat surface, and withdraw fluid into the syringe. *Touch the plunger at the knob only.* | |

# SKILL 5-3
## Removing Medication from an Ampule *(Continued)*

| Excellent | Satisfactory | Needs Practice | | Comments |
|---|---|---|---|---|
| —— | —— | —— | b. Insert the tip of the needle into the ampule and invert the ampule. Keep the needle centered and not touching the sides of the ampule. Withdraw fluid into syringe. *Touch the plunger at the knob only.* | |
| —— | —— | —— | 14. Wait until the needle has been withdrawn to tap the syringe and expel the air carefully by pushing on the plunger. *Check the amount of medication in the syringe with the medication dose and discard any surplus, according to facility policy.* | |
| —— | —— | —— | 15. *Recheck the label with the CMAR/MAR.* | |
| —— | —— | —— | 16. *Engage safety guard on filter needle and remove the needle. Discard the filter needle in a suitable container. Attach appropriate administration device to syringe.* | |
| —— | —— | —— | 17. Discard the ampule in a suitable container. | |
| —— | —— | —— | 18. Lock the medication cart before leaving it. | |
| —— | —— | —— | 19. Perform hand hygiene. | |
| —— | —— | —— | 20. Proceed with administration, based on prescribed route. | |

*Skill Checklists for Taylor's Clinical Nursing Skills:*
*A Nursing Process Approach, 3rd edition*

Name _____   Date _____

Unit _____   Position _____

Instructor/Evaluator: _____   Position _____

SKILL 5-4

# Removing Medication from a Vial

**Goal:** The proper dosage of medication is withdrawn into a syringe using sterile technique.

| Excellent | Satisfactory | Needs Practice | | Comments |
|---|---|---|---|---|
| ___ | ___ | ___ | 1. Gather equipment. Check the medication order against the original order in the medical record, according to facility policy. | |
| ___ | ___ | ___ | 2. Know the actions, special nursing considerations, safe dose ranges, purpose of administration, and adverse effects of the medications to be administered. Consider the appropriateness of the medication for this patient. | |
| ___ | ___ | ___ | 3. Perform hand hygiene. | |
| ___ | ___ | ___ | 4. Move the medication cart to the outside of the patient's room or prepare for administration in the medication area. | |
| ___ | ___ | ___ | 5. Unlock the medication cart or drawer. Enter pass code and scan employee identification, if required. | |
| ___ | ___ | ___ | 6. *Prepare medications for one patient at a time.* | |
| ___ | ___ | ___ | 7. Read the CMAR/MAR and select the proper medication from the patient's medication drawer or unit stock. | |
| ___ | ___ | ___ | 8. Compare the label with the CMAR/MAR. Check expiration dates and perform calculations, if necessary. Scan the bar code on the package, if required. | |
| ___ | ___ | ___ | 9. Remove the metal or plastic cap on the vial that protects the rubber stopper. | |
| ___ | ___ | ___ | 10. *Swab the rubber top with the antimicrobial swab and allow to dry.* | |
| ___ | ___ | ___ | 11. Remove the cap from the needle or blunt cannula by pulling it straight off. Touch the plunger at the knob only. Draw back an amount of air into the syringe that is equal to the specific dose of medication to be withdrawn. Some facilities require use of a filter needle when withdrawing premixed medication from multidose vials. | |
| ___ | ___ | ___ | 12. Hold the vial on a flat surface. Pierce the rubber stopper in the center with the needle tip and inject the measured air into the space above the solution. Do not inject air into the solution. | |
| ___ | ___ | ___ | 13. *Invert the vial. Keep the tip of the needle or blunt cannula below the fluid level.* | |

# Removing Medication from a Vial *(Continued)*

| Excellent | Satisfactory | Needs Practice | | Comments |
|---|---|---|---|---|

| Excellent | Satisfactory | Needs Practice | | |
|---|---|---|---|---|
| ___ | ___ | ___ | 14. Hold the vial in one hand and use the other to withdraw the medication. Touch the plunger at the knob only. *Draw up the prescribed amount of medication while holding the syringe vertically and at eye level.* | |
| ___ | ___ | ___ | 15. If any air bubbles accumulate in the syringe, tap the barrel of the syringe sharply and move the needle past the fluid into the air space to re-inject the air bubble into the vial. Return the needle tip to the solution and continue withdrawal of the medication. | |
| ___ | ___ | ___ | 16. After the correct dose is withdrawn, remove the needle from the vial and carefully replace the cap over the needle. *If a filter needle has been used to draw up the medication, remove it and attach the appropriate administration device.* Some facilities require changing the needle, if one was used to withdraw the medication, before administering the medication. | |
| ___ | ___ | ___ | 17. *Check the amount of medication in the syringe with the medication dose and discard any surplus.* | |
| ___ | ___ | ___ | 18. *Recheck the label with the CMAR/MAR.* | |
| ___ | ___ | ___ | 19. *If a multidose vial is being used, label the vial with the date and time opened, and store the vial containing the remaining medication according to facility policy.* | |
| ___ | ___ | ___ | 20. Lock the medication cart before leaving it. | |
| ___ | ___ | ___ | 21. Perform hand hygiene. | |
| ___ | ___ | ___ | 22. Proceed with administration, based on prescribed route. | |

64

*Skill Checklists for Taylor's Clinical Nursing Skills: A Nursing Process Approach, 3rd edition*

Name _____  Date _____

Unit _____  Position _____

Instructor/Evaluator: _____  Position _____

SKILL 5-5

# Mixing Medications From Two Vials in One Syringe

**Goal:** The proper dosage of medication is withdrawn into a syringe using sterile technique.

| Excellent | Satisfactory | Needs Practice | | Comments |
|---|---|---|---|---|
| —— | —— | —— | 1. Gather equipment. Check medication order against the original order in the medical record, according to facility policy. | |
| —— | —— | —— | 2. Know the actions, special nursing considerations, safe dose ranges, purpose of administration, and adverse effects of the medications to be administered. Consider the appropriateness of the medication for this patient. | |
| —— | —— | —— | 3. Perform hand hygiene. | |
| —— | —— | —— | 4. Move the medication cart to the outside of the patient's room or prepare for administration in the medication area. | |
| —— | —— | —— | 5. Unlock the medication cart or drawer. Enter pass code and scan employee identification, if required. | |
| —— | —— | —— | 6. *Prepare medications for one patient at a time.* | |
| —— | —— | —— | 7. Read the CMAR/MAR and select the proper medications from the patient's medication drawer or unit stock. | |
| —— | —— | —— | 8. Compare the labels with the CMAR/MAR. Check expiration dates and perform calculations, if necessary. Scan the bar code on the package, if required. | |
| —— | —— | —— | 9. If necessary, remove the cap that protects the rubber stopper on each vial. | |
| —— | —— | —— | 10. *If medication is a suspension (e.g., NPH insulin), roll and agitate the vial to mix it well.* | |
| —— | —— | —— | 11. Cleanse the rubber tops with antimicrobial swabs. | |
| —— | —— | —— | 12. Remove cap from needle by pulling it straight off. Touch the plunger at the knob only. Draw back an amount of air into the syringe that is equal to the dose of modified insulin to be withdrawn. | |
| —— | —— | —— | 13. Hold the modified vial on a flat surface. Pierce the rubber stopper in the center with the needle tip and inject the measured air into the space above the solution. Do not inject air into the solution. Withdraw the needle. | |
| —— | —— | —— | 14. Draw back an amount of air into the syringe that is equal to the dose of unmodified insulin to be withdrawn. | |

SKILL 5-5

# SKILL 5-5

## Mixing Medications From Two Vials in One Syringe *(Continued)*

| Excellent | Satisfactory | Needs Practice | | Comments |
|-----------|--------------|----------------|---|----------|
| —— | —— | —— | 15. Hold the unmodified vial on a flat surface. Pierce the rubber stopper in the center with the needle tip and inject the measured air into the space above the solution. Do not inject air into the solution. Keep the needle in the vial. | |
| —— | —— | —— | 16. Invert vial of unmodified insulin. Hold the vial in one hand and use the other to withdraw the medication. Touch the plunger at the knob only. *Draw up the prescribed amount of medication while holding the syringe at eye level and vertically.* Turn the vial over and then remove needle from vial. | |
| —— | —— | —— | 17. Check that there are no air bubbles in the syringe. | |
| —— | —— | —— | 18. *Check the amount of medication in the syringe with the medication dose and discard any surplus.* | |
| —— | —— | —— | 19. *Recheck the vial label with the CMAR/MAR.* | |
| —— | —— | —— | 20. Calculate the endpoint on the syringe for the combined insulin amount by adding the number of units for each dose together. | |
| —— | —— | —— | 21. Insert the needle into the modified vial and invert it, taking care not to push the plunger and inject medication from the syringe into the vial. Invert vial of modified insulin. Hold the vial in one hand and use the other to withdraw the medication. Touch the plunger at the knob only. *Draw up the prescribed amount of medication while holding the syringe at eye level and vertically. Take care to withdraw only the prescribed amount.* Turn the vial over and then remove needle from vial. Carefully recap the needle. Carefully replace the cap over the needle. | |
| —— | —— | —— | 22. *Check the amount of medication in the syringe with the medication dose.* | |
| —— | —— | —— | 23. *Recheck the vial label with the CMAR/MAR.* | |
| —— | —— | —— | 24. *Label the vials with the date and time opened, and store the vials containing the remaining medication according to facility policy.* | |
| —— | —— | —— | 25. Lock medication cart before leaving it. | |
| —— | —— | —— | 26. Perform hand hygiene. | |
| —— | —— | —— | 27. Proceed with administration, based on prescribed route. | |

*Skill Checklists for Taylor's Clinical Nursing Skills:*
*A Nursing Process Approach, 3rd edition*

Name _____ Date _____

Unit _____ Position _____

Instructor/Evaluator: _____ Position _____

| Excellent | Satisfactory | Needs Practice | |
|---|---|---|---|

### SKILL 5-6
# Administering an Intradermal Injection

**Goal:** Medication is safely injected intradermally causing a wheal to appear at the site of injection.

**Comments**

1. Gather equipment. Check each medication order against the original order in the medical record according to facility policy. Clarify any inconsistencies. Check the patient's chart for allergies.

2. Know the actions, special nursing considerations, safe dose ranges, purpose of administration, and adverse effects of the medications to be administered. Consider the appropriateness of the medication for this patient.

3. Perform hand hygiene.

4. Move the medication cart to the outside of the patient's room or prepare for administration in the medication area.

5. Unlock the medication cart or drawer. Enter pass code and scan employee identification, if required.

6. *Prepare medications for one patient at a time.*

7. Read the CMAR/MAR and select the proper medication from the patient's medication drawer or unit stock.

8. Compare the label with the CMAR/MAR. Check expiration dates and perform calculations, if necessary. Scan the bar code on the package, if required.

9. If necessary, withdraw medication from an ampule or vial as described in Skills 5-3 and 5-4.

10. *When all medications for one patient have been prepared, recheck the label with the CMAR/MAR before taking the medications to the patient.*

11. Lock the medication cart before leaving it.

12. Transport medications to the patient's bedside carefully, and keep the medications in sight at all times.

13. *Ensure that the patient receives the medications at the correct time.*

14. Perform hand hygiene and put on PPE, if indicated.

## SKILL 5-6

# Administering an Intradermal Injection *(Continued)*

| Excellent | Satisfactory | Needs Practice | | Comments |
|---|---|---|---|---|
| ___ | ___ | ___ | 15. Identify the patient. Usually, the patient should be identified using two methods. Compare information with the CMAR/MAR. | |
| ___ | ___ | ___ |    a. Check the name and identification number on the patient's identification band. | |
| ___ | ___ | ___ |    b. Ask the patient to state his or her name and birth date, based on facility policy. | |
| ___ | ___ | ___ |    c. If the patient cannot identify him- or herself, verify the patient's identification with a staff member who knows the patient for the second source. | |
| ___ | ___ | ___ | 16. Close the door to the room or pull the bedside curtain. | |
| ___ | ___ | ___ | 17. Complete necessary assessments before administering medications. Check allergy bracelet or ask the patient about allergies. Explain the purpose and action of the medication to the patient. | |
| ___ | ___ | ___ | 18. Scan the patient's bar code on the identification band, if required. | |
| ___ | ___ | ___ | 19. Put on clean gloves. | |
| ___ | ___ | ___ | 20. Select an appropriate administration site. Assist the patient to the appropriate position for the site chosen. Drape as needed to expose only area of site to be used. | |
| ___ | ___ | ___ | 21. Cleanse the site with an antimicrobial swab while wiping with a firm, circular motion and moving outward from the injection site. Allow the skin to dry. | |
| ___ | ___ | ___ | 22. Remove the needle cap with the nondominant hand by pulling it straight off. | |
| ___ | ___ | ___ | 23. Use the nondominant hand to spread the skin taut over the injection site. | |
| ___ | ___ | ___ | 24. Hold the syringe in the dominant hand, between the thumb and forefinger with the bevel of the needle up. | |
| ___ | ___ | ___ | 25. Hold the syringe at a 5- to 15-degree angle from the site. *Place the needle almost flat against the patient's skin, bevel side up, and insert the needle into the skin. Insert the needle only about 1/8 inch with entire bevel under the skin.* | |
| ___ | ___ | ___ | 26. Once the needle is in place, steady the lower end of the syringe. Slide your dominant hand to the end of the plunger. | |
| ___ | ___ | ___ | 27. Slowly inject the agent while watching for a small wheal or blister to appear. | |

## SKILL 5-6
# Administering an Intradermal Injection *(Continued)*

| Excellent | Satisfactory | Needs Practice | | Comments |
|---|---|---|---|---|
| —— | —— | —— | 28. Withdraw the needle quickly at the same angle that it was inserted. Do not recap the used needle. Engage the safety shield or needle guard. | |
| —— | —— | —— | 29. *Do not massage the area after removing needle. Tell patient not to rub or scratch the site. If necessary, gently blot the site with a dry gauze square. Do not apply pressure or rub the site.* | |
| —— | —— | —— | 30. Assist the patient to a position of comfort. | |
| —— | —— | —— | 31. Discard the needle and syringe in the appropriate receptacle. | |
| —— | —— | —— | 32. Remove gloves and additional PPE, if used. Perform hand hygiene. | |
| —— | —— | —— | 33. Document the administration of the medication immediately after administration. | |
| —— | —— | —— | 34. Evaluate the patient's response to medication within appropriate time frame. | |
| —— | —— | —— | 35. Observe the area for signs of a reaction at determined intervals after administration. Inform the patient of the need for inspection. | |

*Skill Checklists for Taylor's Clinical Nursing Skills:*
*A Nursing Process Approach, 3rd edition*

Name _____   Date _____

Unit _____   Position _____

Instructor/Evaluator: _____   Position _____

| Excellent | Satisfactory | Needs Practice | SKILL 5-7 **Administering a Subcutaneous Injection** | Comments |
|---|---|---|---|---|
| | | | **Goal:** The patient safely receives medication via the subcutaneous route. | |
| ____ | ____ | ____ | 1. Gather equipment. Check each medication order against the original order in the medical record, according to facility policy. Clarify any inconsistencies. Check the patient's chart for allergies. | |
| ____ | ____ | ____ | 2. Know the actions, special nursing considerations, safe dose ranges, purpose of administration, and adverse effects of the medications to be administered. Consider the appropriateness of the medication for this patient. | |
| ____ | ____ | ____ | 3. Perform hand hygiene. | |
| ____ | ____ | ____ | 4. Move the medication cart to the outside of the patient's room or prepare for administration in the medication area. | |
| ____ | ____ | ____ | 5. Unlock the medication cart or drawer. Enter pass code and scan employee identification, if required. | |
| ____ | ____ | ____ | 6. *Prepare medications for one patient at a time.* | |
| ____ | ____ | ____ | 7. Read the CMAR/MAR and select the proper medication from the patient's medication drawer or unit stock. | |
| ____ | ____ | ____ | 8. Compare the label with the CMAR/MAR. Check expiration dates and perform calculations, if necessary. Scan the bar code on the package, if required. | |
| ____ | ____ | ____ | 9. If necessary, withdraw medication from an ampule or vial as described in Skills 5-3 and 5-4. | |
| ____ | ____ | ____ | 10. *When all medications for one patient have been prepared, recheck the label with the MAR before taking medications to the patient.* | |
| ____ | ____ | ____ | 11. Lock the medication cart before leaving it. | |
| ____ | ____ | ____ | 12. Transport medications to the patient's bedside carefully, and keep the medications in sight at all times. | |
| ____ | ____ | ____ | 13. *Ensure that the patient receives the medications at the correct time.* | |
| ____ | ____ | ____ | 14. Perform hand hygiene and put on PPE, if indicated. | |

## SKILL 5-7
# Administering a Subcutaneous Injection *(Continued)*

| Excellent | Satisfactory | Needs Practice | | Comments |
|---|---|---|---|---|
| —— | —— | —— | 15. Identify the patient. Usually, the patient should be identified using two methods. Compare information with the CMAR/MAR. | |
| —— | —— | —— | a. Check the name and identification number on the patient's identification band. | |
| —— | —— | —— | b. Ask the patient to state his or her name and birth date, based on facility policy. | |
| —— | —— | —— | c. If the patient cannot identify him- or herself, verify the patient's identification with a staff member who knows the patient for the second source. | |
| —— | —— | —— | 16. Close the door to the room or pull the bedside curtain. | |
| —— | —— | —— | 17. Complete necessary assessments before administering medications. Check the patient's allergy bracelet or ask the patient about allergies. Explain the purpose and action of the medication to the patient. | |
| —— | —— | —— | 18. Scan the patient's bar code on the identification band, if required. | |
| —— | —— | —— | 19. Put on clean gloves. | |
| —— | —— | —— | 20. Select an appropriate administration site. | |
| —— | —— | —— | 21. Assist the patient to the appropriate position for the site chosen. Drape, as needed, to expose only area of site to be used. | |
| —— | —— | —— | 22. Identify the appropriate landmarks for the site chosen. | |
| —— | —— | —— | 23. Cleanse the area around the injection site with an antimicrobial swab. Use a firm, circular motion while moving outward from the injection site. Allow area to dry. | |
| —— | —— | —— | 24. Remove the needle cap with the nondominant hand, pulling it straight off. | |
| —— | —— | —— | 25. Grasp and bunch the area surrounding the injection site or spread the skin taut at the site. | |
| —— | —— | —— | 26. ***Hold the syringe in the dominant hand between the thumb and forefinger. Inject the needle quickly at a 45- to 90-degree angle.*** | |
| —— | —— | —— | 27. After the needle is in place, release the tissue. If you have a large skin fold pinched up, ensure that the needle stays in place as the skin is released. Immediately move your nondominant hand to steady the lower end of the syringe. Slide your dominant hand to the end of the plunger. Avoid moving the syringe. | |
| —— | —— | —— | 28. Inject the medication slowly (at a rate of 10 sec/mL). | |

SKILL 5-7

# Administering a Subcutaneous Injection *(Continued)*

| Excellent | Satisfactory | Needs Practice | | Comments |
|---|---|---|---|---|
| —— | —— | —— | 29. Withdraw the needle quickly at the same angle at which it was inserted, while supporting the surrounding tissue with your nondominant hand. | |
| —— | —— | —— | 30. Using a gauze square, apply gentle pressure to the site after the needle is withdrawn. Do not massage the site. | |
| —— | —— | —— | 31. Do not recap the used needle. Engage the safety shield or needle guard. Discard the needle and syringe in the appropriate receptacle. | |
| —— | —— | —— | 32. Assist the patient to a position of comfort. | |
| —— | —— | —— | 33. Remove gloves and additional PPE, if used. Perform hand hygiene. | |
| —— | —— | —— | 34. Document the administration of the medication immediately after administration. | |
| —— | —— | —— | 35. Evaluate the patient's response to the medication within an appropriate time frame for the particular medication. | |

*Skill Checklists for Taylor's Clinical Nursing Skills:*
*A Nursing Process Approach, 3rd edition*

Name _____  Date _____

Unit _____  Position _____

Instructor/Evaluator: _____  Position _____

SKILL 5-8

# Administering an Intramuscular Injection

**Goal:** The patient safely receives the medication via the intramuscular route using a Z-track method.

| Excellent | Satisfactory | Needs Practice | | Comments |
|---|---|---|---|---|
| — | — | — | 1. Gather equipment. Check each medication order against the original order in the medical record according to facility policy. Clarify any inconsistencies. Check the patient's chart for allergies. | |
| — | — | — | 2. Know the actions, special nursing considerations, safe dose ranges, purpose of administration, and adverse effects of the medications to be administered. Consider the appropriateness of the medication for this patient. | |
| — | — | — | 3. Perform hand hygiene. | |
| — | — | — | 4. Move the medication cart to the outside of the patient's room or prepare for administration in the medication area. | |
| — | — | — | 5. Unlock the medication cart or drawer. Enter pass code and scan employee identification, if required. | |
| — | — | — | 6. *Prepare medications for one patient at a time.* | |
| — | — | — | 7. Read the CMAR/MAR and select the proper medication from the patient's medication drawer or unit stock. | |
| — | — | — | 8. Compare the label with the CMAR/MAR. Check expiration dates and perform calculations, if necessary. Scan the bar code on the package, if required. | |
| — | — | — | 9. If necessary, withdraw medication from an ampule or vial as described in Skills 5-3 and 5-4. | |
| — | — | — | 10. *When all medications for one patient have been prepared, recheck the label with the MAR before taking the medications to the patient.* | |
| — | — | — | 11. Lock the medication cart before leaving it. | |
| — | — | — | 12. Transport medications to the patient's bedside carefully, and keep the medications in sight at all times. | |
| — | — | — | 13. *Ensure that the patient receives the medications at the correct time.* | |
| — | — | — | 14. Perform hand hygiene and put on PPE, if indicated. | |

| Excellent | Satisfactory | Needs Practice | | Comments |
|---|---|---|---|---|
| ___ | ___ | ___ | **15.** Identify the patient. Usually, the patient should be identified using two methods. Compare information with the CMAR/MAR. | |
| ___ | ___ | ___ | a. Check the name and identification number on the patient's identification band. | |
| ___ | ___ | ___ | b. Ask the patient to state his or her name and birth date, based on facility policy. | |
| ___ | ___ | ___ | c. If the patient cannot identify him- or herself, verify the patient's identification with a staff member who knows the patient for the second source. | |
| ___ | ___ | ___ | **16.** Close the door to the room or pull the bedside curtain. | |
| ___ | ___ | ___ | **17.** Complete necessary assessments before administering medications. Check the patient's allergy bracelet or ask the patient about allergies. Explain the purpose and action of the medication to the patient. | |
| ___ | ___ | ___ | **18.** Scan the patient's bar code on the identification band, if required. | |
| ___ | ___ | ___ | **19.** Put on clean gloves. | |
| ___ | ___ | ___ | **20.** Select an appropriate administration site. | |
| ___ | ___ | ___ | **21.** Assist the patient to the appropriate position for the site chosen. Drape, as needed, to expose only the area of site being used. | |
| ___ | ___ | ___ | **22.** *Identify the appropriate landmarks for the site chosen.* | |
| ___ | ___ | ___ | **23.** Cleanse the area around the injection site with an antimicrobial swab. Use a firm, circular motion while moving outward from the injection site. Allow area to dry. | |
| ___ | ___ | ___ | **24.** Remove the needle cap by pulling it straight off. Hold the syringe in your dominant hand between the thumb and forefinger. | |
| ___ | ___ | ___ | **25.** Displace the skin in a Z-track manner by pulling the skin down or to one side about 1 inch (2.5 cm) with your nondominant hand and hold the skin and tissue in this position. (See the Skill Variation in your skills book for administering an intramuscular injection without using the Z-track technique.) | |
| ___ | ___ | ___ | **26.** Quickly dart the needle into the tissue so that the needle is perpendicular to the patient's body. This should ensure that it is given using an angle of injection between 72 and 90 degrees. | |

SKILL 5-8

# Administering an Intramuscular Injection *(Continued)*

| Excellent | Satisfactory | Needs Practice | | Comments |
|---|---|---|---|---|
| —— | —— | —— | 27. As soon as the needle is in place, use the thumb and forefinger of your nondominant hand to hold the lower end of the syringe. Slide your dominant hand to the end of the plunger. Inject the solution slowly (10 sec/mL of medication). | |
| —— | —— | —— | 28. Once the medication has been instilled, wait 10 seconds before withdrawing the needle. | |
| —— | —— | —— | 29. Withdraw the needle smoothly and steadily at the same angle at which it was inserted, supporting tissue around the injection site with your nondominant hand. | |
| —— | —— | —— | 30. *Apply gentle pressure at the site with a dry gauze.* Do not massage the site. | |
| —— | —— | —— | 31. Do not recap the used needle. Engage the safety shield or needle guard, if present. Discard the needle and syringe in the appropriate receptacle. | |
| —— | —— | —— | 32. Assist the patient to a position of comfort. | |
| —— | —— | —— | 33. Remove gloves and additional PPE, if used. Perform hand hygiene. | |
| —— | —— | —— | 34. Document the administration of the medication immediately after administration. | |
| —— | —— | —— | 35. Evaluate the patient's response to medication within an appropriate time frame. Assess site, if possible, within 2 to 4 hours after administration. | |

*Skill Checklists for Taylor's Clinical Nursing Skills:*
*A Nursing Process Approach, 3rd edition*

Name _____  Date _____

Unit _____  Position _____

Instructor/Evaluator: _____  Position _____

| Excellent | Satisfactory | Needs Practice | SKILL 5-9<br>**Administering Continuous Subcutaneous Infusion:**<br>**Applying an Insulin Pump** | |
|---|---|---|---|---|
| | | | **Goal**: The device is applied successfully and medication is administered. | **Comments** |
| ___ | ___ | ___ | 1. Gather equipment. Check each medication order against the original order in the medical record, according to facility policy. Clarify any inconsistencies. Check the patient's chart for allergies. | |
| ___ | ___ | ___ | 2. Know the actions, special nursing considerations, safe dose ranges, purpose of administration, and adverse effects of the medications to be administered. Consider the appropriateness of the medication for this patient. | |
| ___ | ___ | ___ | 3. Perform hand hygiene. | |
| ___ | ___ | ___ | 4. Move the medication cart to the outside of the patient's room or prepare for administration in the medication area. | |
| ___ | ___ | ___ | 5. Unlock the medication cart or drawer. Enter pass code and scan employee identification, if required. | |
| ___ | ___ | ___ | 6. *Prepare medications for one patient at a time.* | |
| ___ | ___ | ___ | 7. Read the CMAR/MAR and select the proper medication from the patient's medication drawer or unit stock. | |
| ___ | ___ | ___ | 8. Compare the label with the CMAR/MAR. Check expiration dates and perform calculations, if necessary. Scan the bar code on the package, if required. | |
| ___ | ___ | ___ | 9. Attach a blunt-ended needle or a small-gauge needle to a syringe. Follow Skill 5-4 to remove insulin from vial, if necessary. Remove enough insulin to last patient 2 to 3 days, plus 30 units for priming tubing. If using prepackaged insulin syringe or cartridge, remove from packaging. | |
| ___ | ___ | ___ | 10. *When all medications for one patient have been prepared, recheck the label with the MAR before taking them to the patient.* | |
| ___ | ___ | ___ | 11. Lock the medication cart before leaving it. | |
| ___ | ___ | ___ | 12. Transport medications to the patient's bedside carefully, and keep the medications in sight at all times. | |
| ___ | ___ | ___ | 13. *Ensure that the patient receives the medications at the correct time.* | |
| ___ | ___ | ___ | 14. Perform hand hygiene and put on PPE, if indicated. | |

| Excellent | Satisfactory | Needs Practice | |
|---|---|---|---|

## SKILL 5-9
# Administering Continuous Subcutaneous Infusion: Applying an Insulin Pump *(Continued)*

**Comments**

—— —— —— 15. Identify the patient. Usually, the patient should be identified using two methods. Compare information with the CMAR/ MAR.

—— —— ——     a. Check the name and identification number on the patient's identification band.

—— —— ——     b. Ask the patient to state his or her name and birth date, based on facility policy.

—— —— ——     c. If the patient cannot identify him- or herself, verify the patient's identification with a staff member who knows the patient.

—— —— —— 16. Close the door to the room or pull the bedside curtain.

—— —— —— 17. Complete necessary assessments before administering medications. Check the patient's allergy bracelet or ask the patient about allergies. Explain the purpose and action of the medication to the patient.

—— —— —— 18. Scan the patient's bar code on the identification band, if required.

—— —— —— 19. Perform hand hygiene. Put on gloves.

—— —— —— 20. Remove the cap from the syringe or insulin cartridge. Attach sterile tubing to syringe or insulin cartridge. Open the pump and place the syringe or cartridge in compartment according to manufacturer's directions. Close the pump.

—— —— —— 21. Initiate priming of the tubing, according to manufacturer's directions. Program the pump according to manufacturer's recommendations following primary care provider's orders. *Check for any bubbles in the tubing.*

—— —— —— 22. Activate the delivery device. Place the needle between prongs of the insertion device with the sharp edge facing out. Push insertion set down until a click is heard.

—— —— —— 23. Select an appropriate administration site.

—— —— —— 24. Assist the patient to the appropriate position for the site chosen. Drape, as needed, to expose only area of site to be used.

—— —— —— 25. Identify the appropriate landmarks for the site chosen.

—— —— —— 26. Cleanse area around injection site with antimicrobial swab. Use a firm, circular motion while moving outward from insertion site. Allow antiseptic to dry.

—— —— —— 27. Remove paper from adhesive backing. Remove the needle guard. Pinch skin at insertion site, press insertion device on site, and press release button to insert needle. Remove triggering device.

| Excellent | Satisfactory | Needs Practice | | SKILL 5-9<br><br>**Administering Continuous Subcutaneous Infusion:<br>Applying an Insulin Pump** *(Continued)* |
|---|---|---|---|---|
| | | | | **Comments** |
| —— | —— | —— | 28. Apply sterile occlusive dressing over insertion site, if not part of insertion device. Attach the pump to patient's clothing, as desired. | |
| —— | —— | —— | 29. Assist the patient to a position of comfort. | |
| —— | —— | —— | 30. Discard the needle and syringe in the appropriate receptacle. | |
| —— | —— | —— | 31. Remove gloves and additional PPE, if used. Perform hand hygiene. | |
| —— | —— | —— | 32. Document the administration of the medication immediately after administration. | |
| —— | —— | —— | 33. Evaluate the patient's response to medication within appropriate time frame. Monitor the patient's blood glucose levels, as appropriate, or as ordered. | |

*Skill Checklists for Taylor's Clinical Nursing Skills:*
*A Nursing Process Approach, 3rd edition*

Name _____     Date _____

Unit _____     Position _____

Instructor/Evaluator: _____     Position _____

| Excellent | Satisfactory | Needs Practice | SKILL 5-10<br>**Administering Medications by Intravenous Bolus or Push Through an Intravenous Infusion**<br><br>**Goal:** The prescribed medication is given to the patient safely via the intravenous route. | Comments |
|:---:|:---:|:---:|---|---|
| — | — | — | 1. Gather equipment. Check medication order against the original order in the medical record, according to facility policy. Clarify any inconsistencies. Check the patient's chart for allergies. Verify the compatibility of the medication and IV fluid. Check a drug resource to clarify whether the medication needs to be diluted before administration. Check the infusion rate. | |
| — | — | — | 2. Know the actions, special nursing considerations, safe dose ranges, purpose of administration, and adverse effects of the medications to be administered. Consider the appropriateness of the medication for this patient. | |
| — | — | — | 3. Perform hand hygiene. | |
| — | — | — | 4. Move the medication cart to the outside of the patient's room or prepare for administration in the medication area. | |
| — | — | — | 5. Unlock the medication cart or drawer. Enter pass code and scan employee identification, if required. | |
| — | — | — | 6. *Prepare medication for one patient at a time.* | |
| — | — | — | 7. Read the CMAR/MAR and select the proper medication from the patient's medication drawer or unit stock. | |
| — | — | — | 8. Compare the label with the CMAR/MAR. Check expiration dates and perform calculations, if necessary. Scan the bar code on the package, if required. | |
| — | — | — | 9. If necessary, withdraw medication from an ampule or vial as described in Skills 5-3 and 5-4. | |
| — | — | — | 10. *Recheck the label with the MAR before taking it to the patient.* | |
| — | — | — | 11. Lock the medication cart before leaving it. | |
| — | — | — | 12. Transport medications and equipment to the patient's bedside carefully, and keep the medications in sight at all times. | |
| — | — | — | 13. *Ensure that the patient receives the medications at the correct time.* | |
| — | — | — | 14. Perform hand hygiene and put on PPE, if indicated. | |

## SKILL 5-10

# Administering Medications by Intravenous Bolus or Push Through an Intravenous Infusion *(Continued)*

| Excellent | Satisfactory | Needs Practice | | Comments |
|---|---|---|---|---|
| —— | —— | —— | 15. Identify the patient. Usually, the patient should be identified using two methods. Compare information with the CMAR/MAR. | |
| —— | —— | —— |    a. Check the name and identification number on the patient's identification band. | |
| —— | —— | —— |    b. Ask the patient to state his or her name and birth date, based on facility policy. | |
| —— | —— | —— |    c. If the patient cannot identify him- or herself, verify the patient's identification with a staff member who knows the patient for the second source. | |
| —— | —— | —— | 16. Close the door to the room or pull the bedside curtain. | |
| —— | —— | —— | 17. Complete necessary assessments before administering medications. Check the patient's allergy bracelet or ask the patient about allergies. Explain the purpose and action of the medication to the patient. | |
| —— | —— | —— | 18. Scan the patient's bar code on the identification band, if required. | |
| —— | —— | —— | 19. *Assess IV site for presence of inflammation or infiltration.* | |
| —— | —— | —— | 20. If IV infusion is being administered via an infusion pump, pause the pump. | |
| —— | —— | —— | 21. Put on clean gloves. | |
| —— | —— | —— | 22. Select injection port on tubing that is closest to venipuncture site. Clean port with antimicrobial swab. | |
| —— | —— | —— | 23. Uncap syringe. Steady port with your nondominant hand while inserting syringe into center of port. | |
| —— | —— | —— | 24. Move your nondominant hand to the section of IV tubing just above the injection port. Fold the tubing between your fingers. | |
| —— | —— | —— | 25. Pull back slightly on plunger just until blood appears in tubing. | |
| —— | —— | —— | 26. *Inject the medication at the recommended rate.* | |
| —— | —— | —— | 27. Release the tubing. Remove the syringe. Do not recap the used needle, if used. Engage the safety shield or needle guard, if present. Release the tubing and allow the IV fluid to flow. Discard the needle and syringe in the appropriate receptacle. | |
| —— | —— | —— | 28. Check IV fluid infusion rate. Restart infusion pump, if appropriate. | |

| Excellent | Satisfactory | Needs Practice | | |
|---|---|---|---|---|
| | | | SKILL 5-10 **Administering Medications by Intravenous Bolus or Push Through an Intravenous Infusion** *(Continued)* | |
| | | | | **Comments** |
| — | — | — | 29. Remove gloves and additional PPE, if used. Perform hand hygiene. | |
| — | — | — | 30. Document the administration of the medication immediately after administration. | |
| — | — | — | 31. Evaluate the patient's response to medication within appropriate time frame. | |

*Skill Checklists for Taylor's Clinical Nursing Skills:*
*A Nursing Process Approach, 3rd edition*

Name _____     Date _____

Unit _____     Position _____

Instructor/Evaluator: _____     Position _____

| Excellent | Satisfactory | Needs Practice | SKILL 5-11 **Administering a Piggyback Intermittent Intravenous Infusion of Medication** | Comments |
|---|---|---|---|---|
| | | | **Goal:** The medication is delivered safely to the patient via the intravenous route using sterile technique. | |
| ___ | ___ | ___ | 1. Gather equipment. Check each medication order against the original order in the medical record, according to facility policy. Clarify any inconsistencies. Check the patient's chart for allergies. | |
| ___ | ___ | ___ | 2. Know the actions, special nursing considerations, safe dose ranges, purpose of administration, and adverse effects of the medications to be administered. Consider the appropriateness of the medication for this patient. | |
| ___ | ___ | ___ | 3. Perform hand hygiene. | |
| ___ | ___ | ___ | 4. Move the medication cart to the outside of the patient's room or prepare for administration in the medication area. | |
| ___ | ___ | ___ | 5. Unlock the medication cart or drawer. Enter pass code and scan employee identification, if required. | |
| ___ | ___ | ___ | 6. *Prepare medications for one patient at a time.* | |
| ___ | ___ | ___ | 7. Read the CMAR/MAR and select the proper medication from the patient's medication drawer or unit stock. | |
| ___ | ___ | ___ | 8. Compare the label with the CMAR/MAR. Check expiration dates. Confirm the prescribed or appropriate infusion rate. Calculate the drip rate if using gravity system. Scan the bar code on the package, if required. | |
| ___ | ___ | ___ | 9. *When all medications for one patient have been prepared, recheck the label with the MAR before taking them to the patient.* | |
| ___ | ___ | ___ | 10. Lock the medication cart before leaving it. | |
| ___ | ___ | ___ | 11. Transport medications to the patient's bedside carefully, and keep the medications in sight at all times. | |
| ___ | ___ | ___ | 12. *Ensure that the patient receives the medications at the correct time.* | |
| ___ | ___ | ___ | 13. Perform hand hygiene and put on PPE, if indicated. | |
| ___ | ___ | ___ | 14. Identify the patient. Usually, the patient should be identified using two methods. Compare information with the CMAR/MAR. | |
| ___ | ___ | ___ | a. Check the name and identification number on the patient's identification band. | |

## SKILL 5-11

# Administering a Piggyback Intermittent
## Intravenous Infusion of Medication *(Continued)*

| Excellent | Satisfactory | Needs Practice | | Comments |
|---|---|---|---|---|
| —— | —— | —— | b. Ask the patient to state his or her name and birth date, based on facility policy. | |
| —— | —— | —— | c. If the patient cannot identify him- or herself, verify the patient's identification with a staff member who knows the patient for the second source. | |
| —— | —— | —— | 15. Close the door to the room or pull the bedside curtain. | |
| —— | —— | —— | 16. Complete necessary assessments before administering medications. Check the patient's allergy bracelet or ask the patient about allergies. Explain the purpose and action of the medication to the patient. | |
| —— | —— | —— | 17. Scan the patient's bar code on the identification band, if required. | |
| —— | —— | —— | 18. Assess the IV site for the presence of inflammation or infiltration. | |
| —— | —— | —— | 19. Close the clamp on the short secondary infusion tubing. Using aseptic technique, remove the cap on the tubing spike and the cap on the port of the medication container, taking care to avoid contaminating either end. | |
| —— | —— | —— | 20. Attach infusion tubing to the medication container by inserting the tubing spike into the port with a firm push and twisting motion, taking care to avoid contaminating either end. | |
| —— | —— | —— | 21. Hang piggyback container on IV pole, positioning it higher than primary IV according to manufacturer's recommendations. Use metal or plastic hook to lower primary IV fluid container. (See the Skill Variation in your skills book for information on administering an intermittent IV medication using a tandem piggyback setup.) | |
| —— | —— | —— | 22. Place label on tubing with appropriate date. | |
| —— | —— | —— | 23. Squeeze drip chamber on tubing and release. Fill to the line or about half full. Open clamp and prime tubing. Close clamp. Place needleless connector on the end of the tubing, using sterile technique, if required. | |
| —— | —— | —— | 24. Use an antimicrobial swab to clean the access port or stopcock above the roller clamp on the primary IV infusion tubing. | |
| —— | —— | —— | 25. Connect piggyback setup to the access port or stopcock. If using, turn the stopcock to the open position. | |

# Administering a Piggyback Intermittent
# Intravenous Infusion of Medication *(Continued)*

| Excellent | Satisfactory | Needs Practice | | Comments |
|---|---|---|---|---|
| —— | —— | —— | 26. Open clamp on the secondary tubing. Set rate for secondary infusion on infusion pump and begin infusion. If using gravity infusion, use the roller clamp on the primary infusion tubing to regulate flow at prescribed delivery rate. Monitor medication infusion at periodic intervals. | |
| —— | —— | —— | 27. Clamp tubing on piggyback set when solution is infused. Follow facility policy regarding disposal of equipment. | |
| —— | —— | —— | 28. Replace primary IV fluid container to original height. *Check primary infusion rate on infusion pump. If using gravity infusion, readjust flow rate of primary IV.* | |
| —— | —— | —— | 29. Remove PPE, if used. Perform hand hygiene. | |
| —— | —— | —— | 30. Document the administration of the medication immediately after administration. | |
| —— | —— | —— | 31. Evaluate the patient's response to medication within appropriate time frame. Monitor IV site at periodic intervals. | |

84

Name _____  Date _____

Unit _____  Position _____

Instructor/Evaluator: _____  Position _____

SKILL 5-12

## Administering an Intermittent Intravenous Infusion of Medication via a Mini-infusion Pump

**Goal:** The medication is delivered via the intravenous route using sterile technique.

| Excellent | Satisfactory | Needs Practice | | Comments |
|---|---|---|---|---|
| ― | ― | ― | 1. Gather equipment. Check each medication order against the original order in the medical record according to facility policy. Clarify any inconsistencies. Check the patient's chart for allergies. | |
| ― | ― | ― | 2. Know the actions, special nursing considerations, safe dose ranges, purpose of administration, and adverse effects of the medications to be administered. Consider the appropriateness of the medication for this patient. | |
| ― | ― | ― | 3. Perform hand hygiene. | |
| ― | ― | ― | 4. Move the medication cart to the outside of the patient's room or prepare for administration in the medication area. | |
| ― | ― | ― | 5. Unlock the medication cart or drawer. Enter pass code and scan employee identification, if required. | |
| ― | ― | ― | 6. *Prepare medications for one patient at a time.* | |
| ― | ― | ― | 7. Read the CMAR/MAR and select the proper medication from the patient's medication drawer or unit stock. | |
| ― | ― | ― | 8. Compare the label with the CMAR/MAR. Check expiration dates. Confirm the prescribed or appropriate infusion rate. Scan the bar code on the package, if required. | |
| ― | ― | ― | 9. *When all medications for one patient have been prepared, recheck the label with the MAR before taking them to the patient.* | |
| ― | ― | ― | 10. Lock the medication cart before leaving it. | |
| ― | ― | ― | 11. Transport medications to the patient's bedside carefully, and keep the medications in sight at all times. | |
| ― | ― | ― | 12. *Ensure that the patient receives the medications at the correct time.* | |
| ― | ― | ― | 13. Perform hand hygiene and put on PPE, if indicated. | |

## SKILL 5-12

# Administering an Intermittent Intravenous Infusion of Medication via a Mini-infusion Pump *(Continued)*

| Excellent | Satisfactory | Needs Practice | | Comments |
|---|---|---|---|---|
| —— | —— | —— | 14. Identify the patient. Usually, the patient should be identified using two methods. Compare information with the MAR/CMAR. | |
| —— | —— | —— |    a. Check the name and identification number on the patient's identification band. | |
| —— | —— | —— |    b. Ask the patient to state his or her name and birth date, based on facility policy. | |
| —— | —— | —— |    c. If the patient cannot identify him- or herself, verify the patient's identification with a staff member who knows the patient for the second source. | |
| —— | —— | —— | 15. Close the door to the room or pull the bedside curtain. | |
| —— | —— | —— | 16. Complete necessary assessments before administering medications. Check the patient's allergy bracelet or ask the patient about allergies. Explain the purpose and action of the medication to the patient. | |
| —— | —— | —— | 17. Scan the patient's bar code on the identification band, if required. | |
| —— | —— | —— | 18. Assess the IV site for the presence of inflammation or infiltration. | |
| —— | —— | —— | 19. Using aseptic technique, remove the cap on the tubing and the cap on the syringe, taking care not to contaminate either end. | |
| —— | —— | —— | 20. Attach infusion tubing to the syringe, taking care not to contaminate either end. | |
| —— | —— | —— | 21. Place label on tubing with appropriate date. | |
| —— | —— | —— | 22. Fill tubing with medication by applying gentle pressure to syringe plunger. Place needleless connector on the end of the tubing, using sterile technique, if required. | |
| —— | —— | —— | 23. Insert syringe into mini-infusion pump according to manufacturer's directions. | |
| —— | —— | —— | 24. Use antimicrobial swab to clean the access port or stopcock below the roller clamp on the primary IV infusion tubing, usually the port closest to the IV insertion site. | |
| —— | —— | —— | 25. Connect the secondary infusion to the primary infusion at the cleansed port. | |
| —— | —— | —— | 26. Program pump to the appropriate rate and begin infusion. Set alarm if recommended by manufacturer. | |

SKILL 5-12

# Administering an Intermittent Intravenous Infusion of Medication via a Mini-infusion Pump (Continued)

| Excellent | Satisfactory | Needs Practice | | Comments |
|---|---|---|---|---|
| —— | —— | —— | 27. Clamp tubing on secondary set when solution is infused. Remove secondary tubing from access port and cap, or replace connector with a new, capped one, if reusing. Follow facility policy regarding disposal of equipment. | |
| —— | —— | —— | 28. Check rate of primary infusion. | |
| —— | —— | —— | 29. Remove PPE, if used. Perform hand hygiene. | |
| —— | —— | —— | 30. Document the administration of the medication immediately after administration. | |
| —— | —— | —— | 31. Evaluate the patient's response to medication within appropriate time frame. Monitor IV site at periodic intervals. | |

*Skill Checklists for Taylor's Clinical Nursing Skills:*
*A Nursing Process Approach, 3rd edition*

Name _____  Date _____

Unit _____  Position _____

Instructor/Evaluator: _____  Position _____

## SKILL 5-13

# Administering an Intermittent Intravenous Infusion of Medication via a Volume-Control Administration Set

**Goal:** The medication is delivered via the intravenous route using sterile technique.

| Excellent | Satisfactory | Needs Practice | | Comments |
|---|---|---|---|---|
| —— | —— | —— | 1. Gather equipment. Check the medication order against the original order in the medical record according to facility policy. Clarify any inconsistencies. Check the patient's chart for allergies. Verify the compatibility of the medication and IV fluid. | |
| —— | —— | —— | 2. Know the actions, special nursing considerations, safe dose ranges, purpose of administration, and adverse effects of the medications to be administered. Consider the appropriateness of the medication for this patient. | |
| —— | —— | —— | 3. Perform hand hygiene. | |
| —— | —— | —— | 4. Move the medication cart to the outside of the patient's room or prepare for administration in the medication area. | |
| —— | —— | —— | 5. Unlock the medication cart or drawer. Enter pass code and scan employee identification, if required. | |
| —— | —— | —— | 6. *Prepare medication for one patient at a time.* | |
| —— | —— | —— | 7. Read the CMAR/MAR and select the proper medication from the patient's medication drawer or unit stock. | |
| —— | —— | —— | 8. Compare the label with the CMAR/MAR. Check expiration dates and perform calculations, if necessary. Confirm the prescribed or appropriate infusion rate. Calculate the drip rate if using gravity system. Scan the bar code on the package, if required. Check the infusion rate. | |
| —— | —— | —— | 9. If necessary, withdraw medication from an ampule or vial as described in Skills 5-3 and 5-4. Attach needleless connector or blunt needle to end of syringe, if necessary. | |
| —— | —— | —— | 10. *When all medications for one patient have been prepared, recheck the label with the CMAR/MAR before taking them to the patient.* | |
| —— | —— | —— | 11. Prepare medication label including name of medication, dose, total volume, including diluent, and time of administration. | |
| —— | —— | —— | 12. Lock the medication cart before leaving it. | |

## SKILL 5-13

# Administering an Intermittent Intravenous Infusion of Medication via a Volume-Control Administration Set *(Continued)*

| Excellent | Satisfactory | Needs Practice | | Comments |
|---|---|---|---|---|
| —— | —— | —— | 13. Transport medications and equipment to the patient's bedside carefully, and keep the medications in sight at all times. | |
| —— | —— | —— | 14. ***Ensure that the patient receives the medications at the correct time.*** | |
| —— | —— | —— | 15. Perform hand hygiene and put on PPE, if indicated. | |
| —— | —— | —— | 16. Identify the patient. Usually, the patient should be identified using two methods. Compare information with the CMAR/MAR. | |
| —— | —— | —— |    a. Check the name and identification number on the patient's identification band. | |
| —— | —— | —— |    b. Ask the patient to state his or her name and birth date, based on facility policy. | |
| —— | —— | —— |    c. If the patient cannot identify him- or herself, verify the patient's identification with a staff member who knows the patient for the second source. | |
| —— | —— | —— | 17. Close the door to the room or pull the bedside curtain. | |
| —— | —— | —— | 18. Complete necessary assessments before administering medications. Check the patient's allergy bracelet or ask the patient about allergies. Explain the purpose and action of the medication to the patient. | |
| —— | —— | —— | 19. Scan the patient's bar code on the identification band, if required. | |
| —— | —— | —— | 20. Assess IV site for presence of inflammation or infiltration. | |
| —— | —— | —— | 21. Fill the volume-control administration set with the prescribed amount of IV fluid by opening the clamp between IV solution and the volume-control administration set. Follow manufacturer's instructions and fill with prescribed amount of IV solution. Close clamp. | |
| —— | —— | —— | 22. Check to make sure the air vent on the volume-control administration set chamber is open. | |
| —— | —— | —— | 23. Use antimicrobial swab to clean access port on volume-control administration set chamber. | |
| —— | —— | —— | 24. Attach the syringe with a twisting motion into the access port while holding the syringe steady. Alternately, insert the needleless device or blunt needle into the port. Inject the medication into the chamber. Gently rotate the chamber. | |
| —— | —— | —— | 25. Attach the medication label to the volume-control device. | |

## SKILL 5-13

# Administering an Intermittent Intravenous Infusion of Medication via a Volume-Control Administration Set *(Continued)*

| Excellent | Satisfactory | Needs Practice | | Comments |
|---|---|---|---|---|
| —— | —— | —— | 26. Use an antimicrobial swab to clean the access port or stop-cock below the roller clamp on the primary IV infusion tubing, usually the port closest to the IV insertion site. | |
| —— | —— | —— | 27. Connect the secondary infusion to the primary infusion at the cleansed port. | |
| —— | —— | —— | 28. The volume-control administration set may be placed on an infusion pump with the appropriate dose programmed into the pump. Alternately, use the roller clamp on the volume-control administration set tubing to adjust the infusion to the prescribed rate. | |
| —— | —— | —— | 29. Discard the syringe in the appropriate receptacle. | |
| —— | —— | —— | 30. Clamp tubing on secondary set when solution is infused. Remove secondary tubing from access port and cap or replace connector with a new, capped one, if reusing. Follow facility policy regarding disposal of equipment. | |
| —— | —— | —— | 31. Check rate of primary infusion. | |
| —— | —— | —— | 32. Remove PPE, if used. Perform hand hygiene. | |
| —— | —— | —— | 33. Document the administration of the medication immediately after administration. | |
| —— | —— | —— | 34. Evaluate the patient's response to medication within appropriate time frame. Monitor IV site at periodic intervals. | |

*Skill Checklists for Taylor's Clinical Nursing Skills:*
*A Nursing Process Approach, 3rd edition*

Name _____   Date _____

Unit _____   Position _____

Instructor/Evaluator: _____   Position _____

## SKILL 5-14

# Introducing Drugs Through a Medication or Drug-Infusion Lock (Intermittent Peripheral Venous Access Device) Using the Saline Flush

**Goal:** The medication is delivered safely to the patient via the intravenous route using sterile technique.

| Excellent | Satisfactory | Needs Practice | | Comments |
|---|---|---|---|---|
| —— | —— | —— | 1. Gather equipment. Check the medication order against the original order in the medical record, according to agency policy. Clarify any inconsistencies. Check the patient's chart for allergies. Check a drug resource to clarify whether medication needs to be diluted before administration. Verify the recommended infusion rate. | |
| —— | —— | —— | 2. Know the actions, special nursing considerations, safe dose ranges, purpose of administration, and adverse effects of the medications to be administered. Consider the appropriateness of the medication for this patient. | |
| —— | —— | —— | 3. Perform hand hygiene. | |
| —— | —— | —— | 4. Move the medication cart to the outside of the patient's room or prepare for administration in the medication area. | |
| —— | —— | —— | 5. Unlock the medication cart or drawer. Enter pass code and scan employee identification, if required. | |
| —— | —— | —— | 6. *Prepare medication for one patient at a time.* | |
| —— | —— | —— | 7. Read the CMAR/MAR and select the proper medication from the patient's medication drawer or unit stock. | |
| —— | —— | —— | 8. Compare the label with the CMAR/MAR. Check expiration dates and perform calculations, if necessary. Scan the bar code on the package, if required. | |
| —— | —— | —— | 9. If necessary, withdraw medication from an ampule or vial as described in Skills 5-3 and 5-4. | |
| —— | —— | —— | 10. *When all medications for one patient have been prepared, recheck the label with the MAR before taking them to the patient.* | |
| —— | —— | —— | 11. Lock the medication cart before leaving it. | |
| —— | —— | —— | 12. Transport medications and equipment to the patient's bedside carefully, and keep the medications in sight at all times. | |
| —— | —— | —— | 13. *Ensure that the patient receives the medications at the correct time.* | |

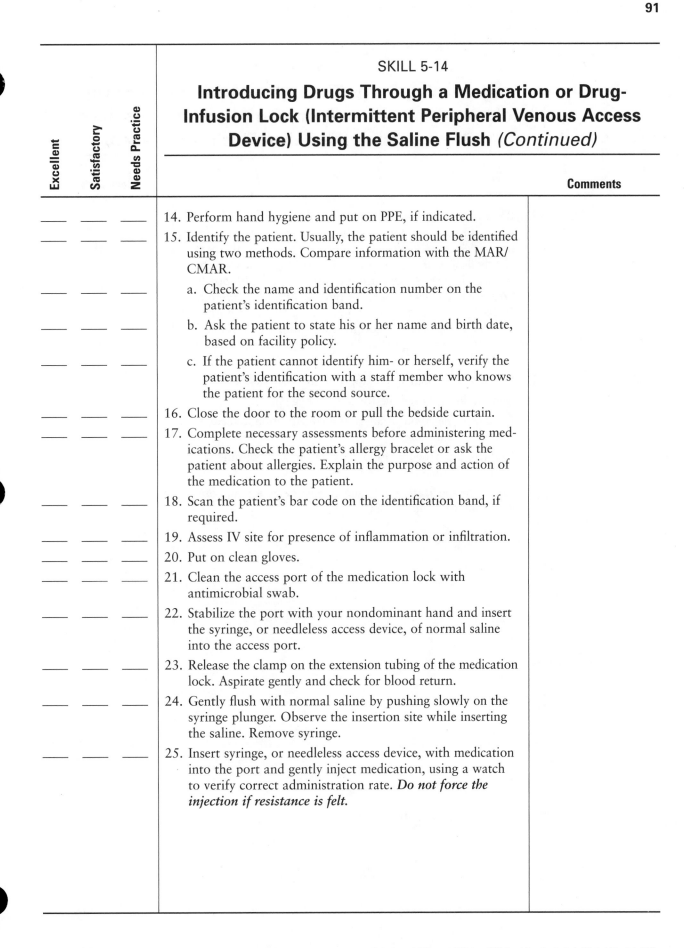

| Excellent | Satisfactory | Needs Practice | SKILL 5-14<br>**Introducing Drugs Through a Medication or Drug-Infusion Lock (Intermittent Peripheral Venous Access Device) Using the Saline Flush** *(Continued)* | Comments |
|---|---|---|---|---|
| —— | —— | —— | 14. Perform hand hygiene and put on PPE, if indicated. | |
| —— | —— | —— | 15. Identify the patient. Usually, the patient should be identified using two methods. Compare information with the MAR/CMAR. | |
| —— | —— | —— | a. Check the name and identification number on the patient's identification band. | |
| —— | —— | —— | b. Ask the patient to state his or her name and birth date, based on facility policy. | |
| —— | —— | —— | c. If the patient cannot identify him- or herself, verify the patient's identification with a staff member who knows the patient for the second source. | |
| —— | —— | —— | 16. Close the door to the room or pull the bedside curtain. | |
| —— | —— | —— | 17. Complete necessary assessments before administering medications. Check the patient's allergy bracelet or ask the patient about allergies. Explain the purpose and action of the medication to the patient. | |
| —— | —— | —— | 18. Scan the patient's bar code on the identification band, if required. | |
| —— | —— | —— | 19. Assess IV site for presence of inflammation or infiltration. | |
| —— | —— | —— | 20. Put on clean gloves. | |
| —— | —— | —— | 21. Clean the access port of the medication lock with antimicrobial swab. | |
| —— | —— | —— | 22. Stabilize the port with your nondominant hand and insert the syringe, or needleless access device, of normal saline into the access port. | |
| —— | —— | —— | 23. Release the clamp on the extension tubing of the medication lock. Aspirate gently and check for blood return. | |
| —— | —— | —— | 24. Gently flush with normal saline by pushing slowly on the syringe plunger. Observe the insertion site while inserting the saline. Remove syringe. | |
| —— | —— | —— | 25. Insert syringe, or needleless access device, with medication into the port and gently inject medication, using a watch to verify correct administration rate. ***Do not force the injection if resistance is felt.*** | |

## SKILL 5-14

# Introducing Drugs Through a Medication or Drug-Infusion Lock (Intermittent Peripheral Venous Access Device) Using the Saline Flush *(Continued)*

| Excellent | Satisfactory | Needs Practice | | Comments |
|---|---|---|---|---|
| —— | —— | —— | 26. Remove the medication syringe from the port. Stabilize the port with your nondominant hand and insert the syringe, or needleless access device, of normal saline into the port. Gently flush with normal saline by pushing slowly on the syringe plunger. *If medication lock is capped with positive pressure valve/device, remove syringe, and then clamp the IV tubing.* Alternately, to gain positive pressure if positive pressure valve/device is not present, clamp the IV tubing as you are still flushing the last of the saline into the medication lock. Remove syringe. | |
| —— | —— | —— | 27. Discard the syringe in the appropriate receptacle. | |
| —— | —— | —— | 28. Remove PPE, if used. Perform hand hygiene. | |
| —— | —— | —— | 29. Document the administration of the medication immediately after administration. | |
| —— | —— | —— | 30. Evaluate the patient's response to medication within appropriate time frame. | |
| —— | —— | —— | 31. Check the medication lock site at least every 8 hours or according to facility policy. | |

*Skill Checklists for Taylor's Clinical Nursing Skills:*
*A Nursing Process Approach, 3rd edition*

Name _____  Date _____

Unit _____  Position _____

Instructor/Evaluator: _____  Position _____

| | | | SKILL 5-15 |
|---|---|---|---|

## SKILL 5-15
## Applying a Transdermal Patch

| Excellent | Satisfactory | Needs Practice | **Goal:** The medication is delivered via the transdermal route. | Comments |
|---|---|---|---|---|
| ___ | ___ | ___ | 1. Gather equipment. Check medication order against the original order in the medical record, according to facility policy. Clarify any inconsistencies. Check the patient's chart for allergies. | |
| ___ | ___ | ___ | 2. Know the actions, special nursing considerations, safe dose ranges, purpose of administration, and adverse effects of the medications to be administered. Consider the appropriateness of the medication for this patient. | |
| ___ | ___ | ___ | 3. Perform hand hygiene. | |
| ___ | ___ | ___ | 4. Move the medication cart to the outside of the patient's room or prepare for administration in the medication area. | |
| ___ | ___ | ___ | 5. Unlock the medication cart or drawer. Enter pass code and scan employee identification, if required. | |
| ___ | ___ | ___ | 6. *Prepare medications for one patient at a time.* | |
| ___ | ___ | ___ | 7. Read the CMAR/MAR and select the proper medication from the patient's medication drawer or unit stock. | |
| ___ | ___ | ___ | 8. Compare the label with the CMAR/MAR. Check expiration dates and perform calculations, if necessary. Scan the bar code on the package, if required. | |
| ___ | ___ | ___ | 9. *When all medications for one patient have been prepared, recheck the label with the CMAR/MAR before taking them to the patient.* | |
| ___ | ___ | ___ | 10. Lock the medication cart before leaving it. | |
| ___ | ___ | ___ | 11. Transport medications to the patient's bedside carefully, and keep the medications in sight at all times. | |
| ___ | ___ | ___ | 12. *Ensure that the patient receives the medications at the correct time.* | |
| ___ | ___ | ___ | 13. Perform hand hygiene and put on PPE, if indicated. | |
| ___ | ___ | ___ | 14. Identify the patient. Usually, the patient should be identified using two methods. Compare information with the CMAR/MAR. | |
| ___ | ___ | ___ |    a. Check the name and identification number on the patient's identification band. | |

| Excellent | Satisfactory | Needs Practice | | Comments |
|---|---|---|---|---|
| | | | SKILL 5-15<br><br>**Applying a Transdermal Patch** *(Continued)* | |

| Excellent | Satisfactory | Needs Practice | | Comments |
|---|---|---|---|---|
| ___ | ___ | ___ | b. Ask the patient to state his or her name and birth date, based on facility policy. | |
| ___ | ___ | ___ | c. If the patient cannot identify him- or herself, verify the patient's identification with a staff member who knows the patient for the second source. | |
| ___ | ___ | ___ | 15. Complete necessary assessments before administering medications. Check the patient's allergy bracelet or ask the patient about allergies. Explain the purpose and action of each medication to the patient. | |
| ___ | ___ | ___ | 16. Scan the patient's bar code on the identification band, if required. | |
| ___ | ___ | ___ | 17. Put on gloves. | |
| ___ | ___ | ___ | 18. Assess the patient's skin where patch is to be placed, looking for any signs of irritation or breakdown. Site should be clean, dry, and free of hair. Rotate application sites. | |
| ___ | ___ | ___ | 19. ***Remove any old transdermal patches from the patient's skin.*** Fold the old patch in half with the adhesive sides sticking together and discard according to facility policy. Gently wash the area where the old patch was with soap and water. | |
| ___ | ___ | ___ | 20. Remove the patch from its protective covering. Initial and write the date and time of administration on the label side of the patch. | |
| ___ | ___ | ___ | 21. Remove the covering on the patch without touching the medication surface. Apply the patch to the patient's skin. Use the palm of your hand to press firmly for about 10 seconds. Do not massage. | |
| ___ | ___ | ___ | 22. Remove gloves and additional PPE, if used. Perform hand hygiene. | |
| ___ | ___ | ___ | 23. Document the administration of the medication immediately after administration. | |
| ___ | ___ | ___ | 24. Evaluate the patient's response to medication within the appropriate time frame. | |

*Skill Checklists for Taylor's Clinical Nursing Skills:*
*A Nursing Process Approach, 3rd edition*

Name _____   Date _____

Unit _____   Position _____

Instructor/Evaluator: _____   Position _____

| Excellent | Satisfactory | Needs Practice | SKILL 5-16 **Instilling Eye Drops** | Comments |
|---|---|---|---|---|
| | | | **Goal:** The medication is delivered successfully into the eye. | |
| ___ | ___ | ___ | 1. Gather equipment. Check medication order against the original order in the medical record, according to facility policy. Clarify any inconsistencies. Check the patient's chart for allergies. | |
| ___ | ___ | ___ | 2. Know the actions, special nursing considerations, safe dose ranges, purpose of administration, and adverse effects of the medications to be administered. Consider the appropriateness of the medication for this patient. | |
| ___ | ___ | ___ | 3. Perform hand hygiene. | |
| ___ | ___ | ___ | 4. Move the medication cart to the outside of the patient's room or prepare for administration in the medication area. | |
| ___ | ___ | ___ | 5. Unlock the medication cart or drawer. Enter pass code and scan employee identification, if required. | |
| ___ | ___ | ___ | 6. *Prepare medications for one patient at a time.* | |
| ___ | ___ | ___ | 7. Read the CMAR/MAR and select the proper medication from the patient's medication drawer or unit stock. | |
| ___ | ___ | ___ | 8. Compare the label with the CMAR/MAR. Check expiration dates and perform calculations, if necessary. Scan the bar code on the package, if required. | |
| ___ | ___ | ___ | 9. *When all medications for one patient have been prepared, recheck the label with the CMAR/MAR before taking them to the patient.* | |
| ___ | ___ | ___ | 10. Lock the medication cart before leaving it. | |
| ___ | ___ | ___ | 11. Transport medications to the patient's bedside carefully, and keep the medications in sight at all times. | |
| ___ | ___ | ___ | 12. *Ensure that the patient receives the medications at the correct time.* | |
| ___ | ___ | ___ | 13. Perform hand hygiene and put on PPE, if indicated. | |
| ___ | ___ | ___ | 14. Identify the patient. Usually, the patient should be identified using two methods. Compare information with the CMAR/MAR. | |
| ___ | ___ | ___ | a. Check the name and identification number on the patient's identification band. | |

SKILL 5-16

# Instilling Eye Drops *(Continued)*

| Excellent | Satisfactory | Needs Practice | | Comments |
|---|---|---|---|---|
| —— | —— | —— | b. Ask the patient to state his or her name and birth date, based on facility policy. | |
| —— | —— | —— | c. If the patient cannot identify him- or herself, verify the patient's identification with a staff member who knows the patient for the second source. | |
| —— | —— | —— | 15. Complete necessary assessments before administering medications. Check the patient's allergy bracelet or ask the patient about allergies. Explain the purpose and action of each medication to the patient. | |
| —— | —— | —— | 16. Scan the patient's bar code on the identification band, if required. | |
| —— | —— | —— | 17. Put on gloves. | |
| —— | —— | —— | 18. Offer tissue to patient. | |
| —— | —— | —— | 19. Cleanse the eyelids and eyelashes of any drainage with a washcloth, cotton balls, or gauze squares moistened with normal saline solution. Use each area of the cleaning surface once, moving from the inner toward the outer canthus. | |
| —— | —— | —— | 20. Tilt the patient's head back slightly if sitting, or place the patient's head over a pillow if lying down. The head may be turned slightly to the affected side to prevent solution or tears from flowing toward the opposite eye. | |
| —— | —— | —— | 21. Remove the cap from the medication bottle, being careful not to touch the inner side of the cap. (See the Skill Variation in your skills book for administering ointment.) | |
| —— | —— | —— | 22. Invert the monodrip plastic container that is commonly used to instill eye drops. Have patient look up and focus on something on the ceiling. | |
| —— | —— | —— | 23. Place thumb or two fingers near margin of lower eyelid immediately below eyelashes, and exert pressure downward over bony prominence of cheek. Lower conjunctival sac is exposed as lower lid is pulled down. | |
| —— | —— | —— | 24. *Hold dropper close to eye, but avoid touching eyelids or lashes.* Squeeze container and allow prescribed number of drops to fall in lower conjunctival sac. | |
| —— | —— | —— | 25. Release lower lid after eye drops are instilled. Ask patient to close eyes gently. | |
| —— | —— | —— | 26. Apply gentle pressure over inner canthus to prevent eye drops from flowing into tear duct. | |
| —— | —— | —— | 27. Instruct patient not to rub affected eye. | |

| Excellent | Satisfactory | Needs Practice | SKILL 5-16 **Instilling Eye Drops** *(Continued)* | Comments |
|---|---|---|---|---|
| ___ | ___ | ___ | 28. Remove gloves. Assist patient to a comfortable position. | |
| ___ | ___ | ___ | 29. Remove additional PPE, if used. Perform hand hygiene. | |
| ___ | ___ | ___ | 30. Document the administration of the medication immediately after administration. | |
| ___ | ___ | ___ | 31. Evaluate the patient's response to medication within appropriate time frame. | |

*Skill Checklists for Taylor's Clinical Nursing Skills:*
*A Nursing Process Approach, 3rd edition*

Name _____   Date _____

Unit _____   Position _____

Instructor/Evaluator: _____   Position _____

SKILL 5-17

# Administering an Eye Irrigation

**Goal:** The eye is cleansed successfully.

| Excellent | Satisfactory | Needs Practice | | Comments |
|---|---|---|---|---|
| — | — | — | 1. Gather equipment. Check the original order in the medical record for the irrigation according to facility policy. Clarify any inconsistencies. Check the patient's chart for allergies. | |
| — | — | — | 2. Perform hand hygiene and put on PPE, if indicated. | |
| — | — | — | 3. Identify the patient. Usually, the patient should be identified using two methods. Compare information with the CMAR/MAR. | |
| — | — | — | a. Check the name and identification number on the patient's identification band. | |
| — | — | — | b. Ask the patient to state his or her name and birth date, based on facility policy. | |
| — | — | — | c. If the patient cannot identify him- or herself, verify the patient's identification with a staff member who knows the patient for the second source. | |
| — | — | — | 4. Explain procedure to patient. | |
| — | — | — | 5. Assemble equipment at patient's bedside. | |
| — | — | — | 6. Have patient sit or lie with head tilted toward side of affected eye. Protect patient and bed with a waterproof pad. | |
| — | — | — | 7. Put on gloves. Clean lids and lashes with washcloth moistened with normal saline or the solution ordered for the irrigation. Wipe from inner canthus to outer canthus. Use a different corner of washcloth with each wipe. | |
| — | — | — | 8. Place curved basin at cheek on the side of the affected eye to receive irrigating solution. If patient is able, ask him or her to support the basin. | |
| — | — | — | 9. Expose lower conjunctival sac and hold upper lid open with your nondominant hand. | |
| — | — | — | 10. Fill the irrigation syringe with the prescribed fluid. *Hold irrigation syringe about 2.5 cm (1 inch) from eye. Direct flow of solution from inner to outer canthus along conjunctival sac.* | |

# Administering an Eye Irrigation (Continued)

| Excellent | Satisfactory | Needs Practice | | Comments |
|---|---|---|---|---|
| —— | —— | —— | 11. Irrigate until the solution is clear or all the solution has been used. *Use only enough force to remove secretions gently from the conjunctiva. Avoid touching any part of the eye with the irrigating tip.* | |
| —— | —— | —— | 12. Pause irrigation and have patient close the eye periodically during procedure. | |
| —— | —— | —— | 13. Dry periorbital area after irrigation with gauze sponge. Offer a towel to the patient if face and neck are wet. | |
| —— | —— | —— | 14. Remove gloves. Assist the patient to a comfortable position. | |
| —— | —— | —— | 15. Remove additional PPE, if used. Perform hand hygiene. | |
| —— | —— | —— | 16. Evaluate the patient's response to medication within appropriate time frame. | |

*Skill Checklists for Taylor's Clinical Nursing Skills:*
*A Nursing Process Approach, 3rd edition*

Name _____    Date _____

Unit _____    Position _____

Instructor/Evaluator: _____    Position _____

| Excellent | Satisfactory | Needs Practice | SKILL 5-18<br>**Instilling Ear Drops** | Comments |
|:---:|:---:|:---:|---|---|
| | | | **Goal:** Drops are administered successfully. | |
| —— | —— | —— | 1. Gather equipment. Check medication order against the original order in the medical record, according to facility policy. Clarify any inconsistencies. Check the patient's chart for allergies. | |
| —— | —— | —— | 2. Know the actions, special nursing considerations, safe dose ranges, purpose of administration, and adverse effects of the medication to be administered. Consider the appropriateness of the medication for this patient. | |
| —— | —— | —— | 3. Perform hand hygiene. | |
| —— | —— | —— | 4. Move the medication cart to the outside of the patient's room or prepare for administration in the medication area. | |
| —— | —— | —— | 5. Unlock the medication cart or drawer. Enter pass code and scan employee identification, if required. | |
| —— | —— | —— | 6. *Prepare medications for one patient at a time.* | |
| —— | —— | —— | 7. Read the CMAR/MAR and select the proper medication from the patient's medication drawer or unit stock. | |
| —— | —— | —— | 8. Compare the label with the CMAR/MAR. Check expiration dates and perform calculations, if necessary. Scan the bar code on the package, if required. | |
| —— | —— | —— | 9. *When all medications for one patient have been prepared, recheck the label with the CMAR/MAR before taking them to the patient.* | |
| —— | —— | —— | 10. Lock the medication cart before leaving it. | |
| —— | —— | —— | 11. Transport medications to the patient's bedside carefully, and keep the medications in sight at all times. | |
| —— | —— | —— | 12. *Ensure that the patient receives the medications at the correct time.* | |
| —— | —— | —— | 13. Perform hand hygiene and put on PPE, if indicated. | |
| —— | —— | —— | 14. Identify the patient. Usually, the patient should be identified using two methods. Compare information with the CMAR/MAR. | |
| —— | —— | —— | a. Check the name and identification number on the patient's identification band. | |

| Excellent | Satisfactory | Needs Practice | SKILL 5-18 **Instilling Ear Drops** *(Continued)* | Comments |
|---|---|---|---|---|
| — | — | — | b. Ask the patient to state his or her name and birth date, based on facility policy. | |
| — | — | — | c. If the patient cannot identify him- or herself, verify the patient's identification with a staff member who knows the patient for the second source. | |
| — | — | — | 15. Complete necessary assessments before administering medications. Check the patient's allergy bracelet or ask the patient about allergies. Explain the purpose and action of each medication to the patient. | |
| — | — | — | 16. Scan the patient's bar code on the identification band, if required. | |
| — | — | — | 17. Put on gloves. | |
| — | — | — | 18. Cleanse external ear of any drainage with cotton ball or washcloth moistened with normal saline. | |
| — | — | — | 19. Place patient on his or her unaffected side in bed, or, if ambulatory, have patient sit with head well tilted to the side so that affected ear is uppermost. | |
| — | — | — | 20. Draw up the amount of solution needed in the dropper. Do not return excess medication to stock bottle. A prepackaged, monodrip plastic container may also be used. | |
| — | — | — | 21. Straighten auditory canal by pulling cartilaginous portion of pinna up and back for an adult. | |
| — | — | — | 22. Hold dropper in the ear with its tip above the auditory canal. Do not touch the dropper to the ear. For an infant or an irrational or confused patient, protect the dropper with a piece of soft tubing to help prevent injury to the ear. | |
| — | — | — | 23. *Allow drops to fall on the side of the canal.* | |
| — | — | — | 24. Release pinna after instilling drops, and have patient maintain the position to prevent escape of medication. | |
| — | — | — | 25. Gently press on the tragus a few times. | |
| — | — | — | 26. If ordered, loosely insert a cotton ball into the ear canal. | |
| — | — | — | 27. Remove gloves. Assist the patient to a comfortable position. | |
| — | — | — | 28. Remove additional PPE, if used. Perform hand hygiene. | |
| — | — | — | 29. Document the administration of the medication immediately after administration. | |
| — | — | — | 30. Evaluate the patient's response to medication within appropriate time frame. | |

*Skill Checklists for Taylor's Clinical Nursing Skills:*
*A Nursing Process Approach, 3rd edition*

Name _____  Date _____

Unit _____  Position _____

Instructor/Evaluator: _____  Position _____

| Excellent | Satisfactory | Needs Practice | SKILL 5-19 **Administering an Ear Irrigation** | Comments |
|:---:|:---:|:---:|---|---|
| | | | **Goal:** The irrigation is administered successfully. | |
| —— | —— | —— | 1. Gather equipment. Check medication order against the original order in the medical record, according to facility policy. Clarify any inconsistencies. Check the patient's chart for allergies. | |
| —— | —— | —— | 2. Know the actions, special nursing considerations, safe dose ranges, purpose of administration, and adverse effects of the medication to be administered. Consider the appropriateness of the medication for this patient. | |
| —— | —— | —— | 3. Perform hand hygiene. | |
| —— | —— | —— | 4. Move the medication cart to the outside of the patient's room or prepare for administration in the medication area. | |
| —— | —— | —— | 5. Unlock the medication cart or drawer. Enter pass code and scan employee identification, if required. | |
| —— | —— | —— | 6. *Prepare medications for one patient at a time.* | |
| —— | —— | —— | 7. Read the CMAR/MAR and select the proper medication from the patient's medication drawer or unit stock. | |
| —— | —— | —— | 8. Compare the label with the CMAR/MAR. Check expiration dates and perform calculations, if necessary. Scan the bar code on the package, if required. | |
| —— | —— | —— | 9. *When all medications for one patient have been prepared, recheck the label with the CMAR/MAR before taking them to the patient.* | |
| —— | —— | —— | 10. Lock the medication cart before leaving it. | |
| —— | —— | —— | 11. Transport medications to the patient's bedside carefully, and keep the medications in sight at all times. | |
| —— | —— | —— | 12. *Ensure that the patient receives the medications at the correct time.* | |
| —— | —— | —— | 13. Perform hand hygiene and put on PPE, if indicated. | |
| —— | —— | —— | 14. Identify the patient. Usually, the patient should be identified using two methods. Compare information with the CMAR/MAR. | |
| —— | —— | —— | a. Check the name and identification number on the patient's identification band. | |

SKILL 5-19

# Administering an Ear Irrigation *(Continued)*

| Excellent | Satisfactory | Needs Practice | | Comments |
|---|---|---|---|---|
| —— | —— | —— | b. Ask the patient to state his or her name and birth date, based on facility policy. | |
| —— | —— | —— | c. If the patient cannot identify him- or herself, verify the patient's identification with a staff member who knows the patient for the second source. | |
| —— | —— | —— | 15. Explain procedure to patient. | |
| —— | —— | —— | 16. Assemble equipment at patient's bedside. | |
| —— | —— | —— | 17. Put on gloves. | |
| —— | —— | —— | 18. Have the patient sit up or lie with head tilted toward side of the affected ear. Protect the patient and bed with a waterproof pad. Have the patient support basin under the ear to receive the irrigating solution. | |
| —— | —— | —— | 19. Clean pinna and meatus of auditory canal, as necessary, with moistened cotton-tipped applicators dipped in warm tap water or the irrigating solution. | |
| —— | —— | —— | 20. Fill bulb syringe with warm solution. If an irrigating container is used, prime the tubing. | |
| —— | —— | —— | 21. Straighten auditory canal by pulling cartilaginous portion of pinna up and back for an adult. | |
| —— | —— | —— | 22. *Direct a steady, slow stream of solution against the roof of the auditory canal, using only enough force to remove secretions. Do not occlude the auditory canal with the irrigating nozzle. Allow solution to flow out unimpeded.* | |
| —— | —— | —— | 23. When irrigation is complete, place a cotton ball loosely in auditory meatus and have patient lie on side of affected ear on a towel or absorbent pad. | |
| —— | —— | —— | 24. Remove gloves. Assist the patient to a comfortable position. | |
| —— | —— | —— | 25. Remove additional PPE, if used. Perform hand hygiene. | |
| —— | —— | —— | 26. Document the administration of the medication immediately after administration. | |
| —— | —— | —— | 27. Evaluate the patient's response to the procedure. Return in 10 to 15 minutes and remove cotton ball and assess drainage. Evaluate the patient's response to medication within appropriate time frame. | |

*Skill Checklists for Taylor's Clinical Nursing Skills:*
*A Nursing Process Approach, 3rd edition*

Name _____  Date _____

Unit _____  Position _____

Instructor/Evaluator: _____  Position _____

| Excellent | Satisfactory | Needs Practice | SKILL 5-20 **Instilling Nose Drops** | Comments |
|---|---|---|---|---|
| | | | **Goal:** The medication is administered successfully into the nose. | |
| ― | ― | ― | 1. Gather equipment. Check medication order against the original order in the medical record, according to facility policy. Clarify any inconsistencies. Check the patient's chart for allergies. | |
| ― | ― | ― | 2. Know the actions, special nursing considerations, safe dose ranges, purpose of administration, and adverse effects of the medication to be administered. Consider the appropriateness of the medication for this patient. | |
| ― | ― | ― | 3. Perform hand hygiene. | |
| ― | ― | ― | 4. Move the medication cart to the outside of the patient's room or prepare for administration in the medication area. | |
| ― | ― | ― | 5. Unlock the medication cart or drawer. Enter pass code and scan employee identification, if required. | |
| ― | ― | ― | 6. *Prepare medications for one patient at a time.* | |
| ― | ― | ― | 7. Read the CMAR/MAR and select the proper medication from the patient's medication drawer or unit stock. | |
| ― | ― | ― | 8. Compare the label with the CMAR/MAR. Check expiration dates and perform calculations, if necessary. Scan the bar code on the package, if required. | |
| ― | ― | ― | 9. *When all medications for one patient have been prepared, recheck the label with the CMAR/MAR before taking them to the patient.* | |
| ― | ― | ― | 10. Lock the medication cart before leaving it. | |
| ― | ― | ― | 11. Transport medications to the patient's bedside carefully, and keep the medications in sight at all times. | |
| ― | ― | ― | 12. *Ensure that the patient receives the medications at the correct time.* | |
| ― | ― | ― | 13. Perform hand hygiene and put on PPE, if indicated. | |
| ― | ― | ― | 14. Identify the patient. Usually, the patient should be identified using two methods. Compare information with the CMAR/MAR. | |
| ― | ― | ― |    a. Check the name and identification number on the patient's identification band. | |

SKILL 5-20

# Instilling Nose Drops (Continued)

| Excellent | Satisfactory | Needs Practice | | Comments |
|---|---|---|---|---|
| — | — | — | b. Ask the patient to state his or her name and birth date, based on facility policy. | |
| — | — | — | c. If the patient cannot identify him- or herself, verify the patient's identification with a staff member who knows the patient for the second source. | |
| — | — | — | 15. Complete necessary assessments before administering medications. Check the patient's allergy bracelet or ask the patient about allergies. Explain the purpose and action of each medication to the patient. | |
| — | — | — | 16. Scan the patient's bar code on the identification band, if required. | |
| — | — | — | 17. Put on gloves. | |
| — | — | — | 18. Provide patient with paper tissues and ask patient to blow his or her nose. | |
| — | — | — | 19. Have patient sit up with head tilted well back. If patient is lying down, tilt head back over a pillow. | |
| — | — | — | 20. Draw sufficient solution into dropper for both nares. Do not return excess solution to a stock bottle. | |
| — | — | — | 21. Ask the patient to breathe through the mouth. Hold tip of nose up and place dropper just above naris, about ⅓ inch. Instill the prescribed number of drops in one naris and then into the other. Protect dropper with a piece of soft tubing if patient is an infant or young child. Avoid touching naris with dropper. | |
| — | — | — | 22. Have patient remain in position with head tilted back for a few minutes. | |
| — | — | — | 23. Remove gloves. Assist the patient to a comfortable position. | |
| — | — | — | 24. Remove additional PPE, if used. Perform hand hygiene. | |
| — | — | — | 25. Document the administration of the medication immediately after administration. | |
| — | — | — | 26. Evaluate the patient's response to the procedure and medication within appropriate time frame. | |

*Skill Checklists for Taylor's Clinical Nursing Skills:*
*A Nursing Process Approach, 3rd edition*

Name _____  Date _____

Unit _____  Position _____

Instructor/Evaluator: _____  Position _____

## SKILL 5-21
# Administering a Vaginal Cream

| Excellent | Satisfactory | Needs Practice | **Goal:** The medication is administered successfully into the vagina. | Comments |
|---|---|---|---|---|
| — | — | — | 1. Gather equipment. Check medication order against the original order in the medical record, according to facility policy. Clarify any inconsistencies. Check the patient's chart for allergies. | |
| — | — | — | 2. Know the actions, special nursing considerations, safe dose ranges, purpose of administration, and adverse effects of the medication to be administered. Consider the appropriateness of the medication for this patient. | |
| — | — | — | 3. Perform hand hygiene. | |
| — | — | — | 4. Move the medication cart to the outside of the patient's room or prepare for administration in the medication area. | |
| — | — | — | 5. Unlock the medication cart or drawer. Enter pass code and scan employee identification, if required. | |
| — | — | — | 6. *Prepare medications for one patient at a time.* | |
| — | — | — | 7. Read the CMAR/MAR and select the proper medication from the patient's medication drawer or unit stock. | |
| — | — | — | 8. Compare the label with the CMAR/MAR. Check expiration dates and perform calculations, if necessary. Scan the bar code on the package, if required. | |
| — | — | — | 9. *When all medications for one patient have been prepared, recheck the label with the MAR before taking them to the patient.* | |
| — | — | — | 10. Lock the medication cart before leaving it. | |
| — | — | — | 11. Transport medications to the patient's bedside carefully, and keep the medications in sight at all times. | |
| — | — | — | 12. *Ensure that the patient receives the medications at the correct time.* | |
| — | — | — | 13. Perform hand hygiene and put on PPE, if indicated. | |
| — | — | — | 14. Identify the patient. Usually, the patient should be identified using two methods. Compare information with the CMAR/MAR. | |
| — | — | — |    a. Check the name and identification number on the patient's identification band. | |

SKILL 5-21

# Administering a Vaginal Cream *(Continued)*

| Excellent | Satisfactory | Needs Practice | | Comments |
|---|---|---|---|---|
| —— | —— | —— | b. Ask the patient to state his or her name and birth date, based on facility policy. | |
| —— | —— | —— | c. If the patient cannot identify herself, verify the patient's identification with a staff member who knows the patient for the second source. | |
| —— | —— | —— | 15. Complete necessary assessments before administering medications. Check the patient's allergy bracelet or ask the patient about allergies. Explain the purpose and action of each medication to the patient. | |
| —— | —— | —— | 16. Scan the patient's bar code on the identification band, if required. | |
| —— | —— | —— | 17. Put on gloves. | |
| —— | —— | —— | 18. Ask the patient to void before inserting the medication. | |
| —— | —— | —— | 19. Position the patient so that she is lying on her back with the knees flexed. Maintain privacy with draping. Provide adequate light to visualize the vaginal opening. | |
| —— | —— | —— | 20. Spread labia with fingers, and cleanse area at vaginal orifice with washcloth and warm water, using a different corner of the washcloth with each stroke. Wipe from above the vaginal orifice downward toward the sacrum (front to back). | |
| —— | —— | —— | 21. Remove gloves and put on new gloves. | |
| —— | —— | —— | 22. Fill vaginal applicator with prescribed amount of cream. (See the Skill Variation in your skills book for administering a vaginal suppository.) | |
| —— | —— | —— | 23. Lubricate applicator with the lubricant, as necessary. | |
| —— | —— | —— | 24. Spread the labia with your nondominant hand and introduce applicator with your dominant hand gently, in a rolling manner, while directing it downward and backward. | |
| —— | —— | —— | 25. After applicator is properly positioned, labia may be allowed to fall in place if necessary to free the hand for manipulating the plunger. Push the plunger to its full length and then gently remove applicator with plunger depressed. | |
| —— | —— | —— | 26. **Ask the patient to remain in the supine position for 5 to 10 minutes after insertion.** Offer the patient a perineal pad to collect drainage. | |
| —— | —— | —— | 27. Dispose of applicator in appropriate receptacle or clean, nondisposable applicator according to manufacturer's directions. | |

| Excellent | Satisfactory | Needs Practice | | Comments |
|---|---|---|---|---|
| | | | **SKILL 5-21**<br>**Administering a Vaginal Cream** *(Continued)* | |
| —— | —— | —— | 28. Remove gloves and additional PPE, if used. Perform hand hygiene. | |
| —— | —— | —— | 29. Document the administration of the medication immediately after administration. | |
| —— | —— | —— | 30. Evaluate the patient's response to medication within appropriate time frame. | |

*Skill Checklists for Taylor's Clinical Nursing Skills:*
*A Nursing Process Approach, 3rd edition*

Name _____  Date _____

Unit _____  Position _____

Instructor/Evaluator: _____  Position _____

| Excellent | Satisfactory | Needs Practice | SKILL 5-22 **Administering a Rectal Suppository** | Comments |
|---|---|---|---|---|
| | | | **Goal:** The medication is administered successfully into the rectum. | |
| —— | —— | —— | 1. Gather equipment. Check medication order against the original order in the medical record, according to facility policy. Clarify any inconsistencies. Check the patient's chart for allergies. | |
| —— | —— | —— | 2. Know the actions, special nursing considerations, safe dose ranges, purpose of administration, and adverse effects of the medication to be administered. Consider the appropriateness of the medication for this patient. | |
| —— | —— | —— | 3. Perform hand hygiene. | |
| —— | —— | —— | 4. Move the medication cart to the outside of the patient's room or prepare for administration in the medication area. | |
| | | | 5. Unlock the medication cart or drawer. Enter pass code and scan employee identification, if required. | |
| —— | —— | —— | 6. *Prepare medications for one patient at a time.* | |
| | | | 7. Read the CMAR/MAR and select the proper medication from the patient's medication drawer or unit stock. | |
| —— | —— | —— | 8. Compare the label with the CMAR/MAR. Check expiration dates and perform calculations, if necessary. Scan the bar code on the package, if required. | |
| —— | —— | —— | 9. *When all medications for one patient have been prepared, recheck the label with the CMAR/MAR before taking them to the patient.* | |
| —— | —— | —— | 10. Lock the medication cart before leaving it. | |
| —— | —— | —— | 11. Transport medications to the patient's bedside carefully, and keep the medications in sight at all times. | |
| —— | —— | —— | 12. *Ensure that the patient receives the medications at the correct time.* | |
| —— | —— | —— | 13. Perform hand hygiene and put on PPE, if indicated. | |
| —— | —— | —— | 14. Identify the patient. Usually, the patient should be identified using two methods. Compare information with the CMAR/MAR. | |
| —— | —— | —— | a. Check the name and identification number on the patient's identification band. | |

| Excellent | Satisfactory | Needs Practice | | |
|---|---|---|---|---|
| | | | ## SKILL 5-22<br>## Administering a Rectal Suppository *(Continued)* | |
| | | | | **Comments** |
| —— | —— | —— | b. Ask the patient to state his or her name and birth date, based on facility policy. | |
| —— | —— | —— | c. If the patient cannot identify him- or herself, verify the patient's identification with a staff member who knows the patient for the second source. | |
| —— | —— | —— | 15. Complete necessary assessments before administering medications. Check the patient's allergy bracelet or ask the patient about allergies. Explain the purpose and action of each medication to the patient. | |
| —— | —— | —— | 16. Scan the patient's bar code on the identification band, if required. | |
| —— | —— | —— | 17. Put on gloves. | |
| —— | —— | —— | 18. Assist the patient to his or her left side in a Sims' position. Drape accordingly to only expose the buttocks. | |
| —— | —— | —— | 19. Remove the suppository from its wrapper. Apply lubricant to the rounded end. Lubricate the index finger of your dominant hand. | |
| —— | —— | —— | 20. Separate the buttocks with your nondominant hand and instruct the patient to breathe slowly and deeply through his or her mouth while the suppository is being inserted. | |
| —— | —— | —— | 21. Using your index finger, insert the suppository, round end first, along the rectal wall. Insert about 3 to 4 inches. | |
| —— | —— | —— | 22. Use toilet tissue to clean any stool or lubricant from around the anus. Release the buttocks. Encourage the patient to remain on his or her side for at least 5 minutes and retain the suppository for the appropriate amount of time for the specific medication. | |
| —— | —— | —— | 23. Remove additional PPE, if used. Perform hand hygiene. | |
| —— | —— | —— | 24. Document the administration of the medication immediately after administration. | |
| —— | —— | —— | 25. Evaluate patient's response to the medication within appropriate time frame. | |

*Skill Checklists for Taylor's Clinical Nursing Skills:*
*A Nursing Process Approach, 3rd edition*

Name _____ Date _____

Unit _____ Position _____

Instructor/Evaluator: _____ Position _____

| Excellent | Satisfactory | Needs Practice | SKILL 5-23<br>**Administering Medication via a**<br>**Metered-Dose Inhaler (MDI)** | |
|---|---|---|---|---|
| | | | **Goal:** The patient receives the medication via an inhaler using the correct technique. | **Comments** |
| —— | —— | —— | 1. Gather equipment. Check each medication order against the original order in the medical record, according to facility policy. Clarify any inconsistencies. Check the patient's chart for allergies. | |
| —— | —— | —— | 2. Know the actions, special nursing considerations, safe dose ranges, purpose of administration, and adverse effects of the medications to be administered. Consider the appropriateness of the medication for this patient. | |
| —— | —— | —— | 3. Perform hand hygiene. | |
| —— | —— | —— | 4. Move the medication cart to the outside of the patient's room or prepare for administration in the medication area. | |
| —— | —— | —— | 5. Unlock the medication cart or drawer. Enter pass code and scan employee identification, if required. | |
| —— | —— | —— | 6. *Prepare medications for one patient at a time.* | |
| —— | —— | —— | 7. Read the CMAR/MAR and select the proper medication from the patient's medication drawer or unit stock. | |
| —— | —— | —— | 8. Compare the label with the CMAR/MAR. Check expiration dates and perform calculations, if necessary. Scan the bar code on the package, if required. | |
| —— | —— | —— | 9. *When all medications for one patient have been prepared, recheck the label with the MAR before taking them to the patient.* | |
| —— | —— | —— | 10. Lock the medication cart before leaving it. | |
| —— | —— | —— | 11. Transport medications to the patient's bedside carefully, and keep the medications in sight at all times. | |
| —— | —— | —— | 12. *Ensure that the patient receives the medications at the correct time.* | |
| —— | —— | —— | 13. Perform hand hygiene and put on PPE, if indicated. | |
| —— | —— | —— | 14. Identify the patient. Usually, the patient should be identified using two methods. Compare information with the CMAR/MAR. | |
| —— | —— | —— |    a. Check the name and identification number on the patient's identification band. | |

| Excellent | Satisfactory | Needs Practice | SKILL 5-23<br>**Administering Medication via a<br>Metered-Dose Inhaler (MDI)** *(Continued)* |
|-----------|--------------|----------------|---|
| | | | **Comments** |
| —— | —— | —— | b. Ask the patient to state his or her name and birth date, based on facility policy. |
| —— | —— | —— | c. If the patient cannot identify him- or herself, verify the patient's identification with a staff member who knows the patient for the second source. |
| —— | —— | —— | 15. Complete necessary assessments before administering medications. Check the patient's allergy bracelet or ask the patient about allergies. Explain what you are going to do and the reason to the patient. |
| —— | —— | —— | 16. Scan the patient's bar code on the identification band, if required. |
| —— | —— | —— | 17. Remove the mouthpiece cover from the MDI and the spacer. Attach the MDI to the spacer. (See the Skill Variation in your skills book for using an MDI without a spacer.) |
| —— | —— | —— | 18. Shake the inhaler and spacer well. |
| —— | —— | —— | 19. Have patient place the spacer's mouthpiece into mouth, grasping securely with teeth and lips. Have patient breathe normally through the spacer. |
| —— | —— | —— | 20. Patient should depress the canister, releasing one puff into the spacer, then inhale slowly and deeply through the mouth. |
| —— | —— | —— | 21. *Instruct patient to hold his or her breath for 5 to 10 seconds, or as long as possible, and then to exhale slowly through pursed lips.* |
| —— | —— | —— | 22. *Wait 1 to 5 minutes, as prescribed, before administering the next puff.* |
| —— | —— | —— | 23. After the prescribed amount of puffs has been administered, have patient remove the MDI from the spacer and replace the caps on both. |
| —— | —— | —— | 24. Have the patient gargle and rinse with tap water after using an MDI, as necessary. Clean the MDI according to the manufacturer's directions. |
| —— | —— | —— | 25. Remove gloves and additional PPE, if used. Perform hand hygiene. |
| —— | —— | —— | 26. Document the administration of the medication immediately after administration. |
| —— | —— | —— | 27. Evaluate the patient's response to medication within appropriate time frame. *Reassess lung sounds, oxygenation saturation if ordered, and respirations.* |

*Skill Checklists for Taylor's Clinical Nursing Skills:*
*A Nursing Process Approach, 3rd edition*

Name _____  Date _____

Unit _____  Position _____

Instructor/Evaluator: _____  Position _____

SKILL 5-24

# Administering Medication via a Small-Volume Nebulizer

**Goal:** The patient receives the medication via a small volume nebulizer using the correct technique.

| Excellent | Satisfactory | Needs Practice | | Comments |
|---|---|---|---|---|
| —— | —— | —— | 1. Gather equipment. Check each medication order against the original order in the medical record, according to facility policy. Clarify any inconsistencies. Check the patient's chart for allergies. | |
| —— | —— | —— | 2. Know the actions, special nursing considerations, safe dose ranges, purpose of administration, and adverse effects of the medications to be administered. Consider the appropriateness of the medication for this patient. | |
| —— | —— | —— | 3. Perform hand hygiene. | |
| —— | —— | —— | 4. Move the medication cart to the outside of the patient's room or prepare for administration in the medication area. | |
| —— | —— | —— | 5. Unlock the medication cart or drawer. Enter pass code and scan employee identification, if required. | |
| —— | —— | —— | 6. *Prepare medications for one patient at a time.* | |
| —— | —— | —— | 7. Read the CMAR/MAR and select the proper medication from the patient's medication drawer or unit stock. | |
| —— | —— | —— | 8. Compare the label with the CMAR/MAR. Check expiration dates and perform calculations, if necessary. Scan the bar code on the package, if required. | |
| —— | —— | —— | 9. *When all medications for one patient have been prepared, recheck the label with the CMAR/MAR before taking them to the patient.* | |
| —— | —— | —— | 10. Lock the medication cart before leaving it. | |
| —— | —— | —— | 11. Transport medications to the patient's bedside carefully, and keep the medications in sight at all times. | |
| —— | —— | —— | 12. *Ensure that the patient receives the medications at the correct time.* | |
| —— | —— | —— | 13. Perform hand hygiene and put on PPE, if indicated. | |
| —— | —— | —— | 14. Identify the patient. Usually, the patient should be identified using two methods. Compare information with the MAR/CMAR. | |
| —— | —— | —— |    a. Check the name and identification number on the patient's identification band. | |

## SKILL 5-24

# Administering Medication via a
# Small-Volume Nebulizer *(Continued)*

| Excellent | Satisfactory | Needs Practice | | Comments |
|---|---|---|---|---|
| —— | —— | —— | b. Ask the patient to state his or her name and birth date, based on facility policy. | |
| —— | —— | —— | c. If the patient cannot identify him- or herself, verify the patient's identification with a staff member who knows the patient for the second source. | |
| —— | —— | —— | 15. Complete necessary assessments before administering medications. Check the patient's allergy bracelet or ask the patient about allergies. Explain what you are going to do, and the reason for doing it, to the patient. | |
| —— | —— | —— | 16. Scan the patient's bar code on the identification band, if required. | |
| —— | —— | —— | 17. Remove the nebulizer cup from the device and open it. Place premeasured unit-dose medication in the bottom section of the cup or use a dropper to place a concentrated dose of medication in cup and add prescribed diluent, if required. | |
| —— | —— | —— | 18. Screw the top portion of the nebulizer cup back in place and attach the cup to the nebulizer. Attach one end of tubing to the stem on the bottom of the nebulizer cuff and the other end to the air compressor or oxygen source. | |
| —— | —— | —— | 19. Turn on the air compressor or oxygen. Check that a fine medication mist is produced by opening the valve. Have patient place mouthpiece into mouth and grasp securely with teeth and lips. | |
| —— | —— | —— | 20. *Instruct patient to inhale slowly and deeply through the mouth. A nose clip may be necessary if the patient is also breathing through the nose. Hold each breath for a slight pause, before exhaling.* | |
| —— | —— | —— | 21. *Continue this inhalation technique until all medication in the nebulizer cup has been aerosolized (usually about 15 minutes). Once the fine mist decreases in amount, gently flick the sides of the nebulizer cup.* | |
| —— | —— | —— | 22. Have the patient gargle and rinse with tap water after using the nebulizer, as necessary. Clean the nebulizer according to the manufacturer's directions. | |
| —— | —— | —— | 23. Remove gloves and additional PPE, if used. Perform hand hygiene. | |
| —— | —— | —— | 24. Document the administration of the medication immediately after administration. | |
| —— | —— | —— | 25. Evaluate patient's response to medication within appropriate time frame. *Reassess lung sounds, oxygenation saturation if ordered, and respirations.* | |

*Skill Checklists for Taylor's Clinical Nursing Skills:*
*A Nursing Process Approach, 3rd edition*

Name _____ Date _____

Unit _____ Position _____

Instructor/Evaluator: _____ Position _____

| Excellent | Satisfactory | Needs Practice | SKILL 5-25<br>**Administering Medication via a<br>Dry Powder Inhaler**<br><br>**Goal:** The patient receives the medication via a dry powder inhaler using the correct technique. | Comments |
|---|---|---|---|---|
| ___ | ___ | ___ | 1. Gather equipment. Check each medication order against the original order in the medical record, according to facility policy. Clarify any inconsistencies. Check the patient's chart for allergies. | |
| ___ | ___ | ___ | 2. Know the actions, special nursing considerations, safe dose ranges, purpose of administration, and adverse effects of the medications to be administered. Consider the appropriateness of the medication for this patient. | |
| ___ | ___ | ___ | 3. Perform hand hygiene. | |
| ___ | ___ | ___ | 4. Move the medication cart to the outside of the patient's room or prepare for administration in the medication area. | |
| ___ | ___ | ___ | 5. Unlock the medication cart or drawer. Enter pass code and scan employee identification, if required. | |
| ___ | ___ | ___ | 6. *Prepare medications for one patient at a time.* | |
| ___ | ___ | ___ | 7. Read the CMAR/MAR and select the proper medication from the patient's medication drawer or unit stock. | |
| ___ | ___ | ___ | 8. Compare the label with the CMAR/MAR. Check expiration dates and perform calculations, if necessary. Scan the bar code on the package, if required. | |
| ___ | ___ | ___ | 9. *When all medications for one patient have been prepared, recheck the label with the CMAR/MAR before taking them to the patient.* | |
| ___ | ___ | ___ | 10. Lock the medication cart before leaving it. | |
| ___ | ___ | ___ | 11. Transport medications to the patient's bedside carefully, and keep the medications in sight at all times. | |
| ___ | ___ | ___ | 12. *Ensure that the patient receives the medications at the correct time.* | |
| ___ | ___ | ___ | 13. Perform hand hygiene and put on PPE, if indicated. | |
| ___ | ___ | ___ | 14. Identify the patient. Usually, the patient should be identified using two methods. Compare information with the CMAR/MAR. | |
| ___ | ___ | ___ |    a. Check the name and identification number on the patient's identification band. | |

| Excellent | Satisfactory | Needs Practice | |
|---|---|---|---|

# Administering Medication via a
# Dry Powder Inhaler (Continued)

**Comments**

b. Ask the patient to state his or her name and birth date, based on facility policy.

c. If the patient cannot identify him- or herself, verify the patient's identification with a staff member who knows the patient for the second source.

15. Complete necessary assessments before administering medications. Check the patient's allergy bracelet or ask the patient about allergies. Explain what you are going to do, and the reason for doing it, to the patient.

16. Scan the patient's bar code on the identification band, if required.

17. Remove the mouthpiece cover or remove from storage container. Load a dose into the device as directed by the manufacturer, if necessary. Alternately, activate the inhaler, if necessary, according to manufacturer's directions.

18. Have the patient breathe out slowly and completely, without breathing into the DPI.

19. *Patient should place teeth over, and seal lips around, the mouthpiece. Do not block the opening with the tongue or teeth.*

20. *Breathe in quickly and deeply through the mouth, for longer than 2 to 3 seconds.*

21. Remove inhaler from mouth. *Instruct patient to hold the breath for 5 to 10 seconds, or as long as possible, and then to exhale slowly through pursed lips.*

22. *Wait 1 to 5 minutes, as prescribed, before administering the next puff.*

23. After the prescribed amount of puffs has been administered, have patient replace the cap or storage container.

24. Have the patient gargle and rinse with tap water after using DPI, as necessary. Clean the DPI according to the manufacturer's directions.

25. Remove gloves and additional PPE, if used. Perform hand hygiene.

26. Document the administration of the medication immediately after administration.

27. Evaluate patient's response to medication within appropriate time frame. *Reassess lung sounds, oxygenation saturation if ordered, and respirations.*

*Skill Checklists for Taylor's Clinical Nursing Skills:*
*A Nursing Process Approach, 3rd edition*

Name _____  Date _____

Unit _____  Position _____

Instructor/Evaluator: _____  Position _____

| Excellent | Satisfactory | Needs Practice | SKILL 6-1<br>**Providing Preoperative Patient Care:**<br>**Hospitalized Patient** | |
|---|---|---|---|---|
| | | | **Goal:** The patient proceeds to surgery physically and psychologically prepared. | **Comments** |
| ___ | ___ | ___ | 1. Check the patient's chart for the type of surgery and review the medical orders. Review the nursing database, history, and physical examination. Check that the baseline data are recorded; report those that are abnormal. | |
| ___ | ___ | ___ | 2. *Check that diagnostic testing has been completed and results are available; identify and report abnormal results.* | |
| ___ | ___ | ___ | 3. Gather the necessary supplies and bring to the bedside stand or overbed table. | |
| ___ | ___ | ___ | 4. Perform hand hygiene and put on PPE, if indicated. | |
| ___ | ___ | ___ | 5. Identify the patient. | |
| ___ | ___ | ___ | 6. Close curtains around bed and close the door to the room, if possible. Explain what you are going to do and why you are going to do it to the patient. | |
| ___ | ___ | ___ | 7. Explore the psychological needs of the patient related to the surgery as well as the family. | |
| ___ | ___ | ___ | a. Establish the therapeutic relationship, encouraging the patient to verbalize concerns or fears. | |
| ___ | ___ | ___ | b. Use active learning skills, answering questions and clarifying any misinformation. | |
| ___ | ___ | ___ | c. Use touch, as appropriate, to convey genuine empathy. | |
| ___ | ___ | ___ | d. Offer to contact spiritual counselor (priest, minister, rabbi) to meet spiritual needs. | |
| ___ | ___ | ___ | 8. *Identify learning needs of patient and family.* Ensure that the informed consent of the patient for the surgery has been signed, witnessed, and dated. Inquire if the patient has any questions regarding the surgical procedure. Check the patient's record to determine if an advance directive has been completed. If an advance directive has not been completed, discuss with the patient the possibility of completing it, as appropriate. If patient has had surgery before, ask about this experience. | |
| ___ | ___ | ___ | 9. Provide teaching about deep breathing exercises. Refer to Skill 6-2. | |
| ___ | ___ | ___ | 10. Provide teaching regarding coughing and splinting (providing support to the incision). Refer to Skill 6-2. | |

| Excellent | Satisfactory | Needs Practice | | Comments |
|---|---|---|---|---|

SKILL 6-1

# Providing Preoperative Patient Care:
## Hospitalized Patient *(Continued)*

| Excellent | Satisfactory | Needs Practice | | Comments |
|---|---|---|---|---|
| — — — | | | 11. Provide teaching regarding incentive spirometer. (Refer to Skill 14-2, Chapter 14, Oxygenation for specific information.) | |
| — — — | | | 12. Provide teaching regarding leg exercises, as appropriate. Refer to Skill 6-3. | |
| — — — | | | 13. Assist the patient in putting on antiembolism stockings (Refer to Skill 9-11, Chapter 9, Activity, for specific information) and demonstrate how the pneumatic compression device operates (Refer to Skill 9-12, Chapter 9, Activity, for specific information). | |
| — — — | | | 14. Provide teaching regarding turning in the bed. | |
| — — — | | |    a. Instruct the patient to use a pillow or bath blanket to splint where the incision will be. Ask the patient to raise his or her left knee and reach across to grasp the right side rail of the bed when turning toward his or her right side. If patient is turning to his or her left side, he or she will bend the right knee and grasp the left side rail. | |
| — — — | | |    b. When turning the patient onto his or her right side, ask the patient to push with bent left leg and pull on the right side rail. Explain to patient that you will place a pillow behind his/her back to provide support, and that the call bell will be placed within easy reach. | |
| — — — | | |    c. Explain to the patient that position change is recommended every 2 hours. | |
| — — — | | | 15. Provide teaching about pain management. | |
| — — — | | |    a. Discuss past experiences with pain and interventions that the patient has used to reduce pain. | |
| — — — | | |    b. Discuss the availability of analgesic medication postoperatively. | |
| — — — | | |    c. Discuss the use of patient controlled analgesia (PCA), as appropriate. Refer to Skill 10-4, Chapter 10, Comfort. | |
| — — — | | |    d. Explore the use of other alternative and nonpharmacologic methods to reduce pain, such as position change, massage, relaxation/diversion, guided imagery, and meditation. | |
| — — — | | | 16. Review equipment that may be used. | |
| — — — | | |    a. Show the patient various equipment, such as IV pumps, electronic blood pressure cuff, tubes, and surgical drains. | |
| — — — | | | 17. Provide skin preparation. | |
| — — — | | |    a. *Ask the patient to bathe or shower with the antiseptic solution. Remind the patient to clean the surgical site.* | |

| Excellent | Satisfactory | Needs Practice | SKILL 6-1
**Providing Preoperative Patient Care: Hospitalized Patient** *(Continued)* |
|---|---|---|---|
| | | | Comments |

| Excellent | Satisfactory | Needs Practice | | Comments |
|---|---|---|---|---|
| — | — | — | 18. Provide teaching about and follow dietary/fluid restrictions. | |
| — | — | — | a. *Explain to the patient that both food and fluid will be restricted before surgery to ensure that the stomach contains a minimal amount of gastric secretions. This restriction is important to reduce the risk of aspiration. Emphasize to the patient the importance of avoiding food and fluids during the prescribed time period, because failure to adhere may necessitate cancellation of the surgery.* | |
| — | — | — | 19. Provide intestinal preparation, as appropriate. In certain situations, the bowel will need to be prepared by administering enemas or laxatives to evacuate the bowel and to reduce the intestinal bacteria. | |
| — | — | — | a. *As needed, provide explanation of the purpose of enemas or laxatives before surgery. If patient will be administering an enema, clarify the steps as needed.* | |
| — | — | — | 20. *Check administration of regularly scheduled medications.* Review with the patient routine medications, over-the-counter medications, and herbal supplements that are taken regularly. Check the physician's orders and review with the patient which medications he or she will be permitted to take the day of surgery. | |
| — | — | — | 21. Remove PPE, if used. Perform hand hygiene. | |

120

*Skill Checklists for Taylor's Clinical Nursing Skills:*
*A Nursing Process Approach, 3rd edition*

Name _____  Date _____

Unit _____  Position _____

Instructor/Evaluator: _____  Position _____

SKILL 6-2

# Deep Breathing Exercises, Coughing, and Splinting

**Goal:** The patient and/or significant other verbalizes an understanding of the instructions and is able to demonstrate the activities.

| Excellent | Satisfactory | Needs Practice | | Comments |
|---|---|---|---|---|
| —— | —— | —— | 1. Check the patient's chart for the type of surgery and review the medical orders. | |
| —— | —— | —— | 2. Gather the necessary supplies and bring to the bedside stand or overbed table. | |
| —— | —— | —— | 3. Perform hand hygiene and put on PPE, if indicated. | |
| —— | —— | —— | 4. Identify the patient. | |
| —— | —— | —— | 5. Close curtains around bed and close the door to the room, if possible. Explain what you are going to do and why you are going to do it to the patient. | |
| —— | —— | —— | 6. Identify the patient's learning needs. Identify the patient's level of knowledge regarding deep breathing exercises, coughing, and splinting of the incision. If the patient has had surgery before, ask about this experience. | |
| —— | —— | —— | 7. Explain the rationale for performing deep breathing exercises, coughing, and splinting of the incision. | |
| —— | —— | —— | 8. Provide teaching about deep breathing exercises. | |
| —— | —— | —— | a. Assist or ask the patient to sit up (semi- or high-Fowler's position) and instruct the patient to place the palms of both hands along the lower anterior rib cage. | |
| —— | —— | —— | b. Instruct the patient to exhale gently and completely. | |
| —— | —— | —— | c. Instruct the patient to breathe in through the nose as deeply as possible and hold breath for 3 seconds. | |
| —— | —— | —— | d. Instruct the patient to exhale through the mouth, pursing the lips like when whistling. | |
| —— | —— | —— | e. Have the patient practice the breathing exercise three times. Instruct the patient that this exercise should be performed every 1 to 2 hours for the first 24 hours after surgery. | |
| —— | —— | —— | 9. Provide teaching regarding coughing and splinting (providing support to the incision). | |
| —— | —— | —— | a. Ask the patient to sit up (semi-Fowler's position) and apply a folded bath blanket or pillow against the part of the body where the incision will be (e.g., abdomen or chest). | |

Copyright © 2011 by Wolters Kluwer Health | Lippincott Williams & Wilkins. *Skill Checklists for Taylor's Clinical Nursing Skills: A Nursing Process Approach*, 3rd edition, by Pamela Lynn and Marilee LeBon.

## SKILL 6-2

# Deep Breathing Exercises, Coughing, and Splinting *(Continued)*

| Excellent | Satisfactory | Needs Practice | | Comments |
|---|---|---|---|---|
| —— | —— | —— | b. Instruct the patient to inhale and exhale through the nose three times. | |
| —— | —— | —— | c. Ask the patient to take a deep breath and hold it for 3 seconds and then cough out three short breaths. | |
| —— | —— | —— | d. Ask the patient to take a breath through the mouth and strongly cough again two times. | |
| —— | —— | —— | e. Instruct the patient that he or she should perform these actions every 2 hours when awake after surgery. | |
| —— | —— | —— | 10. Validate patient's understanding of information. Ask the patient to give a return demonstration. Ask the patient if he or she has any questions. Encourage the patient to practice the activities and ask questions, if necessary. | |
| —— | —— | —— | 11. Remove PPE, if used. Perform hand hygiene. | |

*Skill Checklists for Taylor's Clinical Nursing Skills:*
*A Nursing Process Approach, 3rd edition*

Name _____ Date _____

Unit _____ Position _____

Instructor/Evaluator: _____ Position _____

## SKILL 6-3
# Leg Exercises

| Excellent | Satisfactory | Needs Practice | **Goal:** The patient the patient and/or significant other verbalizes an understanding of the instructions related to leg exercises and is able to demonstrate the activities. | Comments |
|:---:|:---:|:---:|---|---|
| —— | —— | —— | 1. Check the patient's chart for the type of surgery and review the medical orders. | |
| —— | —— | —— | 2. Gather the necessary supplies and bring to the bedside stand or overbed table. | |
| —— | —— | —— | 3. Perform hand hygiene and put on PPE, if indicated. | |
| —— | —— | —— | 4. Identify the patient. | |
| —— | —— | —— | 5. Close curtains around bed and close the door to the room, if possible. Explain what you are going to do and why you are going to do it to the patient. | |
| —— | —— | —— | 6. Identify the patient's learning needs. Identify the patient's level of knowledge regarding leg exercises. If the patient has had surgery before, ask about this experience. | |
| —— | —— | —— | 7. Explain the rationale for performing leg exercises. | |
| —— | —— | —— | 8. Provide teaching regarding leg exercises. | |
| —— | —— | —— |    a. Assist or ask the patient to sit up (semi-Fowler's position) and explain to the patient that you will first demonstrate, and then coach him/her to exercise one leg at a time. | |
| | | |    b. Straighten the patient's knee, raise the foot, extend the lower leg, and hold this position for a few seconds. Lower the entire leg. Practice this exercise with the other leg. | |
| —— | —— | —— |    c. Assist or ask the patient to point the toes of both legs toward the foot of the bed, then relax them. Next, flex or pull the toes toward the chin. | |
| —— | —— | —— |    d. Assist or ask the patient to keep legs extended and to make circles with both ankles, first circling to the left and then to the right. Instruct the patient to repeat these exercises three times. | |
| —— | —— | —— | 9. Validate the patient's understanding of information. Ask the patient to give a return demonstration. Ask the patient if he or she has any questions. Encourage the patient to practice the activities and ask questions, if necessary. | |
| —— | —— | —— | 10. Remove PPE, if used. Perform hand hygiene. | |

*Skill Checklists for Taylor's Clinical Nursing Skills:*
*A Nursing Process Approach, 3rd edition*

Name _____  Date _____

Unit _____  Position _____

Instructor/Evaluator: _____  Position _____

| Excellent | Satisfactory | Needs Practice | SKILL 6-4 **Providing Preoperative Patient Care: Hospitalized Patient (Day of Surgery)** | |
|---|---|---|---|---|
| | | | **Goal:** The patient will be prepared physically and psychologically to proceed to surgery. | **Comments** |
| ____ | ____ | ____ | 1. Check the patient's chart for the type of surgery and review the medical orders. Review the nursing database, history, and physical examination. Check that the baseline data are recorded; report those that are abnormal. | |
| ____ | ____ | ____ | 2. Gather the necessary supplies and bring to the bedside stand or overbed table. | |
| ____ | ____ | ____ | 3. Perform hand hygiene and put on PPE, if indicated. | |
| ____ | ____ | ____ | 4. Identify the patient. | |
| ____ | ____ | ____ | 5. Close curtains around bed and close the door to the room, if possible. Explain what you are going to do and why you are going to do it to the patient. | |
| ____ | ____ | ____ | 6. Check that preoperative consent forms are signed, witnessed, and correct; that advance directives are in the medical record (as applicable); and that the patient's chart is in order. | |
| ____ | ____ | ____ | 7. *Check vital signs.* Notify primary care provider and surgeon of any pertinent changes (e.g., rise or drop in blood pressure, elevated temperature, cough, symptoms of infection). | |
| ____ | ____ | ____ | 8. Provide hygiene and oral care. Assess for loose teeth and caps. Remind patient of food and fluid restrictions before surgery. | |
| ____ | ____ | ____ | 9. Instruct the patient to remove all personal clothing, including underwear, and put on a hospital gown. | |
| ____ | ____ | ____ | 10. Ask patient to remove cosmetics, jewelry including body-piercing, nail polish, and prostheses (e.g., contact lenses, false eyelashes, dentures, and so forth). Some facilities allow a wedding band to be left in place depending on the type of surgery, provided it is secured to the finger with tape. | |
| ____ | ____ | ____ | 11. If possible, give valuables to family member or place valuables in appropriate area, such as the hospital safe, if this is not possible. They should not be placed in narcotics drawer. | |
| ____ | ____ | ____ | 12. *Have patient empty bladder and bowel before surgery.* | |

| Excellent | Satisfactory | Needs Practice | SKILL 6-4<br>**Providing Preoperative Patient Care:**<br>**Hospitalized Patient (Day of Surgery)** *(Continued)* | |
|---|---|---|---|---|
| | | | | **Comments** |
| —— | —— | —— | 13. Attend to any special preoperative orders, such as starting an IV line. | |
| —— | —— | —— | 14. Complete preoperative checklist and record of patient's preoperative preparation. | |
| —— | —— | —— | 15. Question patient regarding the location of the operative site. Document the location in the medical record according to facility policy. The actual site will be marked on the patient when the patient arrives in the preoperative holding area by the licensed independent practitioner who will be directly involved in the procedure (The Joint Commission, 2008). | |
| —— | —— | —— | 16. *Administer preoperative medication as prescribed by physician/anesthesia provider.* | |
| —— | —— | —— | 17. Raise side rails of bed; place bed in lowest position. Instruct patient to remain in bed or on stretcher. If necessary, use a safety belt. | |
| —— | —— | —— | 18. Help move the patient from the bed to the transport stretcher, if necessary. Reconfirm patient identification and ensure that all preoperative events and measures are documented. | |
| —— | —— | —— | 19. Tell the patient's family where the patient will be taken after surgery and the location of the waiting area where the surgeon will come to explain the outcome of the surgery. If possible, take the family to the waiting area. | |
| —— | —— | —— | 20. After the patient leaves for the operating room, prepare the room and make a postoperative bed for the patient. Anticipate any necessary equipment based on the type of surgery and the patient's history. | |
| —— | —— | —— | 21. Remove PPE, if used. Perform hand hygiene. | |

*Skill Checklists for Taylor's Clinical Nursing Skills:*
*A Nursing Process Approach, 3rd edition*

Name _____   Date _____

Unit _____   Position _____

Instructor/Evaluator: _____   Position _____

| Excellent | Satisfactory | Needs Practice | |
|---|---|---|---|
| | | | **SKILL 6-5**<br>**Providing Postoperative Care When**<br>**Patient Returns to Room** |

**Goal:** The patient will recover from the surgery with postoperative risks minimized by frequent assessments.

**Comments**

**Immediate Care**

| Excellent | Satisfactory | Needs Practice | | Comments |
|---|---|---|---|---|
| ___ | ___ | ___ | 1. When patient returns from the PACU, obtain a report from the PACU nurse and review the operating room and PACU data. | |
| ___ | ___ | ___ | 2. Perform hand hygiene and put on PPE, if indicated. | |
| ___ | ___ | ___ | 3. Identify the patient. | |
| ___ | ___ | ___ | 4. Close curtains around bed and close the door to the room, if possible. Explain what you are going to do and why you are going to do it to the patient. | |
| ___ | ___ | ___ | 5. *Place patient in safe position (semi- or high Fowler's or side-lying). Note level of consciousness.* | |
| ___ | ___ | ___ | 6. *Obtain vital signs. Monitor and record vital signs frequently.* Assessment order may vary, but usual frequency includes taking vital signs every 15 minutes the first hour, every 30 minutes the next 2 hours, every hour for 4 hours, and finally every 4 hours. | |
| ___ | ___ | ___ | 7. Assess the patient's respiratory status. (Refer to Skill 2-4, in Chapter 2, Health Assessment.) Measure the patient's oxygen saturation level. | |
| ___ | ___ | ___ | 8. Assess the patient's cardiovascular status. (Refer to Skill 2-5, in Chapter 2, Health Assessment.) | |
| ___ | ___ | ___ | 9. Assess the patient's neurovascular status, based on the type of surgery performed. (Refer to Skill 2-7, in Chapter 2, Health Assessment.) | |
| ___ | ___ | ___ | 10. Provide for warmth, using heated or extra blankets, as necessary. Assess skin color and condition. | |
| ___ | ___ | ___ | 11. Check dressings for color, odor, presence of drains, and amount of drainage. Mark the drainage on the dressing by circling the amount, and include the time. Turn the patient to assess visually under the patient for bleeding from the surgical site. | |
| ___ | ___ | ___ | 12. Verify that all tubes and drains are patent and equipment is operative; note amount of drainage in collection device. If an indwelling urinary (Foley) catheter is in place, note urinary output. | |

| Excellent | Satisfactory | Needs Practice | | |
|---|---|---|---|---|
| | | | **SKILL 6-5**<br>**Providing Postoperative Care When**<br>**Patient Returns to Room** *(Continued)* | |
| | | | | **Comments** |
| —— | —— | —— | 13. Verify and maintain IV infusion at correct rate. | |
| —— | —— | —— | 14. Assess for pain and relieve it by administering medications ordered by the physician. If the patient has been instructed in use of PCA for pain management, review its use. Check record to verify if analgesic medication was administered in the PACU. | |
| —— | —— | —— | 15. Provide for a safe environment. Keep bed in low position with side rails up, based on facility policy. Have call bell within patient's reach. | |
| —— | —— | —— | 16. Remove PPE, if used. Perform hand hygiene. | |
| | | | **Ongoing Care** | |
| —— | —— | —— | 17. Promote optimal respiratory function. | |
| —— | —— | —— | a. Assess respiratory rate, depth, quality, color, and capillary refill. Ask if the patient is experiencing any difficulty breathing. | |
| —— | —— | —— | b. Assist with coughing and deep breathing exercises (Refer to Skill 6-2). | |
| —— | —— | —— | c. Assist with incentive spirometry (Refer to Skill 14-2). | |
| —— | —— | —— | d. Assist with early ambulation. | |
| —— | —— | —— | e. Provide frequent position change. | |
| —— | —— | —— | f. Administer oxygen as ordered. | |
| —— | —— | —— | g. Monitor pulse oximetry (Refer to Skill 14-1). | |
| —— | —— | —— | 18. Promote optimal cardiovascular function: | |
| —— | —— | —— | a. Assess apical rate, rhythm, and quality and compare with peripheral pulses, color, and blood pressure. Ask if the patient has any chest pains or shortness of breath. | |
| —— | —— | —— | b. Provide frequent position changes. | |
| —— | —— | —— | c. Assist with early ambulation. | |
| —— | —— | —— | d. Apply antiembolism stockings or pneumatic compression devices, if ordered and not in place. If in place, assess for integrity. | |
| —— | —— | —— | e. Provide leg and range-of-motion exercises if not contraindicated (Refer to Skill 6-3). | |
| —— | —— | —— | 19. Promote optimal neurologic function: | |
| —— | —— | —— | a. Assess level of consciousness, motor, and sensation. | |
| —— | —— | —— | b. Determine the level of orientation to person, place, and time. | |
| —— | —— | —— | c. Test motor ability by asking the patient to move each extremity. | |

| Excellent | Satisfactory | Needs Practice | | |
|---|---|---|---|---|
| | | | **SKILL 6-5** <br><br> **Providing Postoperative Care When Patient Returns to Room** *(Continued)* | |
| | | | | **Comments** |
| —— | —— | —— | d. Evaluate sensation by asking the patient if he or she can feel your touch on an extremity. | |
| —— | —— | —— | 20. Promote optimal renal and urinary function and fluid and electrolyte status. Assess intake and output, evaluate for urinary retention and monitor serum electrolyte levels. | |
| —— | —— | —— | a. Promote voiding by offering bedpan at regular intervals, noting the frequency, amount, and if any burning or urgency symptoms. | |
| —— | —— | —— | b. Monitor urinary catheter drainage if present. | |
| —— | —— | —— | c. Measure intake and output. | |
| —— | —— | —— | 21. Promote optimal gastrointestinal function and meet nutritional needs: | |
| —— | —— | —— | a. Assess abdomen for distention and firmness. Ask if patient feels nauseated, any vomiting, and if passing flatus. | |
| —— | —— | —— | b. Auscultate for bowel sounds. | |
| —— | —— | —— | c. Assist with diet progression; encourage fluid intake; monitor intake. | |
| —— | —— | —— | d. Medicate for nausea and vomiting, as ordered by physician. | |
| —— | —— | —— | 22. Promote optimal wound healing. | |
| —— | —— | —— | a. Assess condition of wound for presence of drains and any drainage. | |
| —— | —— | —— | b. Use surgical asepsis for dressing changes. | |
| —— | —— | —— | c. Inspect all skin surfaces for beginning signs of pressure ulcer development and use pressure-relieving supports to minimize potential skin breakdown. | |
| —— | —— | —— | 23. Promote optimal comfort and relief from pain. | |
| —— | —— | —— | a. Assess for pain (location and intensity using scale). | |
| —— | —— | —— | b. Provide for rest and comfort; provide extra blankets, as needed, for warmth. | |
| —— | —— | —— | c. Administer pain medications, as needed, or other nonpharmacologic methods. | |
| —— | —— | —— | 24. Promote optimal meeting of psychosocial needs: | |
| —— | —— | —— | a. Provide emotional support to patient and family, as needed. | |
| —— | —— | —— | b. Explain procedures and offer explanations regarding postoperative recovery, as needed, to both patient and family members. | |

Name _____     Date _____

Unit _____     Position _____

Instructor/Evaluator: _____     Position _____

| Excellent | Satisfactory | Needs Practice | SKILL 6-6 **Applying a Forced-Air Warming Device** | Comments |
|---|---|---|---|---|
| | | | **Goal:** The patient returns to and maintain a temperature of 97.7°F to 99.5°F (36.5°C to 37.5°C). | |
| —— | —— | —— | 1. Check patient's chart for the medical order for the use of a forced-air warming device. | |
| —— | —— | —— | 2. Gather the necessary supplies and bring to the bedside stand or overbed table. | |
| —— | —— | —— | 3. Perform hand hygiene and put on PPE, if indicated. | |
| —— | —— | —— | 4. Identify the patient. | |
| —— | —— | —— | 5. Close curtains around bed and close the door to the room, if possible. Explain what you are going to do and why you are going to do it to the patient. | |
| —— | —— | —— | 6. *Assess patient's temperature.* | |
| —— | —— | —— | 7. Plug forced-air warming device into electrical outlet. Place blanket over patient, with plastic side up. Keep air-hose inlet at foot of bed. | |
| —— | —— | —— | 8. Securely insert air hose into inlet. Place a lightweight fabric blanket over forced-air blanket, according to manufacturer's instructions. Turn machine on and adjust temperature of air to desired effect. | |
| —— | —— | —— | 9. Remove PPE, if used. Perform hand hygiene. | |
| —— | —— | —— | 10. *Monitor patient's temperature at least every 30 minutes while using the forced-air device. If rewarming a patient with hypothermia, do not raise temperature more than 1°C/hour to prevent a rapid vasodilation effect.* | |
| —— | —— | —— | 11. Discontinue use of forced-air device once patient's temperature is adequate and patient can maintain the temperature without assistance. | |
| —— | —— | —— | 12. Remove device and clean according to agency policy and manufacturer's instructions. | |

*Skill Checklists for Taylor's Clinical Nursing Skills:*
*A Nursing Process Approach, 3rd edition*

Name _____ Date _____

Unit _____ Position _____

Instructor/Evaluator: _____ Position _____

SKILL 7-1

# Giving a Bed Bath

| Excellent | Satisfactory | Needs Practice | **Goal:** The patient will vocalize feeling clean and fresh. | Comments |
|---|---|---|---|---|
| | ✓ | | 1. Review chart for any limitations in physical activity. | |
| | ✓ | | 2. Bring necessary equipment to the bedside stand or overbed table. | |
| | ✓ | | 3. Perform hand hygiene and put on gloves and/or other PPE, if indicated. | |
| | ✓ | | 4. Identify the patient. Discuss procedure with the patient and assess the patient's ability to assist in the bathing process, as well as personal hygiene preferences. | |
| | ✓ | | 5. Close curtains around bed and close the door to the room, if possible. Adjust the room temperature, if necessary. | |
| | ✓ | | 6. Remove sequential compression devices and antiembolism stockings from lower extremities according to agency protocol. | |
| | ✓ | | 7. Offer patient bedpan or urinal. | |
| | ✓ | | 8. Remove gloves and perform hand hygiene. | |
| | ✓ | | 9. Adjust the bed to a comfortable working height; usually elbow height of the caregiver (VISN 8 Patient Safety Center, 2009). | |
| | ✓ | | 10. Put on gloves. Lower side rail nearer to you and assist patient to side of bed where you will work. Have patient lie on his or her back. | |
| | ✓ | | 11. Loosen top covers and remove all except the top sheet. Place bath blanket over patient and then remove top sheet while patient holds bath blanket in place. If linen is to be reused, fold it over a chair. Place soiled linen in laundry bag. Take care to prevent linen from coming in contact with your clothing. | |
| | ✓ | | 12. Remove patient's gown and keep bath blanket in place. If patient has an IV line and is not wearing a gown with snap sleeves, remove gown from other arm first. *Lower the IV container and pass gown over the tubing and the container. Rehang the container and check the drip rate.* | |

| Excellent | Satisfactory | Needs Practice | SKILL 7-1<br>**Giving a Bed Bath** *(Continued)* | Comments |
|---|---|---|---|---|
| | ✓ | | 13. *Raise side rails.* Fill basin with a sufficient amount of comfortably warm water (110°F to 115°F). Add the skin cleanser, if appropriate, according to manufacturer's directions. Change as necessary throughout the bath. Lower side rail closer to you when you return to the bedside to begin the bath. | |
| | ✓ | | 14. Put on gloves, if necessary. Fold the washcloth like a mitt on your hand so that there are no loose ends. | |
| | ✓ | | 15. Lay a towel across patient's chest and on top of bath blanket. | |
| | ✓ | | 16. *With no cleanser on the washcloth, wipe one eye from the inner part of the eye, near the nose, to the outer part. Rinse or turn the cloth before washing the other eye.* | |
| | ✓ | | 17. Bathe patient's face, neck, and ears. Apply appropriate emollient. | |
| | ✓ | | 18. Expose patient's far arm and place towel lengthwise under it. Using firm strokes, wash hand, arm, and axilla, lifting the arm as necessary to access axillary region. Rinse, if necessary, and dry. Apply appropriate emollient. | |
| | ✓ | | 19. Place a folded towel on the bed next to the patient's hand and put basin on it. Soak the patient's hand in basin. Wash, rinse if necessary, and dry hand. Apply appropriate emollient. | |
| | ✓ | | 20. Repeat Actions 18 and 19 for the arm nearer you. An option for the shorter nurse or one susceptible to back strain might be to bathe one side of the patient and move to the other side of the bed to complete the bath. | |
| | ✓ | | 21. Spread a towel across patient's chest. Lower bath blanket to patient's umbilical area. Wash, rinse, if necessary, and dry chest. Keep chest covered with towel between the wash and rinse. Pay special attention to the folds of skin under the breasts. | |
| | ✓ | | 22. Lower bath blanket to the perineal area. Place a towel over patient's chest. | |
| | ✓ | | 23. Wash, rinse, if necessary, and dry abdomen. Carefully inspect and clean umbilical area and any abdominal folds or creases. | |
| | ✓ | | 24. Return bath blanket to original position and expose far leg. Place towel under far leg. Using firm strokes, wash, rinse, if necessary, and dry leg from ankle to knee and knee to groin. Apply appropriate emollient. | |

| Excellent | Satisfactory | Needs Practice | | |
|---|---|---|---|---|

## SKILL 7-1
## Giving a Bed Bath *(Continued)*

| | | | | Comments |
|---|---|---|---|---|

|  |  |  |  |
|---|---|---|---|
| ___ | ✓ | ___ | 25. Wash, rinse if necessary, and dry the foot. Pay particular attention to the areas between toes. Apply appropriate emollient. |
| ___ | ✓ | ___ | 26. Repeat Actions 21 and 22 for the other leg and foot. |
| ___ | ✓ | ___ | 27. Make sure patient is covered with bath blanket. Change water and washcloth at this point or earlier, if necessary. |
| ___ | ✓ | ___ | 28. Assist patient to prone or side-lying position. Put on gloves, if not applied earlier. Position bath blanket and towel to expose only the back and buttocks. |
| ___ | ✓ | ___ | 29. Wash, rinse, if necessary, and dry back and buttocks area. *Pay particular attention to cleansing between gluteal folds, and observe for any redness or skin breakdown in the sacral area.* |
| ___ | ✓ | ___ | 30. If not contraindicated, give patient a backrub, as described in Chapter 10. Back massage may be given also after perineal care. Apply appropriate emollient and/or skin barrier product. |
| ___ | ✓ | ___ | 31. Raise the side rail. Refill basin with clean water. Discard washcloth and towel. Remove gloves and put on clean gloves. |
| ___ | ✓ | ___ | 32. Clean perineal area or set patient up so that he or she can complete perineal self-care. If the patient is unable, lower the side rail and complete perineal care, following guidelines in the accompanying Skill Variation. Apply skin barrier, as indicated. Raise side rail, remove gloves, and perform hand hygiene. |
| ___ | ___ | ✓ | 33. Help patient put on a clean gown and assist with the use of other personal toiletries, such as deodorant or cosmetics. |
| ___ | ✓ | ___ | 34. Protect pillow with towel and groom patient's hair. |
| ___ | ✓ | ___ | 35. *When finished, make sure the patient is comfortable, with the side rails up and the bed in the lowest position.* |
| ___ | ___ | ✓ | 36. Change bed linens, as described in Skills 7-8 and 7-9. Dispose of soiled linens according to agency policy. Remove gloves and any other PPE, if used. Perform hand hygiene. |

*Skill Checklists for Taylor's Clinical Nursing Skills:*
*A Nursing Process Approach, 3rd edition*

Name _____  Date _____

Unit _____  Position _____

Instructor/Evaluator: _____  Position _____

## SKILL 7-2

# Assisting the Patient With Oral Care

**Goal:** The patient has a clean mouth and clean teeth, exhibits a positive body image, and verbalizes the importance of oral care.

| Excellent | Satisfactory | Needs Practice | | Comments |
|---|---|---|---|---|
| — | — | — | 1. Perform hand hygiene and put on gloves if assisting with oral care, and/or other PPE, if indicated. | |
| — | — | — | 2. Identify the patient. Explain procedure to the patient. | |
| — | — | — | 3. Assemble equipment on overbed table within patient's reach. | |
| — | — | — | 4. Close the room door or curtains. Place the bed at an appropriate and comfortable working height; usually elbow height of the caregiver (VISN 8 Patient Safety Center, 2009). | |
| — | — | — | 5. Lower side rail and assist patient to sitting position, if permitted, or turn patient onto side. Place towel across patient's chest. Raise bed to a comfortable working position. | |
| — | — | — | 6. Encourage patient to brush own teeth, or assist, if necessary. | |
| — | — | — | a. Moisten toothbrush and apply toothpaste to bristles. | |
| — | — | — | b. Place brush at a 45-degree angle to gum line and brush from gum line to crown of each tooth. Brush outer and inner surfaces. Brush back and forth across biting surface of each tooth. | |
| — | — | — | c. Brush tongue gently with toothbrush. | |
| — | — | — | d. Have patient rinse vigorously with water and spit into emesis basin. Repeat until clear. Suction may be used as an alternative for removal of fluid and secretions from mouth. | |
| — | — | — | 7. Assist patient to floss teeth, if appropriate: | |
| — | — | — | a. Remove approximately 6 inches of dental floss from container or use a plastic floss holder. Wrap the floss around the index fingers, keeping about 1 to 1.5 inches of floss taut between the fingers. | |
| — | — | — | b. Insert floss gently between teeth, moving it back and forth downward to the gums. | |

SKILL 7-2

# Assisting the Patient With Oral Care *(Continued)*

| Excellent | Satisfactory | Needs Practice | | Comments |
|---|---|---|---|---|
| —— | —— | —— | c. Move the floss up and down, first on one side of a tooth and then on the side of the other tooth, until the surfaces are clean. Repeat in the spaces between all teeth. | |
| —— | —— | —— | d. Instruct patient to rinse mouth well with water after flossing. | |
| —— | —— | —— | 8. Offer mouthwash if patient prefers. | |
| —— | —— | —— | 9. Offer lip balm or petroleum jelly. | |
| —— | —— | —— | 10. Remove equipment. Remove gloves and discard. Raise side rail and lower bed. Assist patient to a position of comfort. | |
| —— | —— | —— | 11. Remove any other PPE, if used. Perform hand hygiene. | |

*Skill Checklists for Taylor's Clinical Nursing Skills:*
*A Nursing Process Approach, 3rd edition*

Name _____   Date _____

Unit _____   Position _____

Instructor/Evaluator: _____   Position _____

## SKILL 7-3

# Providing Oral Care for the Dependent Patient

**Goal:** The patient has a clean mouth and clean teeth; is free from impaired oral mucous membranes; demonstrates improvement in body image; and verbalizes, if able, an understanding about the importance of oral care.

| Excellent | Satisfactory | Needs Practice | | Comments |
|---|---|---|---|---|
| —— | —— | —— | 1. Perform hand hygiene and put on PPE, if indicated. | |
| —— | —— | —— | 2. Identify the patient. Explain procedure to patient. | |
| —— | —— | —— | 3. Assemble equipment on overbed table within reach. | |
| —— | —— | —— | 4. Close the room door or curtains. Place the bed at an appropriate and comfortable working height, usually elbow height of the caregiver (VISN 8 Patient Safety Center, 2009). Lower one side rail and position patient on the side, with head tilted forward. Place towel across patient's chest and emesis basin in position under chin. Put on gloves. | |
| —— | —— | —— | 5. Gently open the patient's mouth by applying pressure to lower jaw at the front of the mouth. Remove dentures, if present. (Refer to Skill 7-4.) Brush the teeth and gums carefully with toothbrush and paste. Lightly brush the tongue. | |
| —— | —— | —— | 6. Use toothette dipped in water to rinse the oral cavity. If desired, insert the rubber tip of the irrigating syringe into patient's mouth and rinse gently with a small amount of water. ***Position patient's head to allow for return of water or use suction apparatus to remove the water from oral cavity.*** | |
| —— | —— | —— | 7. Clean the dentures before replacing. (See Skill 7-4.) | |
| —— | —— | —— | 8. Apply lubricant to patient's lips. | |
| —— | —— | —— | 9. Remove equipment and return patient to a position of comfort. Remove your gloves. Raise side rail and lower bed. | |
| —— | —— | —— | 10. Remove additional PPE, if used. Perform hand hygiene. | |

*Skill Checklists for Taylor's Clinical Nursing Skills:*
*A Nursing Process Approach, 3rd edition*

Name _____    Date _____

Unit _____    Position _____

Instructor/Evaluator: _____    Position _____

| Excellent | Satisfactory | Needs Practice | SKILL 7-4<br>**Providing Denture Care** | Comments |
|:---:|:---:|:---:|---|---|
| | | | **Goal:** The patient will have a clean mouth and clean dentures, exhibit a positive body image, and verbalize the importance of oral care. | |
| ___ | ___ | ___ | 1. Perform hand hygiene and put on PPE, if indicated. | |
| ___ | ___ | ___ | 2. Identify patient. Explain procedure to patient. | |
| ___ | ___ | ___ | 3. Assemble equipment on overbed table within reach. | |
| ___ | ___ | ___ | 4. Provide privacy for patient. | |
| ___ | ___ | ___ | 5. Lower side rail and assist patient to sitting position, if permitted, or turn patient onto side. Place towel across patient's chest. Raise bed to a comfortable working position, usually elbow height of the caregiver (VISN 8 Patient Safety Center, 2009). Put on gloves. | |
| ___ | ___ | ___ | 6. Apply gentle pressure with 4 × 4 gauze to grasp upper denture plate and remove it. Place it immediately in denture cup. Lift lower dentures with gauze, using slight rocking motion. Remove, and place in denture cup. | |
| ___ | ___ | ___ | 7. Place paper towels or washcloth in sink while brushing. Using the toothbrush and paste, brush all surfaces gently but thoroughly. If patient prefers, add denture cleaner to cup with water and follow directions on preparation. | |
| ___ | ___ | ___ | 8. Rinse thoroughly with water. Apply denture adhesive, if appropriate. | |
| ___ | ___ | ___ | 9. Use a toothbrush and paste to gently clean gums, mucous membranes, and tongue. Offer water and/or mouthwash so patient can rinse mouth before replacing dentures. | |
| ___ | ___ | ___ | 10. Insert upper denture in mouth and press firmly. Insert lower denture. Check that the dentures are securely in place and comfortable. | |
| ___ | ___ | ___ | 11. If the patient desires, dentures can be stored in the denture cup in cold water, instead of returning to the mouth. Label the cup and place in the patient's bedside table. | |
| ___ | ___ | ___ | 12. Remove equipment and return patient to a position of comfort. Remove your gloves. Raise side rail and lower bed. | |
| ___ | ___ | ___ | 13. Remove additional PPE, if used. Perform hand hygiene. | |

*Skill Checklists for Taylor's Clinical Nursing Skills:*
*A Nursing Process Approach, 3rd edition*

Name _____   Date _____

Unit _____   Position _____

Instructor/Evaluator: _____   Position _____

## SKILL 7-5

# Removing Contact Lenses

**Goal:** The lenses are removed without trauma to the eye and stored safely.

| Excellent | Satisfactory | Needs Practice | | Comments |
|---|---|---|---|---|
| —— | —— | —— | 1. Perform hand hygiene and put on PPE, if indicated. | |
| —— | —— | —— | 2. Identify the patient. Explain the procedure to the patient. | |
| —— | —— | —— | 3. Assemble equipment on overbed table within reach. | |
| —— | —— | —— | 4. Close curtains around bed and close the door to the room, if possible. | |
| —— | —— | —— | 5. Assist patient to supine position. Elevate bed. Lower side rail closest to you. | |
| —— | —— | —— | 6. If containers are not already labeled, do so now. Place 5 mL of normal saline in each container. | |
| —— | —— | —— | 7. Put on gloves. Remove soft contact lens: | |
| —— | —— | —— |   a. Have the patient look forward. Retract the lower lid with one hand. Using the pad of the index finger of the other hand, move the lens down to the sclera. | |
| —— | —— | —— |   b. Using the pads of the thumb and index finger, grasp the lens with a gentle pinching motion and remove. | |
| | | |   (See the Skill Variation in your skills book for figures showing other techniques for removing both hard and soft lenses.) | |
| | | | 8. Place the first lens in its designated cup in the storage case before removing the second lens. | |
| —— | —— | —— | 9. Repeat actions to remove other contact lens. | |
| —— | —— | —— | 10. If patient is awake and has glasses at bedside, offer patient glasses. | |
| —— | —— | —— | 11. Remove equipment and return patient to a position of comfort. Remove your gloves. Raise side rail and lower bed. | |
| —— | —— | —— | 12. Remove additional PPE, if used. Perform hand hygiene. | |

*Skill Checklists for Taylor's Clinical Nursing Skills:*
*A Nursing Process Approach, 3rd edition*

Name _____     Date _____

Unit _____     Position _____

Instructor/Evaluator: _____     Position _____

## SKILL 7-6
## Shampooing a Patient's Hair in Bed

**Goal:** The patient's hair is cleaned with minimal discomfort to the patient.

| Excellent | Satisfactory | Needs Practice | | Comments |
|---|---|---|---|---|
| ___ | ___ | ___ | 1. Review chart for any limitations in physical activity, or contraindications to the procedure. | |
| ___ | ___ | ___ | 2. Perform hand hygiene. Put on PPE, as indicated. | |
| ___ | ___ | ___ | 3. Identify the patient. Explain the procedure to the patient. | |
| ___ | ___ | ___ | 4. Assemble equipment on overbed table within reach. | |
| ___ | ___ | ___ | 5. Close curtains around bed and close the door to the room, if possible. | |
| ___ | ___ | ___ | 6. Lower the head of the bed. Remove pillow and place protective pad under patient's head and shoulders. | |
| ___ | ___ | ___ | 7. *Fill the pitcher with warm water (43°C to 46°C [110°F to 115°F]).* Position the patient at the top of the bed, in a supine position. Have the patient lift his or her head and place shampoo board underneath patient's head. If necessary, pad the edge of the board with a small towel. | |
| ___ | ___ | ___ | 8. Place a drain container underneath the drain of the shampoo board. | |
| ___ | ___ | ___ | 9. Put on gloves. If the patient is able, have him or her hold a folded washcloth at the forehead. Pour pitcher of warm water slowly over patient's head, making sure that all hair is saturated. Refill pitcher, if needed. | |
| ___ | ___ | ___ | 10. Apply a small amount of shampoo to patient's hair. *Massage deep into the scalp, avoiding any cuts, lesions, or sore spots.* | |
| ___ | ___ | ___ | 11. Rinse with warm water (43°C to 46°C [110°F to 115°F]) until all shampoo is out of hair. Repeat shampoo, if necessary. | |
| ___ | ___ | ___ | 12. If patient has thick hair or requests it, apply a small amount of conditioner to hair and massage throughout. Avoid any cuts, lesions, or sore spots. | |
| ___ | ___ | ___ | 13. If drain container is small, empty before rinsing hair. Rinse with warm water (43°C to 46°C [110°F to 115°F]) until all conditioner is out of hair. | |
| ___ | ___ | ___ | 14. Remove shampoo board. Place towel around patient's hair. | |

## SKILL 7-6
# Shampooing a Patient's Hair in Bed *(Continued)*

| Excellent | Satisfactory | Needs Practice | | Comments |
|---|---|---|---|---|
| ___ | ___ | ___ | 15. Pat hair dry, avoiding any cuts, lesions, or sore spots. Remove protective padding but keep one dry protective pad under patient's hair. | |
| ___ | ___ | ___ | 16. Gently brush hair, removing tangles as needed. | |
| ___ | ___ | ___ | 17. Blow-dry hair on a cool setting, if allowed and if patient wishes. If not, consider covering the patient's head with a dry towel, until hair is dry. | |
| ___ | ___ | ___ | 18. Change patient's gown and remove protective pad. Replace pillow. | |
| ___ | ___ | ___ | 19. Remove equipment and return patient to a position of comfort. Remove your gloves. Raise side rail and lower bed. | |
| ___ | ___ | ___ | 20. Remove additional PPE, if used. Perform hand hygiene. | |

*Skill Checklists for Taylor's Clinical Nursing Skills:
A Nursing Process Approach, 3rd edition*

Name _____  Date _____

Unit _____  Position _____

Instructor/Evaluator: _____  Position _____

| Excellent | Satisfactory | Needs Practice | SKILL 7-7 **Assisting the Patient to Shave** | Comments |
|---|---|---|---|---|
| | | | **Goal:** The patient skin is free of hair without evidence of trauma to the skin. | |
| ___ | ___ | ___ | 1. Perform hand hygiene. Put on PPE, as indicated. | |
| ___ | ___ | ___ | 2. Identify patient. Explain procedure to the patient. | |
| ___ | ___ | ___ | 3. Assemble equipment on overbed table within reach. | |
| ___ | ___ | ___ | 4. Close curtains around bed and close the door to the room, if possible. | |
| ___ | ___ | ___ | 5. Cover patient's chest with a towel or waterproof pad. Fill bath basin with warm (43°C to 46°C [110°F to 115°F]) water. Put on gloves. Moisten the area to be shaved with a washcloth. | |
| ___ | ___ | ___ | 6. Dispense shaving cream into palm of hand. Apply cream to area to be shaved in a layer about 0.5 inch thick. | |
| ___ | ___ | ___ | 7. With one hand, pull the skin taut at the area to be shaved. Using a smooth stroke, begin shaving. *If shaving the face,* shave with the direction of hair growth in downward, short strokes. *If shaving a leg,* shave against the hair in upward, short strokes. *If shaving an underarm,* pull skin taut and use short, upward strokes. | |
| ___ | ___ | ___ | 8. Wash off residual shaving cream. | |
| ___ | ___ | ___ | 9. If patient requests, apply aftershave or lotion to area shaved. | |
| ___ | ___ | ___ | 10. Remove equipment and return patient to a position of comfort. Remove your gloves. Raise side rail and lower bed. | |
| ___ | ___ | ___ | 11. Remove additional PPE, if used. Perform hand hygiene. | |

*Skill Checklists for Taylor's Clinical Nursing Skills:*
*A Nursing Process Approach, 3rd edition*

Name _____   Date _____

Unit _____   Position _____

Instructor/Evaluator: _____   Position _____

## SKILL 7-8

# Making an Unoccupied Bed

| Excellent | Satisfactory | Needs Practice | | Comments |
|---|---|---|---|---|
| | | | **Goal**: The bed linens are changed without injury to the patient or nurse. | |
| ― | ― | ― | 1. Assemble equipment and arrange on a bedside chair in the order in which items will be used. | |
| ― | ― | ― | 2. Perform hand hygiene. Put on PPE, as indicated. | |
| ― | ― | ― | 3. Adjust the bed to a comfortable working height, usually elbow height of the caregiver (VISN 8 Patient Safety Center, 2009). Drop the side rails. | |
| ― | ― | ― | 4. Disconnect call bell or any tubes from bed linens. | |
| ― | ― | ― | 5. Put on gloves. Loosen all linen as you move around the bed, from the head of the bed on the far side to the head of the bed on the near side. | |
| ― | ― | ― | 6. Fold reusable linens, such as sheets, blankets, or spread, in place on the bed in fourths and hang them over a clean chair. | |
| ― | ― | ― | 7. Snugly roll all the soiled linen inside the bottom sheet and place directly into the laundry hamper. ***Do not place on floor or furniture. Do not hold soiled linens against your uniform.*** | |
| ― | ― | ― | 8. If possible, shift mattress up to head of bed. If mattress is soiled, clean and dry according to facility policy before applying new sheets. | |
| ― | ― | ― | 9. Remove your gloves, unless indicated for transmission precautions. Place the bottom sheet with its center fold in the center of the bed. Open the sheet and fan-fold to the center. | |
| ― | ― | ― | 10. If using, place the drawsheet with its center fold in the center of the bed and positioned so it will be located under the patient's midsection. Open the drawsheet and fan-fold to the center of the mattress. If a protective pad is used, place it over the drawsheet in the proper area and open to the centerfold. Not all agencies use drawsheets routinely. The nurse may decide to use one. In some institutions, the protective pad doubles as a drawsheet. | |
| ― | ― | ― | 11. Pull the bottom sheet over the corners at the head and foot of the mattress. (See the Skill Variation in your skills book for using a flat bottom sheet instead of a fitted sheet.) Tuck the drawsheet securely under the mattress. | |

SKILL 7-8

# Making an Unoccupied Bed *(Continued)*

| Excellent | Satisfactory | Needs Practice | | Comments |
|---|---|---|---|---|
| —— | —— | —— | 12. Move to the other side of the bed to secure bottom linens. Pull the bottom sheet tightly and secure over the corners at the head and foot of the mattress. Pull the drawsheet tightly and tuck it securely under the mattress. | |
| —— | —— | —— | 13. Place the top sheet on the bed with its center fold in the center of the bed and with the hem even with the head of the mattress. Unfold the top sheet. Follow same procedure with top blanket or spread, placing the upper edge about 6 inches below the top of the sheet. | |
| —— | —— | —— | 14. Tuck the top sheet and blanket under the foot of the bed on the near side. Miter the corners. | |
| —— | —— | —— | 15. Fold the upper 6 inches of the top sheet down over the spread and make a cuff. | |
| —— | —— | —— | 16. Move to the other side of the bed and follow the same procedure for securing top sheets under the foot of the bed and making a cuff. | |
| —— | —— | —— | 17. Place the pillows on the bed. Open each pillowcase in the same manner as you opened other linens. Gather the pillowcase over one hand toward the closed end. Grasp the pillow with the hand inside the pillowcase. Keep a firm hold on the top of the pillow and pull the cover onto the pillow. Place the pillow at the head of the bed. | |
| —— | —— | —— | 18. Fan-fold or pie-fold the top linens. | |
| —— | —— | —— | 19. Secure the signal device on the bed, according to agency policy. | |
| —— | —— | —— | 20. Raise side rail and lower bed. | |
| —— | —— | —— | 21. Dispose of soiled linen according to agency policy. | |
| —— | —— | —— | 22. Remove any other PPE, if used. Perform hand hygiene. | |

*Skill Checklists for Taylor's Clinical Nursing Skills:*
*A Nursing Process Approach, 3rd edition*

Name _____  Date _____

Unit _____  Position _____

Instructor/Evaluator: _____  Position _____

## SKILL 7-9

# Making an Occupied Bed

**Goal:** The bed linens are applied without injury to the patient or nurse.

| Excellent | Satisfactory | Needs Practice | | Comments |
|-----------|--------------|----------------|---|----------|
| —— | —— | —— | 1. Check chart for limitations on patient's physical activity. | |
| —— | —— | —— | 2. Assemble equipment and arrange on bedside chair in the order the items will be used. | |
| —— | —— | —— | 3. Perform hand hygiene. Put on PPE, as indicated. | |
| —— | —— | —— | 4. Identify the patient. Explain what you are going to do. | |
| —— | —— | —— | 5. Close curtains around bed and close the door to the room, if possible. | |
| —— | —— | —— | 6. Adjust the bed to a comfortable working height, usually elbow height of the caregiver (VISN 8 Patient Safety Center, 2009). | |
| —— | —— | —— | 7. Lower side rail nearest you, leaving the opposite side rail up. Place bed in flat position unless contraindicated. | |
| —— | —— | —— | 8. Put on gloves. Check bed linens for patient's personal items. *Disconnect the call bell or any tubes/drains from bed linens.* | |
| —— | —— | —— | 9. Place a bath blanket over patient. Have patient hold on to bath blanket while you reach under it and remove top linens. Leave top sheet in place if a bath blanket is not used. Fold linen that is to be reused over the back of a chair. Discard soiled linen in laundry bag or hamper. *Do not place on floor or furniture. Do not hold soiled linens against your uniform.* | |
| —— | —— | —— | 10. If possible, and another person is available to assist, grasp mattress securely and shift it up to head of bed. | |
| —— | —— | —— | 11. Assist patient to turn toward opposite side of the bed, and reposition pillow under patient's head. | |
| —— | —— | —— | 12. Loosen all bottom linens from head, foot, and side of bed. | |
| —— | —— | —— | 13. Fan-fold soiled linens as close to patient as possible. | |
| —— | —— | —— | 14. Use clean linen and make the near side of the bed. Place the bottom sheet with its center fold in the center of the bed. Open the sheet and fan-fold to the center, positioning it under the old linens. Pull the bottom sheet over the corners at the head and foot of the mattress. | |

| Excellent | Satisfactory | Needs Practice | | Comments |
|---|---|---|---|---|

# Making an Occupied Bed *(Continued)*

|  |  |  |  |
|---|---|---|---|
| ___ ___ ___ | 15. | If using, place the drawsheet with its center fold in the center of the bed and positioned so it will be located under the patient's midsection. Open the drawsheet and fan-fold to the center of the mattress. Tuck the drawsheet securely under the mattress. If a protective pad is used, place it over the drawsheet in the proper area and open to the center fold. Not all agencies use drawsheets routinely. The nurse may decide to use one. | |
| ___ ___ ___ | 16. | Raise side rail. Assist patient to roll over the folded linen in the middle of the bed toward you. Reposition pillow and bath blanket or top sheet. Move to other side of the bed and lower side rail. | |
| ___ ___ ___ | 17. | Loosen and remove all bottom linen. Discard soiled linen in laundry bag or hamper. *Do not place on floor or furniture. Do not hold soiled linens against your uniform.* | |
| ___ ___ ___ | 18. | Ease clean linen from under the patient. Pull the bottom sheet taut and secure at the corners at the head and foot of the mattress. Pull the drawsheet tight and smooth. Tuck the drawsheet securely under the mattress. | |
| ___ ___ ___ | 19. | Assist patient to turn back to the center of bed. Remove pillow and change pillowcase. Open each pillowcase in the same manner as you opened other linens. Gather the pillowcase over one hand toward the closed end. Grasp the pillow with the hand inside the pillowcase. Keep a firm hold on the top of the pillow and pull the cover onto the pillow. Place the pillow under the patient's head. | |
| ___ ___ ___ | 20. | Apply top linen, sheet and blanket, if desired, so that it is centered. Fold the top linens over at the patient's shoulders to make a cuff. Have patient hold on to top linen and remove the bath blanket from underneath. | |
| ___ ___ ___ | 21. | Secure top linens under foot of mattress and miter corners. (Refer to Skill Variation in Skill 7-8.) Loosen top linens over patient's feet by grasping them in the area of the feet and pulling gently toward foot of bed. | |
| ___ ___ ___ | 22. | Return patient to a position of comfort. Remove your gloves. Raise side rail and lower bed. Reattach call bell. | |
| ___ ___ ___ | 23. | Dispose of soiled linens according to agency policy. | |
| ___ ___ ___ | 24. | Remove any other PPE, if used. Perform hand hygiene. | |

*Skill Checklists for Taylor's Clinical Nursing Skills:*
*A Nursing Process Approach, 3rd edition*

Name _____     Date _____

Unit _____     Position _____

Instructor/Evaluator: _____     Position _____

SKILL 8-1

# Cleaning a Wound and Applying a Dry, Sterile Dressing

**Goal:** The wound is cleaned and protected with a dressing without contaminating the wound area, without causing trauma to the wound, and without causing the patient to experience pain or discomfort.

| Excellent | Satisfactory | Needs Practice | | Comments |
|---|---|---|---|---|
| —— | —— | —— | 1. Review the medical orders for wound care or the nursing plan of care related to wound care. | |
| —— | —— | —— | 2. Gather the necessary supplies and bring to the bedside stand or overbed table. | |
| —— | —— | —— | 3. Perform hand hygiene and put on PPE, if indicated. | |
| —— | —— | —— | 4. Identify the patient. | |
| —— | —— | —— | 5. Close curtains around bed and close door to room if possible. Explain what you are going to do and why you are going to do it to the patient. | |
| —— | —— | —— | 6. Assess the patient for possible need for nonpharmacologic pain-reducing interventions or analgesic medication before wound care dressing change. Administer appropriate prescribed analgesic. Allow enough time for analgesic to achieve its effectiveness. | |
| —— | —— | —— | 7. Place a waste receptacle or bag at a convenient location for use during the procedure. | |
| —— | —— | —— | 8. Adjust bed to comfortable working height, usually elbow height of the caregiver (VISN 8, 2009). | |
| —— | —— | —— | 9. Assist the patient to a comfortable position that provides easy access to the wound area. Use the bath blanket to cover any exposed area other than the wound. Place a waterproof pad under the wound site. | |
| —— | —— | —— | 10. Check the position of drains, tubes, or other adjuncts before removing the dressing. Put on clean, disposable gloves and loosen tape on the old dressings. If necessary, use an adhesive remover to help get the tape off. | |
| —— | —— | —— | 11. Carefully remove the soiled dressings. If there is resistance, use a silicone-based adhesive remover to help remove the tape. If any part of the dressing sticks to the underlying skin, use small amounts of sterile saline to help loosen and remove. | |

# Cleaning a Wound and Applying a Dry, Sterile Dressing (Continued)

| Excellent | Satisfactory | Needs Practice | | Comments |
|---|---|---|---|---|
| —— | —— | —— | 12. After removing the dressing, note the presence, amount, type, color, and odor of any drainage on the dressings. Place soiled dressings in the appropriate waste receptacle. Remove your gloves and dispose of them in an appropriate waste receptacle. | |
| —— | —— | —— | 13. Inspect the wound site for size, appearance, and drainage. Assess if any pain is present. Check the status of sutures, adhesive closure strips, staples, and drains or tubes, if present. Note any problems to include in your documentation. | |
| —— | —— | —— | 14. *Using sterile technique, prepare a sterile work area and open the needed supplies.* | |
| —— | —— | —— | 15. Open the sterile cleaning solution. Depending on the amount of cleaning needed, the solution might be poured directly over gauze sponges over a container for small cleaning jobs, or into a basin for more complex or larger cleaning. | |
| —— | —— | —— | 16. Put on sterile gloves. | |
| —— | —— | —— | 17. Clean the wound. *Clean the wound from top to bottom and from the center to the outside. Following this pattern, use new gauze for each wipe, placing the used gauze in the waste receptacle. Alternately, spray the wound from top to bottom with a commercially prepared wound cleanser.* | |
| —— | —— | —— | 18. Once the wound is cleaned, dry the area using a gauze sponge in the same manner. Apply ointment or perform other treatments, as ordered. | |
| —— | —— | —— | 19. If a drain is in use at the wound location, clean around the drain. Refer to Skills 8-7, 8-8, 8-9, and 8-10. | |
| —— | —— | —— | 20. Apply a layer of dry, sterile dressing over the wound. Forceps may be used to apply the dressing. | |
| —— | —— | —— | 21. Place a second layer of gauze over the wound site. | |
| —— | —— | —— | 22. Apply a surgical or abdominal pad (ABD) over the gauze at the site as the outermost layer of the dressing. | |
| —— | —— | —— | 23. Remove and discard gloves. Apply tape, Montgomery straps or roller gauze to secure the dressings. Alternately, many commercial wound products are self adhesive and do not require additional tape. | |

| Excellent | Satisfactory | Needs Practice | SKILL 8-1<br>**Cleaning a Wound and Applying a Dry, Sterile Dressing** *(Continued)* | |
|---|---|---|---|---|
| | | | | **Comments** |
| —— | —— | —— | 24. After securing the dressing, label dressing with date and time. Remove all remaining equipment; place the patient in a comfortable position, with side rails up and bed in the lowest position. | |
| —— | —— | —— | 25. Remove PPE, if used. Perform hand hygiene. | |
| —— | —— | —— | 26. Check all wound dressings every shift. More frequent checks may be needed if the wound is more complex or dressings become saturated quickly. | |

*Skill Checklists for Taylor's Clinical Nursing Skills:*
*A Nursing Process Approach, 3rd edition*

Name _____   Date _____

Unit _____   Position _____

Instructor/Evaluator: _____   Position _____

| Excellent | Satisfactory | Needs Practice | SKILL 8-2 **Applying a Saline-Moistened Dressing** | Comments |
|:---:|:---:|:---:|---|---|
| | | | **Goal:** The procedure is accomplished without contaminating the wound area, without causing trauma to the wound, and without causing the patient to experience pain or discomfort. | |
| ___ | ___ | ___ | 1. Review the medical orders for wound care or the nursing plan of care related to wound care. | |
| ___ | ___ | ___ | 2. Gather the necessary supplies and bring to the bedside stand or overbed table. | |
| ___ | ___ | ___ | 3. Perform hand hygiene and put on PPE, if indicated. | |
| ___ | ___ | ___ | 4. Identify the patient. | |
| ___ | ___ | ___ | 5. Close curtains around bed and close door to room if possible. Explain what you are going to do and why you are going to do it to the patient. | |
| ___ | ___ | ___ | 6. Assess the patient for possible need for nonpharmacologic pain-reducing interventions or analgesic medication before wound care dressing change. Administer appropriate prescribed analgesic. Allow enough time for analgesic to achieve its effectiveness. | |
| ___ | ___ | ___ | 7. Place a waste receptacle or bag at a convenient location for use during the procedure. | |
| ___ | ___ | ___ | 8. Adjust bed to comfortable working height, usually elbow height of the caregiver (VISN 8, 2009). | |
| ___ | ___ | ___ | 9. Assist the patient to a comfortable position that provides easy access to the wound area. Position the patient so the wound cleanser or irrigation solution will flow from the clean end of the wound toward the dirtier end, if being used (see Skill 8-1 for wound cleansing and Skill 8-4 for irrigation techniques). Use the bath blanket to cover any exposed area other than the wound. Place a waterproof pad under the wound site. | |
| ___ | ___ | ___ | 10. Put on clean gloves. Carefully and gently remove the soiled dressings. If there is resistance, use a silicone-based adhesive remover to help remove the tape. If any part of the dressing sticks to the underlying skin, use small amounts of sterile saline to help loosen and remove. | |
| ___ | ___ | ___ | 11. After removing the dressing, note the presence, amount, type, color, and odor of any drainage on the dressings. Place soiled dressings in the appropriate waste receptacle. | |

| Excellent | Satisfactory | Needs Practice | SKILL 8-2<br>**Applying a Saline-Moistened Dressing** *(Continued)* | Comments |
|:---:|:---:|:---:|---|---|
| —— | —— | —— | 12. Assess the wound for appearance, stage, the presence of eschar, granulation tissue, **epithelialization**, undermining, tunneling, necrosis, **sinus tract,** and drainage. Assess the appearance of the surrounding tissue. Measure the wound. Refer to Fundamentals Review 8-3. | |
| —— | —— | —— | 13. Remove your gloves and put them in the receptacle. | |
| —— | —— | —— | 14. Using sterile technique, open the supplies and dressings. Place the fine-mesh gauze into the basin and pour the ordered solution over the mesh to saturate it. | |
| —— | —— | —— | 15. Put on the sterile gloves. Alternately, clean gloves (clean technique) may be used to clean a chronic wound. | |
| —— | —— | —— | 16. Clean the wound. Refer to Skill 8-1. Alternately, irrigate the wound, as ordered or required (see Skill 8-4). | |
| —— | —— | —— | 17. Dry the surrounding skin with sterile gauze dressings. | |
| —— | —— | —— | 18. Apply a skin protectant to the surrounding skin if needed. | |
| —— | —— | —— | 19. If not already on, put on sterile gloves. Squeeze excess fluid from the gauze dressing. Unfold and fluff the dressing. | |
| —— | —— | —— | 20. Gently press to loosely pack the moistened gauze into the wound. If necessary, use the forceps or cotton-tipped applicators to press the gauze into all wound surfaces. | |
| —— | —— | —— | 21. Apply several dry, sterile gauze pads over the wet gauze. | |
| —— | —— | —— | 22. Place the ABD pad over the gauze. | |
| —— | —— | —— | 23. Remove and discard gloves. Apply tape, Montgomery straps or roller gauze to secure the dressings. Alternately, many commercial wound products are self adhesive and do not require additional tape. | |
| —— | —— | —— | 24. After securing the dressing, label dressing with date and time. Remove all remaining equipment; place the patient in a comfortable position, with side rails up and bed in the lowest position. | |
| —— | —— | —— | 25. Remove PPE, if used. Perform hand hygiene. | |
| —— | —— | —— | 26. Check all wound dressings every shift. More frequent checks may be needed if the wound is more complex or dressings become saturated quickly. | |

*Skill Checklists for Taylor's Clinical Nursing Skills:*
*A Nursing Process Approach, 3rd edition*

Name _____  Date _____

Unit _____  Position _____

Instructor/Evaluator: _____  Position _____

## SKILL 8-3
# Applying a Hydrocolloid Dressing

**Goal:** The procedure is accomplished without contaminating the wound area, without causing trauma to the wound, and without causing the patient to experience pain or discomfort.

| Excellent | Satisfactory | Needs Practice | | Comments |
|---|---|---|---|---|
| ___ | ___ | ___ | 1. Review the medical orders for wound care or the nursing plan of care related to wound care. | |
| ___ | ___ | ___ | 2. Gather the necessary supplies and bring to the bedside stand or overbed table. | |
| ___ | ___ | ___ | 3. Perform hand hygiene and put on PPE, if indicated. | |
| ___ | ___ | ___ | 4. Identify the patient. | |
| ___ | ___ | ___ | 5. Close curtains around bed and close door to room if possible. Explain what you are going to do and why you are going to do it to the patient. | |
| ___ | ___ | ___ | 6. Assess the patient for possible need for nonpharmacologic pain-reducing interventions or analgesic medication before wound care dressing change. Administer appropriate prescribed analgesic. Allow enough time for analgesic to achieve its effectiveness before beginning procedure. | |
| ___ | ___ | ___ | 7. Place a waste receptacle or bag at a convenient location for use during the procedure. | |
| ___ | ___ | ___ | 8. Adjust bed to comfortable working height, usually elbow height of the caregiver (VISN 8, 2009). | |
| ___ | ___ | ___ | 9. Assist the patient to a comfortable position that provides easy access to the wound area. Position the patient so the wound cleanser or irrigation solution will flow from the clean end of the wound toward the dirtier end, if being used (See Skill 8-1 for wound cleansing and Skill 8-4 for irrigation techniques). Use the bath blanket to cover any exposed area other than the wound. Place a waterproof pad under the wound site. | |
| ___ | ___ | ___ | 10. Put on clean gloves. Carefully and gently remove the soiled dressings. If there is resistance, use a silicone-based adhesive remover to help remove the tape. If any part of the dressing sticks to the underlying skin, use small amounts of sterile saline to help loosen and remove. | |
| ___ | ___ | ___ | 11. After removing the dressing, note the presence, amount, type, color, and odor of any drainage on the dressings. Place soiled dressings in the appropriate waste receptacle. | |

## SKILL 8-3
## Applying a Hydrocolloid Dressing *(Continued)*

| Excellent | Satisfactory | Needs Practice | | Comments |
|---|---|---|---|---|
| —— | —— | —— | 12. Assess the wound for appearance, stage, the presence of eschar, granulation tissue, epithelialization, undermining, tunneling, necrosis, sinus tract, and drainage. Assess the appearance of the surrounding tissue. Measure the wound. Refer to Fundamentals Review 8-3. | |
| —— | —— | —— | 13. Remove your gloves and put them in the receptacle. | |
| —— | —— | —— | 14. Set up a sterile field, if indicated, and wound cleaning supplies. Put on sterile gloves. Alternately, clean gloves (clean technique) may be used when cleaning a chronic wound. | |
| —— | —— | —— | 15. Clean the wound. Refer to Skill 8-1. Alternately, irrigate the wound, as ordered or required (see Skill 8-4). | |
| —— | —— | —— | 16. Dry the surrounding skin with gauze dressings. | |
| —— | —— | —— | 17. Apply a skin protectant to the surrounding skin. | |
| —— | —— | —— | 18. Cut the dressing to size, if indicated, using sterile scissors. Size the dressing generously, allowing at least a 1″ margin of healthy skin around the wound to be covered with the dressing. | |
| —— | —— | —— | 19. Remove the release paper from the adherent side of the dressing. Apply the dressing to the wound without stretching the dressing. Smooth wrinkles as the dressing is applied. | |
| —— | —— | —— | 20. If necessary, secure the dressing edges with tape. Apply additional skin barrier to the areas to be covered with tape, if necessary. Dressings that are near the anus need to have the edges taped. Apply additional skin barrier to the areas to be covered with tape, if necessary. | |
| —— | —— | —— | 21. After securing the dressing, label dressing with date and time. Remove all remaining equipment; place the patient in a comfortable position, with side rails up and bed in the lowest position. | |
| —— | —— | —— | 22. Remove PPE, if used. Perform hand hygiene. | |
| —— | —— | —— | 23. Check all wound dressings every shift. More frequent checks may be needed if the wound is more complex or dressings become saturated quickly. | |

*Skill Checklists for Taylor's Clinical Nursing Skills:*
*A Nursing Process Approach, 3rd edition*

Name _____ Date _____

Unit _____ Position _____

Instructor/Evaluator: _____ Position _____

| | | | SKILL 8-4 | |
|---|---|---|---|---|

### SKILL 8-4
# Performing Irrigation of a Wound

| Excellent | Satisfactory | Needs Practice | **Goal:** The wound is cleaned without contamination or trauma and without causing the patient to experience pain or discomfort. | **Comments** |
|---|---|---|---|---|
| ___ | ___ | ___ | 1. Review the medical orders for wound care or the nursing plan of care related to wound care. | |
| ___ | ___ | ___ | 2. Gather the necessary supplies and bring to the bedside stand or overbed table. | |
| ___ | ___ | ___ | 3. Perform hand hygiene and put on PPE, if indicated. | |
| ___ | ___ | ___ | 4. Identify the patient. | |
| ___ | ___ | ___ | 5. Close curtains around bed and close door to room if possible. Explain what you are going to do and why you are going to do it to the patient. | |
| ___ | ___ | ___ | 6. Assess the patient for possible need for nonpharmacologic pain-reducing interventions or analgesic medication before wound care and/or dressing change. Administer appropriate prescribed analgesic. Allow enough time for analgesic to achieve its effectiveness before beginning procedure. | |
| ___ | ___ | ___ | 7. Place a waste receptacle or bag at a convenient location for use during the procedure. | |
| ___ | ___ | ___ | 8. Adjust bed to comfortable working height, usually elbow height of the caregiver (VISN 8, 2009). | |
| ___ | ___ | ___ | 9. Assist the patient to a comfortable position that provides easy access to the wound area. Position the patient so the irrigation solution will flow from the clean end of the wound toward the dirtier end. Use the bath blanket to cover any exposed area other than the wound. Place a waterproof pad under the wound site. | |
| ___ | ___ | ___ | 10. Put on a gown, mask, and eye protection. | |
| ___ | ___ | ___ | 11. Put on clean gloves. Carefully and gently remove the soiled dressings. If there is resistance, use a silicone-based adhesive remover to help remove the tape. If any part of the dressing sticks to the underlying skin, use small amounts of sterile saline to help loosen and remove. | |
| ___ | ___ | ___ | 12. After removing the dressing, note the presence, amount, type, color, and odor of any drainage on the dressings. Place soiled dressings in the appropriate waste receptacle. | |

SKILL 8-4

# Performing Irrigation of a Wound *(Continued)*

| Excellent | Satisfactory | Needs Practice | | Comments |
|---|---|---|---|---|
| —— | —— | —— | 13. Assess the wound for appearance, stage, the presence of eschar, granulation tissue, epithelialization, undermining, tunneling, necrosis, sinus tract, and drainage. Assess the appearance of the surrounding tissue. Measure the wound. Refer to Fundamentals Review 8-3. | |
| —— | —— | —— | 14. Remove your gloves and put them in the receptacle. | |
| —— | —— | —— | 15. Set up a sterile field, if indicated, and wound cleaning supplies. Pour warmed sterile irrigating solution into the sterile container. Put on the sterile gloves. Alternately, clean gloves (clean technique) may be used when irrigating a chronic wound. | |
| —— | —— | —— | 16. Position the sterile basin below the wound to collect the irrigation fluid. | |
| —— | —— | —— | 17. Fill the irrigation syringe with solution. *Using your nondominant hand, gently apply pressure to the basin against the skin below the wound to form a seal with the skin.* | |
| —— | —— | —— | 18. *Gently direct a stream of solution into the wound. Keep the tip of the syringe at least 1" above the upper tip of the wound. When using a catheter tip, insert it gently into the wound until it meets resistance. Gently flush all wound areas.* | |
| —— | —— | —— | 19. Watch for the solution to flow smoothly and evenly. When the solution from the wound flows out clear, discontinue irrigation. | |
| —— | —— | —— | 20. Dry the surrounding skin with gauze dressings. | |
| —— | —— | —— | 21. Apply a skin protectant to the surrounding skin. | |
| —— | —— | —— | 22. Apply a new dressing to the wound (see Skills 8-1, 8-2, 8-3). | |
| —— | —— | —— | 23. Remove and discard gloves. Apply tape, Montgomery straps, or roller gauze to secure the dressings. Alternately, many commercial wound products are self adhesive and do not require additional tape. | |
| —— | —— | —— | 24. After securing the dressing, label dressing with date and time. Remove all remaining equipment; place the patient in a comfortable position, with side rails up and bed in the lowest position. | |
| —— | —— | —— | 25. Remove remaining PPE. Perform hand hygiene. | |
| —— | —— | —— | 26. Check all wound dressings every shift. More frequent checks may be needed if the wound is more complex or dressings become saturated quickly. | |

*Skill Checklists for Taylor's Clinical Nursing Skills:*
*A Nursing Process Approach, 3rd edition*

Name _____  Date _____

Unit _____  Position _____

Instructor/Evaluator: _____  Position _____

## SKILL 8-5
## Collecting a Wound Culture

**Goal:** The culture is obtained without evidence of contamination, without exposing the patient to additional pathogens, and without causing discomfort for the patient.

| Excellent | Satisfactory | Needs Practice | | Comments |
|---|---|---|---|---|
| ___ | ___ | ___ | 1. Review the medical orders for obtaining a wound culture. | |
| ___ | ___ | ___ | 2. Gather the necessary supplies and bring to the bedside stand or overbed table. | |
| ___ | ___ | ___ | 3. Perform hand hygiene and put on PPE, if indicated. | |
| ___ | ___ | ___ | 4. Identify the patient. | |
| ___ | ___ | ___ | 5. Close curtains around bed and close door to room if possible. Explain what you are going to do and why you are going to do it to the patient. | |
| ___ | ___ | ___ | 6. Assess the patient for possible need for nonpharmacologic pain-reducing interventions or analgesic medication before obtaining the wound culture. Administer appropriate prescribed analgesic. Allow enough time for analgesic to achieve its effectiveness before beginning procedure. | |
| ___ | ___ | ___ | 7. Place an appropriate waste receptacle within easy reach for use during the procedure. | |
| ___ | ___ | ___ | 8. Adjust bed to comfortable working height, usually elbow height of the caregiver (VISN 8, 2009). | |
| ___ | ___ | ___ | 9. Assist the patient to a comfortable position that provides easy access to the wound. If necessary, drape the patient with the bath blanket to expose only the wound area. Place a waterproof pad under the wound site. Check the culture label against the patient's identification bracelet. | |
| ___ | ___ | ___ | 10. If there is a dressing in place on the wound, put on clean gloves. Carefully and gently remove the soiled dressings. If there is resistance, use a silicone-based adhesive remover to help remove the tape. If any part of the dressing sticks to the underlying skin, use small amounts of sterile saline to help loosen and remove. | |
| ___ | ___ | ___ | 11. After removing the dressing, note the presence, amount, type, color, and odor of any drainage on the dressings. Place soiled dressings in the appropriate waste receptacle. | |

| Excellent | Satisfactory | Needs Practice | | Comments |
|---|---|---|---|---|
| | | | **SKILL 8-5**<br>**Collecting a Wound Culture** *(Continued)* | |
| — — — | | | 12. Assess the wound for appearance, stage, the presence of eschar, granulation tissue, epithelialization, undermining, tunneling, necrosis, sinus tract, and drainage. Assess the appearance of the surrounding tissue. Measure the wound. Refer to Fundamentals Review 8-3. | |
| — — — | | | 13. Remove your gloves and put them in the receptacle. | |
| — — — | | | 14. Set up a sterile field, if indicated, and wound cleaning supplies. Put on the sterile gloves. Alternately, clean gloves (clean technique) may be used when cleaning a chronic wound. | |
| — — — | | | 15. Clean the wound. Refer to Skill 8-1. Alternately, irrigate the wound, as ordered or required (see Skill 8-4). | |
| — — — | | | 16. Dry the surrounding skin with gauze dressings. Put on clean gloves. | |
| — — — | | | 17. Twist the cap to loosen the swab on the Culturette tube, or open the separate swab and remove the cap from the culture tube. *Keep the swab and inside of the culture tube sterile.* | |
| — — — | | | 18. If contact with the wound is necessary to separate wound margins to permit insertion of the swab deep into the wound, put a sterile glove on one hand to manipulate the wound margins. Clean gloves may be appropriate for contact with pressure ulcers and chronic wounds. | |
| — — — | | | 19. *Carefully insert the swab into the wound. Press and rotate the swab several times over the wound surfaces. Avoid touching the swab to intact skin at the wound edges. Use another swab if collecting a specimen from another site.* | |
| — — — | | | 20. Place the swab back in the culture tube. *Do not touch the outside of the tube with the swab.* Secure the cap. Some swab containers have an ampule of medium at the bottom of the tube. It might be necessary to crush this ampule to activate. Follow the manufacturer's instructions for use. | |
| — — — | | | 21. Remove gloves and discard them accordingly. | |
| — — — | | | 22. Put on gloves. Place a dressing on the wound, as appropriate, based on medical orders and/or the nursing plan of care. Refer to Skills 8-1 through 8-3. Remove gloves. | |
| — — — | | | 23. After securing the dressing, label dressing with date and time. Remove all remaining equipment; place the patient in a comfortable position, with side rails up and bed in the lowest position. | |
| — — — | | | 24. Label the specimen according to your institution's guidelines and send it to the laboratory in a biohazard bag. | |
| — — — | | | 25. Remove PPE, if used. Perform hand hygiene. | |

Skill Checklists for Taylor's Clinical Nursing Skills:
A Nursing Process Approach, 3rd edition

Name _____ Date _____

Unit _____ Position _____

Instructor/Evaluator: _____ Position _____

SKILL 8-6

# Applying Montgomery Straps

| Excellent | Satisfactory | Needs Practice | **Goal:** The patient's skin is free from irritation and injury. | Comments |
|---|---|---|---|---|
| —— | —— | —— | 1. Review the medical orders for wound care or the nursing plan of care related to wound care. | |
| —— | —— | —— | 2. Gather the necessary supplies and bring to the bedside stand or overbed table. | |
| —— | —— | —— | 3. Perform hand hygiene and put on PPE, if indicated. | |
| —— | —— | —— | 4. Identify the patient. | |
| —— | —— | —— | 5. Close curtains around bed and close door to room if possible. Explain what you are going to do and why you are going to do it to the patient. | |
| —— | —— | —— | 6. Assess the patient for possible need for nonpharmacologic pain-reducing interventions or analgesic medication before wound care dressing change. Administer appropriate prescribed analgesic. Allow enough time for analgesic to achieve its effectiveness before beginning procedure. | |
| —— | —— | —— | 7. Place a waste receptacle at a convenient location for use during the procedure. | |
| —— | —— | —— | 8. Adjust bed to comfortable working height, usually elbow height of the caregiver (VISN 8, 2009). | |
| —— | —— | —— | 9. Assist the patient to a comfortable position that provides easy access to the wound area. Use a bath blanket to cover any exposed area other than the wound. Place a waterproof pad under the wound site. | |
| —— | —— | —— | 10. Perform wound care and a dressing change as outlined in Skills 8-1 through 8-4, as ordered. | |
| —— | —— | —— | 11. Put on clean gloves. Clean the skin on either side of the wound with the gauze, moistened with normal saline. Dry the skin. | |
| —— | —— | —— | 12. *Apply a skin protectant to the skin where the straps will be placed.* | |
| —— | —— | —— | 13. Remove gloves. | |
| —— | —— | —— | 14. Cut the skin barrier to the size of the tape or strap. Apply the skin barrier to the patient's skin, near the dressing. Apply the sticky side of each tape or strap to the skin barrier sheet, so the openings for the strings are at the edge of the dressing. Repeat for the other side. | |

SKILL 8-6

# Applying Montgomery Straps *(Continued)*

| Excellent | Satisfactory | Needs Practice | | Comments |
|---|---|---|---|---|
| —— | —— | —— | 15. Thread a separate string through each pair of holes in the straps. Tie one end of the string in the hole. Fasten the other end with the opposing tie, like a shoelace. ***Do not secure too tightly.*** Repeat according to the number of straps needed. If commercially prepared straps are used, tie strings like a shoelace. Note date and time of application on strap. | |
| —— | —— | —— | 16. After securing the dressing, label dressing with date and time. Remove all remaining equipment; place the patient in a comfortable position, with side rails up and bed in the lowest position. | |
| —— | —— | —— | 17. Remove additional PPE, if used. Perform hand hygiene. | |
| —— | —— | —— | 18. Check all wound dressings every shift. More frequent checks may be needed if the wound is more complex or dressings become saturated quickly. | |
| —— | —— | —— | 19. Replace the ties and straps whenever they are soiled, or every 2 to 3 days. Straps can be reapplied onto skin barrier. Skin barrier can remain in place up to 7 days. Use a silicone-based adhesive remover to help remove the skin barrier. | |

*Skill Checklists for Taylor's Clinical Nursing Skills:*
*A Nursing Process Approach, 3rd edition*

Name _____ Date _____

Unit _____ Position _____

Instructor/Evaluator: _____ Position _____

| | | | SKILL 8-7 **Caring for a Penrose Drain** | |
|---|---|---|---|---|

SKILL 8-7

# Caring for a Penrose Drain

**Goal:** The Penrose drain remains patent and intact; the care is accomplished without contaminating the wound area, or causing trauma to the wound; and without causing the patient to experience pain or discomfort.

| Excellent | Satisfactory | Needs Practice | | Comments |
|---|---|---|---|---|
| ___ | ___ | ___ | 1. Review the medical orders for wound care or the nursing plan of care related to wound/drain care. | |
| ___ | ___ | ___ | 2. Gather the necessary supplies and bring to the bedside stand or overbed table. | |
| ___ | ___ | ___ | 3. Perform hand hygiene and put on PPE, if indicated. | |
| ___ | ___ | ___ | 4. Identify the patient. | |
| ___ | ___ | ___ | 5. Close curtains around bed and close door to room if possible. Explain what you are going to do and why you are going to do it to the patient. | |
| ___ | ___ | ___ | 6. Assess the patient for possible need for nonpharmacologic pain-reducing interventions or analgesic medication before wound care dressing change. Administer appropriate prescribed analgesic. Allow enough time for analgesic to achieve its effectiveness before beginning procedure. | |
| ___ | ___ | ___ | 7. Place a waste receptacle at a convenient location for use during the procedure. | |
| ___ | ___ | ___ | 8. Adjust bed to comfortable working height, usually elbow height of the caregiver (VISN 8, 2009). | |
| ___ | ___ | ___ | 9. Assist the patient to a comfortable position that provides easy access to the drain and/or wound area. Use a bath blanket to cover any exposed area other than the wound. Place a waterproof pad under the wound site. | |
| ___ | ___ | ___ | 10. Put on clean gloves. Check the position of the drain or drains before removing the dressing. Carefully and gently remove the soiled dressings. If there is resistance, use a silicone-based adhesive remover to help remove the tape. If any part of the dressing sticks to the underlying skin, use small amounts of sterile saline to help loosen and remove. | |
| ___ | ___ | ___ | 11. After removing the dressing, note the presence, amount, type, color, and odor of any drainage on the dressings. Place soiled dressings in the appropriate waste receptacle. | |
| ___ | ___ | ___ | 12. Inspect the drain site for appearance and drainage. Assess if any pain is present. | |

## SKILL 8-7
# Caring for a Penrose Drain *(Continued)*

| Excellent | Satisfactory | Needs Practice | | Comments |
|---|---|---|---|---|
| —— | —— | —— | 13. Using sterile technique, prepare a sterile work area and open the needed supplies. | |
| —— | —— | —— | 14. Open the sterile cleaning solution. Pour the cleansing solution into the basin. Add the gauze sponges. | |
| —— | —— | —— | 15. Put on sterile gloves. | |
| —— | —— | —— | 16. Cleanse the drain site with the cleaning solution. Use the forceps and the moistened gauze or cotton-tipped applicators. *Start at the drain insertion site, moving in a circular motion toward the periphery. Use each gauze sponge or applicator only once. Discard and use new gauze if additional cleansing is needed.* | |
| —— | —— | —— | 17. Dry the skin with a new gauze pad in the same manner. Apply skin protectant to the skin around the drain; extend out to include the area of skin that will be taped. Place a presplit drain sponge under the drain. Closely observe the safety pin in the drain. If the pin or drain is crusted, replace the pin with a new sterile pin. *Take care not to dislodge the drain.* | |
| —— | —— | —— | 18. Apply gauze pads over the drain. Apply ABD pads over the gauze. | |
| —— | —— | —— | 19. Remove and discard gloves. Apply tape, Montgomery straps, or roller gauze to secure the dressings. | |
| —— | —— | —— | 20. After securing the dressing, label dressing with date and time. Remove all remaining equipment; place the patient in a comfortable position, with side rails up and bed in the lowest position. | |
| —— | —— | —— | 21. Remove additional PPE, if used. Perform hand hygiene. | |
| —— | —— | —— | 22. Check all wound dressings every shift. More frequent checks may be needed if the wound is more complex or dressings become saturated quickly. | |

*Skill Checklists for Taylor's Clinical Nursing Skills:*
*A Nursing Process Approach, 3rd edition*

Name _____  Date _____

Unit _____  Position _____

Instructor/Evaluator: _____  Position _____

SKILL 8-8

# Caring for a T-Tube Drain

**Goal:** The drain remains patent and intact; drain care is accomplished without contaminating the wound area and/or without causing trauma to the wound; and the patient does not experience pain or discomfort.

| Excellent | Satisfactory | Needs Practice | | Comments |
|---|---|---|---|---|
| —— | —— | —— | 1. Review the medical orders for wound care or the nursing plan of care related to wound/drain care. | |
| —— | —— | —— | 2. Gather the necessary supplies and bring to the bedside stand or overbed table. | |
| —— | —— | —— | 3. Perform hand hygiene and put on PPE, if indicated. | |
| —— | —— | —— | 4. Identify the patient. | |
| —— | —— | —— | 5. Close curtains around bed and close door to room if possible. Explain what you are going to do and why you are going to do it to the patient. | |
| —— | —— | —— | 6. Assess the patient for possible need for nonpharmacologic pain-reducing interventions or analgesic medication before wound care dressing change. Administer appropriate prescribed analgesic. Allow enough time for analgesic to achieve its effectiveness before beginning procedure. | |
| —— | —— | —— | 7. Place a waste receptacle at a convenient location for use during the procedure. | |
| —— | —— | —— | 8. Adjust bed to comfortable working height, usually elbow height of the caregiver (VISN 8, 2009). | |
| —— | —— | —— | 9. Assist the patient to a comfortable position that provides easy access to the drain and/or wound area. Use a bath blanket to cover any exposed area other than the wound. Place a waterproof pad under the wound site. | |

**Emptying Drainage**

| Excellent | Satisfactory | Needs Practice | | Comments |
|---|---|---|---|---|
| —— | —— | —— | 10. Put on clean gloves; put on mask or face shield if indicated. | |
| —— | —— | —— | 11. Using sterile technique, open a gauze pad, making a sterile field with the outer wrapper. | |
| —— | —— | —— | 12. Place the graduated collection container under the outlet valve of the drainage bag. *Without touching the outlet, pull the cap off and empty the bag's contents completely into the container. Use the gauze to wipe the outlet, and replace the cap.* | |

| Excellent | Satisfactory | Needs Practice | | Comments |
|---|---|---|---|---|
| | | | **SKILL 8-8**<br>**Caring for a T-Tube Drain** *(Continued)* | |

| Excellent | Satisfactory | Needs Practice | | Comments |
|---|---|---|---|---|
| —— | —— | —— | 13. Carefully measure and note the characteristics of the drainage. Discard the drainage according to facility policy. | |
| —— | —— | —— | 14. Remove gloves and perform hand hygiene. | |
| | | | **Cleaning the Drain Site** | |
| —— | —— | —— | 15. Put on clean gloves. Check the position of the drain or drains before removing the dressing. Carefully and gently remove the soiled dressings. If there is resistance, use a silicone-based adhesive remover to help remove the tape. If any part of the dressing sticks to the underlying skin, use small amounts of sterile saline to help loosen and remove. Do not reach over the drain site. | |
| —— | —— | —— | 16. After removing the dressing, note the presence, amount, type, color, and odor of any drainage on the dressings. Place soiled dressings in the appropriate waste receptacle. Remove gloves and dispose of in appropriate waste receptacle. | |
| —— | —— | —— | 17. Inspect the drain site for appearance and drainage. Assess if any pain is present. | |
| —— | —— | —— | 18. Using sterile technique, prepare a sterile work area and open the needed supplies. | |
| —— | —— | —— | 19. Open the sterile cleaning solution. Pour the cleansing solution into the basin. Add the gauze sponges. | |
| —— | —— | —— | 20. Put on sterile gloves. | |
| —— | —— | —— | 21. Cleanse the drain site with the cleaning solution. Use the forceps and the moistened gauze or cotton-tipped applicators. *Start at the drain insertion site, moving in a circular motion toward the periphery. Use each gauze sponge only once. Discard and use new gauze if additional cleansing is needed.* | |
| —— | —— | —— | 22. Dry with new sterile gauze in the same manner. Apply skin protectant to the skin around the drain; extend out to include the area of skin that will be taped. | |
| —— | —— | —— | 23. Place a presplit drain sponge under the drain. Apply gauze pads over the drain. Remove and discard gloves. | |
| —— | —— | —— | 24. Secure the dressings with tape as needed. Alternatively, before removing gloves, place a transparent dressing over the tube and insertion site. *Be careful not to kink the tubing.* | |

SKILL 8-8

# Caring for a T-Tube Drain *(Continued)*

| Excellent | Satisfactory | Needs Practice | | Comments |
|---|---|---|---|---|
| —— | —— | —— | 25. After securing the dressing, label dressing with date and time. Remove all remaining equipment; place the patient in a comfortable position, with side rails up and bed in the lowest position. | |
| —— | —— | —— | 26. Remove additional PPE, if used. Perform hand hygiene. | |
| —— | —— | —— | 27. Check drain status at least every four hours. Check all wound dressings every shift. More frequent checks may be needed if the wound is more complex or dressings become saturated quickly. | |

*Skill Checklists for Taylor's Clinical Nursing Skills:*
*A Nursing Process Approach, 3rd edition*

Name _____  Date _____

Unit _____  Position _____

Instructor/Evaluator: _____  Position _____

| Excellent | Satisfactory | Needs Practice | SKILL 8-9 **Caring for a Jackson-Pratt Drain** | |
|---|---|---|---|---|
| | | | **Goal:** The drain is patent and intact. | **Comments** |
| —— | —— | —— | 1. Review the medical orders for wound care or the nursing plan of care related to wound/drain care. | |
| —— | —— | —— | 2. Gather the necessary supplies and bring to the bedside stand or overbed table. | |
| —— | —— | —— | 3. Perform hand hygiene and put on PPE, if indicated. | |
| —— | —— | —— | 4. Identify the patient. | |
| —— | —— | —— | 5. Close curtains around bed and close door to room if possible. Explain what you are going to do and why you are going to do it to the patient. | |
| —— | —— | —— | 6. Assess the patient for possible need for nonpharmacologic pain-reducing interventions or analgesic medication before wound care dressing change. Administer appropriate prescribed analgesic. Allow enough time for analgesic to achieve its effectiveness before beginning procedure. | |
| —— | —— | —— | 7. Place a waste receptacle at a convenient location for use during the procedure. | |
| —— | —— | —— | 8. Adjust bed to comfortable working height, usually elbow height of the caregiver (VISN 8, 2009). | |
| —— | —— | —— | 9. Assist the patient to a comfortable position that provides easy access to the drain and/or wound area. Use a bath blanket to cover any exposed area other than the wound. Place a waterproof pad under the wound site. | |
| —— | —— | —— | 10. Put on clean gloves; put on mask or face shield if indicated. | |
| —— | —— | —— | 11. Place the graduated collection container under the outlet of the drain. Without contaminating the outlet valve, pull the cap off. The chamber will expand completely as it draws in air. *Empty the chamber's contents completely into the container. Use the gauze pad to clean the outlet. Fully compress the chamber with one hand and replace the cap with your other hand.* | |
| —— | —— | —— | 12. Check the patency of the equipment. Make sure the tubing is free from twists and kinks. | |

SKILL 8-9

# Caring for a Jackson-Pratt Drain *(Continued)*

| Excellent | Satisfactory | Needs Practice | | Comments |
|---|---|---|---|---|
| —— | —— | —— | 13. Secure the Jackson-Pratt drain to the patient's gown below the wound with a safety pin, making sure that there is no tension on the tubing. | |
| —— | —— | —— | 14. Carefully measure and record the character, color, and amount of the drainage. Discard the drainage according to facility policy. Remove gloves. | |
| —— | —— | —— | 15. Put on clean gloves. If the drain site has a dressing, re-dress the site as outlined in Skill 8-8. Include cleaning of the sutures with the gauze pad moistened with normal saline. Dry sutures with gauze before applying new dressing. | |
| —— | —— | —— | 16. If the drain site is open to air, observe the sutures that secure the drain to the skin. Look for signs of pulling, tearing, swelling, or infection of the surrounding skin. Gently clean the sutures with the gauze pad moistened with normal saline. Dry with a new gauze pad. Apply skin protectant to the surrounding skin if needed. | |
| —— | —— | —— | 17. Remove and discard gloves. Remove all remaining equipment; place the patient in a comfortable position, with side rails up and bed in the lowest position. | |
| —— | —— | —— | 18. Remove additional PPE, if used. Perform hand hygiene. | |
| —— | —— | —— | 19. Check drain status at least every four hours. Check all wound dressings every shift. More frequent checks may be needed if the wound is more complex or dressings become saturated quickly. | |

*Skill Checklists for Taylor's Clinical Nursing Skills:*
*A Nursing Process Approach, 3rd edition*

Name _____   Date _____

Unit _____   Position _____

Instructor/Evaluator: _____   Position _____

| Excellent | Satisfactory | Needs Practice | SKILL 8-10<br>**Caring for a Hemovac Drain** | |
|---|---|---|---|---|
| | | | **Goal:** The drain is patent and intact. | **Comments** |
| —— | —— | —— | 1. Review the medical orders for wound care or the nursing plan of care related to wound/drain care. | |
| —— | —— | —— | 2. Gather the necessary supplies and bring to the bedside stand or overbed table. | |
| —— | —— | —— | 3. Perform hand hygiene and put on PPE, if indicated. | |
| —— | —— | —— | 4. Identify the patient. | |
| —— | —— | —— | 5. Close curtains around bed and close door to room if possible. Explain what you are going to do and why you are going to do it to the patient. | |
| —— | —— | —— | 6. Assess the patient for possible need for nonpharmacologic pain-reducing interventions or analgesic medication before wound care dressing change. Administer appropriate prescribed analgesic. Allow enough time for analgesic to achieve its effectiveness before beginning procedure. | |
| —— | —— | —— | 7. Place a waste receptacle at a convenient location for use during the procedure. | |
| —— | —— | —— | 8. Adjust bed to comfortable working height, usually elbow height of the caregiver (VISN 8, 2009). | |
| —— | —— | —— | 9. Assist the patient to a comfortable position that provides easy access to the drain and/or wound area. Use a bath blanket to cover any exposed area other than the wound. Place a waterproof pad under the wound site. | |
| —— | —— | —— | 10. Put on clean gloves; put on mask or face shield if indicated. | |
| —— | —— | —— | 11. Place the graduated collection container under the outlet of the drain. Without contaminating the outlet, pull the cap off. The chamber will expand completely as it draws in air. *Empty the chamber's contents completely into the container. Use the gauze pad to clean the outlet. Fully compress the chamber by pushing the top and bottom together with your hands. Keep the device tightly compressed while you apply the cap.* | |
| —— | —— | —— | 12. Check the patency of the equipment. Make sure the tubing is free from twists and kinks. | |

# Caring for a Hemovac Drain *(Continued)*

| Excellent | Satisfactory | Needs Practice | | Comments |
|---|---|---|---|---|
| —— | —— | —— | 13. Secure the Hemovac drain to the patient's gown below the wound with a safety pin, making sure that there is no tension on the tubing. | |
| —— | —— | —— | 14. Carefully measure and record the character, color, and amount of the drainage. Discard the drainage according to facility policy. | |
| —— | —— | —— | 15. Put on clean gloves. If the drain site has a dressing, re-dress the site as outlined in Skill 8-8. Include cleaning of the sutures with the gauze pad moistened with normal saline. Dry sutures with gauze before applying new dressing. | |
| —— | —— | —— | 16. If the drain site is open to air, observe the sutures that secure the drain to the skin. Look for signs of pulling, tearing, swelling, or infection of the surrounding skin. Gently clean the sutures with the gauze pad moistened with normal saline. Dry with a new gauze pad. Apply skin protectant to the surrounding skin if needed. | |
| —— | —— | —— | 17. Remove and discard gloves. Remove all remaining equipment; place the patient in a comfortable position, with side rails up and bed in the lowest position. | |
| —— | —— | —— | 18. Remove additional PPE, if used. Perform hand hygiene. | |
| —— | —— | —— | 19. Check drain status at least every four hours. Check all wound dressings every shift. More frequent checks may be needed if the wound is more complex or dressings become saturated quickly. | |

*Skill Checklists for Taylor's Clinical Nursing Skills:*
*A Nursing Process Approach, 3rd edition*

Name _____ Date _____

Unit _____ Position _____

Instructor/Evaluator: _____ Position _____

### SKILL 8-11

# Applying Negative Pressure Wound Therapy

**Goal:** The therapy is accomplished without contaminating the wound area, without causing trauma to the wound, and without causing the patient to experience pain or discomfort.

| Excellent | Satisfactory | Needs Practice | | Comments |
|---|---|---|---|---|
| ⎯⎯ | ⎯⎯ | ⎯⎯ | 1. Review the medical order for the application of NPWT therapy, including the ordered pressure setting for the device. | |
| ⎯⎯ | ⎯⎯ | ⎯⎯ | 2. Gather the necessary supplies and bring to the bedside stand or overbed table. | |
| ⎯⎯ | ⎯⎯ | ⎯⎯ | 3. Perform hand hygiene and put on PPE, if indicated. | |
| ⎯⎯ | ⎯⎯ | ⎯⎯ | 4. Identify the patient. | |
| ⎯⎯ | ⎯⎯ | ⎯⎯ | 5. Close curtains around bed and close door to room if possible. Explain what you are going to do and why you are going to do it to the patient. | |
| ⎯⎯ | ⎯⎯ | ⎯⎯ | 6. Assess the patient for possible need for nonpharmacologic pain-reducing interventions or analgesic medication before wound care dressing change. Administer appropriate prescribed analgesic. Allow enough time for analgesic to achieve its effectiveness before beginning procedure. | |
| ⎯⎯ | ⎯⎯ | ⎯⎯ | 7. Adjust bed to comfortable working height, usually elbow height of the caregiver (VISN 8, 2009). | |
| ⎯⎯ | ⎯⎯ | ⎯⎯ | 8. Assist the patient to a comfortable position that provides easy access to the wound area. Position the patient so the irrigation solution will flow from the clean end of the wound toward the dirty end. Expose the area and drape the patient with a bath blanket if needed. Put a waterproof pad under the wound area. | |
| ⎯⎯ | ⎯⎯ | ⎯⎯ | 9. Have the disposal bag or waste receptacle within easy reach for use during the procedure. | |
| ⎯⎯ | ⎯⎯ | ⎯⎯ | 10. Using sterile technique, prepare a sterile field and add all the sterile supplies needed for the procedure to the field. Pour warmed, sterile irrigating solution into the sterile container. | |
| ⎯⎯ | ⎯⎯ | ⎯⎯ | 11. Put on a gown, mask, and eye protection. | |
| ⎯⎯ | ⎯⎯ | ⎯⎯ | 12. Put on clean gloves. Carefully and gently remove the dressing. If there is resistance, use a silicone-based adhesive remover to help remove the drape. *Note the number of pieces of foam removed from the wound. Compare with the documented number from the previous dressing change.* | |

# Applying Negative Pressure Wound Therapy *(Continued)*

| Excellent | Satisfactory | Needs Practice | | Comments |
|---|---|---|---|---|
| —— | —— | —— | 13. Discard the dressings in the receptacle. Remove your gloves and put them in the receptacle. | |
| —— | —— | —— | 14. Put on sterile gloves. Using sterile technique, irrigate the wound (see Skill 8-4). | |
| —— | —— | —— | 15. Clean the area around the skin with normal saline. Dry the surrounding skin with a sterile gauze sponge. | |
| —— | —— | —— | 16. Assess the wound for appearance, stage, the presence of eschar, granulation tissue, epithelialization, undermining, tunneling, necrosis, sinus tract, and drainage. Assess the appearance of the surrounding tissue. Measure the wound. Refer to Fundamentals Review 8-3. | |
| —— | —— | —— | 17. *Wipe intact skin around the wound with a skin-protectant wipe and allow it to dry well.* | |
| —— | —— | —— | 18. Remove gloves if they become contaminated and discard them into the receptacle. | |
| —— | —— | —— | 19. Put on a new pair of sterile gloves, if necessary. *Using sterile scissors, cut the foam to the shape and measurement of the wound. Do not cut foam over the wound.* More than one piece of foam may be necessary if the first piece is cut too small. Carefully place the foam in the wound. *Ensure foam-to-foam contact if more than one piece is required. Note the number of pieces of foam placed in the wound.* | |
| —— | —— | —— | 20. Trim and place the V.A.C. Drape to cover the foam dressing and an additional 3 to 5 cm border of intact periwound tissue. V.A.C. Drape may be cut into multiple pieces for easier handling. | |
| —— | —— | —— | 21. Choose an appropriate site to apply the T.R.A.C. Pad. | |
| —— | —— | —— | 22. Pinch the Drape and cut a 2-cm hole through the Drape. Apply the T.R.A.C. Pad. Remove V.A.C. Canister from package and insert into the V.A.C. Therapy Unit until it locks into place. Connect T.R.A.C. Pad tubing to canister tubing and check that the clamps on each tube are open. Turn on the power to the V.A.C. Therapy Unit and select the prescribed therapy setting. | |
| —— | —— | —— | 23. Assess the dressing to ensure seal integrity. The dressing should be collapsed, shrinking to the foam and skin. | |
| —— | —— | —— | 24. Remove and discard gloves. Apply tape, Montgomery straps or roller gauze to secure the dressings. Alternately, many commercial wound products are self adhesive and do not require additional tape. | |

## SKILL 8-11
# Applying Negative Pressure Wound Therapy (Continued)

| Excellent | Satisfactory | Needs Practice | | Comments |
|---|---|---|---|---|
| —— | —— | —— | 25. Label dressing with date and time. Remove all remaining equipment; place the patient in a comfortable position, with side rails up and bed in the lowest position. | |
| —— | —— | —— | 26. Remove PPE, if used. Perform hand hygiene. | |
| —— | —— | —— | 27. Check all wound dressings every shift. More frequent checks may be needed if the wound is more complex or dressings become saturated quickly. | |

*Skill Checklists for Taylor's Clinical Nursing Skills:*
*A Nursing Process Approach, 3rd edition*

Name _____   Date _____

Unit _____   Position _____

Instructor/Evaluator: _____   Position _____

| Excellent | Satisfactory | Needs Practice | SKILL 8-12<br>**Removing Sutures** | Comments |
|---|---|---|---|---|
| | | | **Goal:** The sutures are removed without contaminating the incisional area, without causing trauma to the wound, and without causing the patient to experience pain or discomfort. | |
| ___ | ___ | ___ | 1. Review the medical orders for suture removal. | |
| ___ | ___ | ___ | 2. Gather the necessary supplies and bring to the bedside stand or overbed table. | |
| ___ | ___ | ___ | 3. Perform hand hygiene and put on PPE, if indicated. | |
| ___ | ___ | ___ | 4. Identify the patient. | |
| ___ | ___ | ___ | 5. Close curtains around bed and close door to room if possible. Explain what you are going to do and why you are going to do it to the patient. Describe the sensation of suture removal as a pulling or slightly uncomfortable experience. | |
| ___ | ___ | ___ | 6. Assess the patient for possible need for nonpharmacologic pain-reducing interventions or analgesic medication before beginning the procedure. Administer appropriate prescribed analgesic. Allow enough time for analgesic to achieve its effectiveness before beginning procedure. | |
| ___ | ___ | ___ | 7. Place a waste receptacle at a convenient location for use during the procedure. | |
| ___ | ___ | ___ | 8. Adjust bed to comfortable working height, usually elbow height of the caregiver (VISN 8, 2009). | |
| ___ | ___ | ___ | 9. Assist the patient to a comfortable position that provides easy access to the incision area. Use a bath blanket to cover any exposed area other than the incision. Place a waterproof pad under the incision site. | |
| ___ | ___ | ___ | 10. Put on clean gloves. Carefully and gently remove the soiled dressings. If there is resistance, use a silicone-based adhesive remover to help remove the tape. If any part of the dressing sticks to the underlying skin, use small amounts of sterile saline to help loosen and remove. Inspect the incision area. | |
| ___ | ___ | ___ | 11. Clean the incision using the wound cleanser and gauze, according to facility policies and procedures. | |
| ___ | ___ | ___ | 12. Using the forceps, grasp the knot of the first suture and gently lift the knot up off the skin. | |

| Excellent | Satisfactory | Needs Practice | SKILL 8-12<br>**Removing Sutures** *(Continued)* | Comments |
|---|---|---|---|---|
| —— | —— | —— | 13. Using the scissors, cut one side of the suture below the knot, close to the skin. Grasp the knot with the forceps and pull the cut suture through the skin. ***Avoid pulling the visible portion of the suture through the underlying tissue.*** | |
| —— | —— | —— | 14. Remove every other suture to be sure the wound edges are healed. If they are, remove the remaining sutures as ordered. Dispose of sutures according to facility policy. | |
| —— | —— | —— | 15. If wound closure strips are to be applied, apply skin protectant to skin around incision. ***Do not apply to incision.*** Apply adhesive closure strips. Take care to handle the strips by the paper backing. | |
| —— | —— | —— | 16. Reapply the dressing, depending on the medical orders and facility policy. | |
| —— | —— | —— | 17. Remove gloves and discard. Remove all remaining equipment; place the patient in a comfortable position, with side rails up and bed in the lowest position. | |
| —— | —— | —— | 18. Remove additional PPE, if used. Perform hand hygiene. | |
| —— | —— | —— | 19. Assess all wounds every shift. More frequent checks may be needed if the wound is more complex. | |

*Skill Checklists for Taylor's Clinical Nursing Skills:*
*A Nursing Process Approach, 3rd edition*

Name _____  Date _____

Unit _____  Position _____

Instructor/Evaluator: _____  Position _____

| Excellent | Satisfactory | Needs Practice | SKILL 8-13 **Removing Surgical Staples** | Comments |
|---|---|---|---|---|
| | | | **Goal:** The staples are removed without contaminating the incisional area, without causing trauma to the wound, and without causing the patient to experience pain or discomfort. | |
| ___ | ___ | ___ | 1. Review the medical orders for staple removal. | |
| ___ | ___ | ___ | 2. Gather the necessary supplies and bring to the bedside stand or overbed table. | |
| ___ | ___ | ___ | 3. Perform hand hygiene and put on PPE, if indicated. | |
| ___ | ___ | ___ | 4. Identify the patient. | |
| ___ | ___ | ___ | 5. Close curtains around bed and close door to room if possible. Explain what you are going to do and why you are going to do it to the patient. Describe the sensation of staple removal as a pulling experience. | |
| ___ | ___ | ___ | 6. Assess the patient for possible need for nonpharmacologic pain-reducing interventions or analgesic medication before beginning the procedure. Administer appropriate prescribed analgesic. Allow enough time for analgesic to achieve its effectiveness before beginning procedure. | |
| ___ | ___ | ___ | 7. Place a waste receptacle at a convenient location for use during the procedure. | |
| ___ | ___ | ___ | 8. Adjust bed to comfortable working height, usually elbow height of the caregiver (VISN 8). | |
| ___ | ___ | ___ | 9. Assist the patient to a comfortable position that provides easy access to the incision area. Use a bath blanket to cover any exposed area other than the incision. Place a waterproof pad under the incision site. | |
| ___ | ___ | ___ | 10. Put on clean gloves. Carefully and gently remove the soiled dressings. If there is resistance, use a silicone-based adhesive remover to help remove the tape. If any part of the dressing sticks to the underlying skin, use small amounts of sterile saline to help loosen and remove. Inspect the incision area. | |
| ___ | ___ | ___ | 11. Clean the incision using the wound cleanser and gauze, according to facility policies and procedures. | |
| ___ | ___ | ___ | 12. Grasp the staple remover. *Position the staple remover under the staple to be removed. Firmly close the staple remover. The staple will bend in the middle and the edges will pull up out of the skin.* | |

| Excellent | Satisfactory | Needs Practice | | Comments |
|-----------|--------------|----------------|---|----------|

## SKILL 8-13
# Removing Surgical Staples *(Continued)*

| Excellent | Satisfactory | Needs Practice | | Comments |
|-----------|--------------|----------------|---|----------|
| —— | —— | —— | 13. Remove every other staple to be sure the wound edges are healed. If they are, remove the remaining staples as ordered. Dispose of staples in the sharps container. | |
| —— | —— | —— | 14. If wound closure strips are to be applied, apply skin protectant to skin around incision. ***Do not apply to incision.*** Apply adhesive closure strips. Take care to handle the strips by the paper backing. | |
| —— | —— | —— | 15. Reapply the dressing, depending on the medical orders and facility policy. | |
| —— | —— | —— | 16. Remove gloves and discard. Remove all remaining equipment; place the patient in a comfortable position, with side rails up and bed in the lowest position. | |
| —— | —— | —— | 17. Remove additional PPE, if used. Perform hand hygiene. | |
| —— | —— | —— | 18. Assess all wounds every shift. More frequent checks may be needed if the wound is more complex. | |

*Skill Checklists for Taylor's Clinical Nursing Skills:*
*A Nursing Process Approach, 3rd edition*

Name _____ Date _____

Unit _____ Position _____

Instructor/Evaluator: _____ Position _____

## SKILL 8-14

# Applying an External Heating Pad

**Excellent** **Satisfactory** **Needs Practice**

**Goal:** Desired outcome depends on the patient's nursing diagnosis.

**Comments**

| Excellent | Satisfactory | Needs Practice | | |
|---|---|---|---|---|
| —— | —— | —— | 1. Review the medical order for the application of heat therapy, including frequency, type of therapy, body area to be treated, and length of time for the application. | |
| —— | —— | —— | 2. Gather the necessary supplies and bring to the bedside stand or overbed table. | |
| —— | —— | —— | 3. Perform hand hygiene and put on PPE, if indicated. | |
| —— | —— | —— | 4. Identify the patient. | |
| —— | —— | —— | 5. Close curtains around bed and close door to room if possible. Explain what you are going to do and why you are going to do it to the patient. | |
| —— | —— | —— | 6. Adjust bed to comfortable working height, usually elbow height of the caregiver (VISN 8, 2009). | |
| —— | —— | —— | 7. Assist the patient to a comfortable position that provides easy access to the area where the heat will be applied; use a bath blanket to cover any other exposed area. | |
| —— | —— | —— | 8. Assess the condition of the skin where the heat is to be applied. | |
| —— | —— | —— | 9. Check that the water in the electronic unit is at the appropriate level. Fill the unit two-thirds full or to the fill mark, with distilled water, if necessary. Check the temperature setting on the unit to ensure it is within the safe range. | |
| —— | —— | —— | 10. Attach pad tubing to electronic unit tubing. | |
| —— | —— | —— | 11. Plug in the unit and warm the pad before use. Apply the heating pad to the prescribed area. Secure with gauze bandage or tape. | |
| —— | —— | —— | 12. *Assess the condition of the skin and the patient's response to the heat at frequent intervals, according to facility policy. Do not exceed the prescribed length of time for the application of heat.* | |

| Excellent | Satisfactory | Needs Practice | SKILL 8-14<br><br>**Applying an External Heating Pad** *(Continued)* | |
|:---:|:---:|:---:|---|---|
| | | | | **Comments** |
| —— | —— | —— | 13. Remove gloves and discard. Remove all remaining equipment; place the patient in a comfortable position, with side rails up and bed in the lowest position. | |
| —— | —— | —— | 14. Remove additional PPE, if used. Perform hand hygiene. | |
| —— | —— | —— | 15. Remove after the prescribed amount of time. Reassess the patient and area of application, noting the effect and presence of adverse effects. | |

*Skill Checklists for Taylor's Clinical Nursing Skills:*
*A Nursing Process Approach, 3rd edition*

Name _____   Date _____

Unit _____   Position _____

Instructor/Evaluator: _____   Position _____

SKILL 8-15

# Applying a Warm Compress

**Goal:** The patient displays signs of improvement, such as decreased inflammation, decreased muscle spasms, or decreased pain that indicate problems have been relieved.

| Excellent | Satisfactory | Needs Practice | | Comments |
|---|---|---|---|---|
| ___ | ___ | ___ | 1. Review the medical order for the application of a moist warm compress, including frequency, and length of time for the application. | |
| ___ | ___ | ___ | 2. Gather the necessary supplies and bring to the bedside stand or overbed table. | |
| ___ | ___ | ___ | 3. Perform hand hygiene and put on PPE, if indicated. | |
| ___ | ___ | ___ | 4. Identify the patient. | |
| ___ | ___ | ___ | 5. Assess the patient for possible need for nonpharmacologic pain-reducing interventions or analgesic medication before beginning the procedure. Administer appropriate analgesic, consulting physician's orders, and allow enough time for analgesic to achieve its effectiveness before beginning procedure. | |
| ___ | ___ | ___ | 6. Close curtains around bed and close door to room if possible. Explain what you are going to do and why you are going to do it to the patient. | |
| ___ | ___ | ___ | 7. If using an electronic heating device, check that the water in the unit is at the appropriate level. Fill the unit two-thirds full with distilled water, or to the fill mark, if necessary. Check the temperature setting on the unit to ensure it is within the safe range (Refer to Skill 8-14). | |
| ___ | ___ | ___ | 8. Assist the patient to a comfortable position that provides easy access to the area. Use a bath blanket to cover any exposed area other than the intended site. Place a waterproof pad under the site. | |
| ___ | ___ | ___ | 9. Place a waste receptacle at a convenient location for use during the procedure. | |
| ___ | ___ | ___ | 10. Pour the warmed solution into the container and drop the gauze for the compress into the solution. Alternately, if commercially packaged pre-warmed gauze is used, open packaging. | |
| ___ | ___ | ___ | 11. Put on clean gloves. Assess the application site for inflammation, skin color, and ecchymosis. | |

## SKILL 8-15
# Applying a Warm Compress *(Continued)*

| Excellent | Satisfactory | Needs Practice | | Comments |
|---|---|---|---|---|
| —— | —— | —— | 12. *Retrieve the compress from the warmed solution, squeezing out any excess moisture. Alternately, remove pre-warmed gauze from open package. Apply the compress by gently and carefully molding it to the intended area. Ask patient if the application feels too hot.* | |
| —— | —— | —— | 13. Cover the site with a single layer of gauze and with a clean dry bath towel; secure in place if necessary. | |
| —— | —— | —— | 14. Place the Aquathermia or heating device, if used, over the towel. | |
| —— | —— | —— | 15. Remove gloves and discard them appropriately. Perform hand hygiene and remove additional PPE, if used. | |
| —— | —— | —— | 16. *Monitor the time the compress is in place to prevent burns and skin/tissue damage. Monitor the condition of the patient's skin and the patient's response at frequent intervals.* | |
| —— | —— | —— | 17. After the prescribed time for the treatment (up to 30 minutes), remove the external heating device (if used) and put on gloves. | |
| —— | —— | —— | 18. Carefully remove the compress while assessing the skin condition around the site and observing the patient's response to the heat application. Note any changes in the application area. | |
| —— | —— | —— | 19. Remove gloves. Place the patient in a comfortable position. Lower the bed. Dispose of any other supplies appropriately. | |
| —— | —— | —— | 20. Remove additional PPE, if used. Perform hand hygiene. | |

*Skill Checklists for Taylor's Clinical Nursing Skills:*
*A Nursing Process Approach, 3rd edition*

Name _____ Date _____

Unit _____ Position _____

Instructor/Evaluator: _____ Position _____

| Excellent | Satisfactory | Needs Practice | SKILL 8-16 **Assisting With a Sitz Bath** | Comments |
|---|---|---|---|---|
| | | | **Goal:** The patient states an increase in comfort. | |
| —— | —— | —— | 1. Review the medical order for the application of a Sitz bath, including frequency, and length of time for the application. | |
| —— | —— | —— | 2. Gather the necessary supplies and bring to the bedside stand or overbed table. | |
| —— | —— | —— | 3. Perform hand hygiene and put on PPE, if indicated. | |
| —— | —— | —— | 4. Identify the patient. | |
| —— | —— | —— | 5. Close curtains around bed and close door to room if possible. | |
| —— | —— | —— | 6. Put on gloves. Assemble equipment; at the bedside if using a bedside commode or in bathroom. | |
| —— | —— | —— | 7. Raise lid of toilet or commode. Place bowl of sitz bath, with drainage ports to rear and infusion port in front, in the toilet. Fill bowl of sitz bath about halfway full with tepid to warm water (37°–46°C [98°–115°F]). | |
| —— | —— | —— | 8. Clamp tubing on bag. Fill bag with same temperature water as mentioned above. Hang bag above patient's shoulder height on the IV pole. | |
| —— | —— | —— | 9. Assist patient to sit on toilet or commode and provide any extra draping if needed. Insert tubing into infusion port of sitz bath. Slowly unclamp tubing and allow sitz bath to fill. | |
| —— | —— | —— | 10. Clamp tubing once sitz bath is full. Instruct patient to open clamp when water in bowl becomes cool. *Ensure that call bell is within reach. Instruct patient to call if she feels light-headed or dizzy or has any problems. Instruct patient not to try standing without assistance.* | |
| —— | —— | —— | 11. Remove gloves and perform hand hygiene. | |
| —— | —— | —— | 12. When patient is finished (in about 15–20 minutes, or prescribed time), put on clean gloves. Assist the patient to stand and gently pat perineal area dry. Remove gloves. Assist patient to bed or chair. Ensure that call bell is within reach. | |
| —— | —— | —— | 13. Put on gloves. Empty and disinfect Sitz bath bowl according to agency policy. | |
| —— | —— | —— | 14. Remove gloves and any additional PPE, if used. Perform hand hygiene. | |

**178**

Name _____  Date _____

Unit _____  Position _____

Instructor/Evaluator: _____  Position _____

SKILL 8-17

# Applying Cold Therapy

| Excellent | Satisfactory | Needs Practice | **Goal:** The patient reports a relief of pain and increased comfort. | Comments |
|---|---|---|---|---|
| —— | —— | —— | 1. Review the medical order or nursing plan of care for the application of cold therapy, including frequency, type of therapy, body area to be treated, and length of time for the application. | |
| —— | —— | —— | 2. Gather the necessary supplies and bring to the bedside stand or overbed table. | |
| —— | —— | —— | 3. Perform hand hygiene and put on PPE, if indicated. | |
| —— | —— | —— | 4. Identify the patient. Determine if the patient has had any previous adverse reaction to hypothermia therapy. | |
| —— | —— | —— | 5. Close curtains around bed and close door to room if possible. Explain what you are going to do and why you are going to do it to the patient. | |
| —— | —— | —— | 6. Assess the condition of the skin where the ice is to be applied. | |
| —— | —— | —— | 7. Assist the patient to a comfortable position that provides easy access to the area to be treated. Expose the area and drape the patient with a bath blanket if needed. Put the waterproof pad under the wound area, if necessary. | |
| —— | —— | —— | 8. Prepare device: Fill the bag, collar, or glove about three-fourths full with ice. *Remove any excess air from the device.* Securely fasten the end of the bag or collar; tie the glove closed, checking for holes and leakage of water. Prepare commercially prepared ice pack if appropriate. | |
| —— | —— | —— | 9. *Cover the device with a towel or washcloth.* (If the device has a cloth exterior, this is not necessary.) | |
| —— | —— | —— | 10. Position cooling device on top of designated area and lightly secure in place as needed. | |
| —— | —— | —— | 11. *Remove the ice and assess the site for redness after 30 seconds. Ask the patient about the presence of burning sensations.* | |
| —— | —— | —— | 12. Replace the device snugly against the site if no problems are evident. Secure it in place with gauze wrap, ties, or tape. | |

SKILL 8-17

# Applying Cold Therapy *(Continued)*

| Excellent | Satisfactory | Needs Practice | | Comments |
|:---:|:---:|:---:|---|---|
| —— | —— | —— | 13. Reassess the treatment area every 5 minutes or according to facility policy. | |
| —— | —— | —— | 14. *After 20 minutes or the prescribed amount of time, remove the ice and dry the skin.* | |
| —— | —— | —— | 15. Remove PPE, if used. Perform hand hygiene. | |

*Skill Checklists for Taylor's Clinical Nursing Skills:*
*A Nursing Process Approach, 3rd edition*

Name _____   Date _____

Unit _____   Position _____

Instructor/Evaluator: _____   Position _____

| Excellent | Satisfactory | Needs Practice | SKILL 9-1<br>**Assisting a Patient With Turning in Bed** | |
|---|---|---|---|---|
| | | | **Goal:** The activity takes place without injury to patient or nurse. | **Comments** |
| ___ | ___ | ___ | 1. Review the physician's orders and nursing plan of care for patient activity. Identify any movement limitations and the ability of the patient to assist with turning. Consult patient handling algorithm, if available, to plan appropriate approach to moving the patient. | |
| ___ | ___ | ___ | 2. Gather any positioning aids or supports, if necessary. | |
| ___ | ___ | ___ | 3. Perform hand hygiene. Put on PPE, as indicated. | |
| ___ | ___ | ___ | 4. Identify the patient. Explain the procedure to the patient. | |
| ___ | ___ | ___ | 5. Close the curtains around bed and close the door to the room, if possible. Position at least one nurse on either side of the bed. Place pillows, wedges, or any other support to be used for positioning within easy reach. Place the bed at an appropriate and comfortable working height, usually elbow height of the caregiver (VISN 8 Patient Safety Center, 2009). Lower both side rails. | |
| ___ | ___ | ___ | 6. If not already in place, position a friction-reducing sheet under the patient. | |
| ___ | ___ | ___ | 7. Using the friction-reducing sheet, move the patient to the edge of the bed, opposite the side to which he or she will be turned. Raise the side rails. | |
| ___ | ___ | ___ | 8. If the patient is able, have the patient grasp the side rail on the side of the bed toward which he or she is turning. Alternately, place the patient's arms across his or her chest and cross his or her far leg over the leg nearest you. | |
| ___ | ___ | ___ | 9. If available, activate the bed mechanism to inflate the side of the bed behind the patient's back. | |
| ___ | ___ | ___ | 10. *The nurse on the side of the bed toward which the patient is turning should stand opposite the patient's center with his or her feet spread about shoulder width and with one foot ahead of the other. Tighten your gluteal and abdominal muscles and flex your knees. Use your leg muscles to do the pulling. The other nurse should position his or her hands on the patient's shoulder and hip, assisting to roll the patient to the side. Instruct the patient to pull on the bed rail at the same time. Use the friction-reducing sheet to gently pull the patient over on his or her side.* | |

SKILL 9-1

# Assisting a Patient With Turning in Bed *(Continued)*

| Excellent | Satisfactory | Needs Practice | | Comments |
|---|---|---|---|---|
| —— | —— | —— | 11. Use a pillow or other support behind the patient's back. Pull the shoulder blade forward and out from under the patient. | |
| —— | —— | —— | 12. Make the patient comfortable and position in proper alignment, using pillows or other supports under the leg and arm, as needed. Readjust the pillow under the patient's head. Elevate the head of the bed as needed for comfort. | |
| —— | —— | —— | 13. *Place the bed in the lowest position, with the side rails up. Make sure the call bell and other necessary items are within easy reach.* | |
| —— | —— | —— | 14. Clean transfer aids, per facility policy, if not indicated for single patient use. Remove gloves and other PPE, if used. Perform hand hygiene. | |

*Skill Checklists for TAYLOR's Clinical Nursing Skills:*
*A Nursing Process Approach, 3rd edition*

Name _____   Date _____

Unit _____   Position _____

Instructor/Evaluator: _____   Position _____

| Excellent | Satisfactory | Needs Practice | SKILL 9-2 **Moving a Patient Up in Bed With the Assistance of Another Nurse** | |
|---|---|---|---|---|
| | | | **Goal:** The patient remains free from injury and maintains proper body alignment. | **Comments** |
| ___ | ___ | ___ | 1. Review the medical record and nursing plan of care for conditions that may influence the patient's ability to move or to be positioned. Assess for tubes, IV lines, incisions, or equipment that may alter the positioning procedure. Identify any movement limitations. Consult patient handling algorithm, if available, to plan appropriate approach to moving the patient. | |
| ___ | ___ | ___ | 2. Perform hand hygiene and put on PPE, if indicated. | |
| ___ | ___ | ___ | 3. Identify the patient. Explain the procedure to the patient. | |
| ___ | ___ | ___ | 4. Close curtains around bed and close the door to the room, if possible. Place the bed at an appropriate and comfortable working height, usually elbow height of the caregiver (VISN 8 Patient Safety Center, 2009). Adjust the head of the bed to a flat position or as low as the patient can tolerate. Placing the bed in slight Trendelenburg position aids movement, if the patient is able to tolerate it. | |
| ___ | ___ | ___ | 5. Remove all pillows from under the patient. Leave one at the head of the bed, leaning upright against the headboard. | |
| ___ | ___ | ___ | 6. Position at least one nurse on either side of the bed, and lower both side rails. | |
| ___ | ___ | ___ | 7. If a friction-reducing sheet (or device) is not in place under the patient, place one under the patient's midsection. | |
| ___ | ___ | ___ | 8. Ask the patient (if able) to bend his or her legs and put his or her feet flat on the bed to assist with the movement. | |
| ___ | ___ | ___ | 9. Have the patient fold the arms across the chest. Have the patient (if able) lift the head with chin on chest. | |
| ___ | ___ | ___ | 10. One nurse should be positioned on each side of the bed, at the patient's midsection with feet spread shoulder width apart and one foot slightly in front of the other. | |
| ___ | ___ | ___ | 11. If available on bed, engage mechanism to make the bed surface firmer for repositioning. | |
| ___ | ___ | ___ | 12. Grasp the friction-reducing sheet securely, close to the patient's body. | |
| ___ | ___ | ___ | 13. Flex your knees and hips. Tighten your abdominal and gluteal muscles and keep your back straight. | |

SKILL 9-2

# Moving a Patient Up in Bed With the Assistance of Another Nurse *(Continued)*

| Excellent | Satisfactory | Needs Practice | | Comments |
|---|---|---|---|---|
| —— | —— | —— | 14. Shift your weight back and forth from your back leg to your front leg and count to three. On the count of three, move the patient up in bed. If possible, the patient can assist with the move by pushing with the legs. Repeat the process, if necessary, to get the patient to the right position. | |
| —— | —— | —— | 15. *Assist the patient to a comfortable position and readjust the pillows and supports, as needed. Return bed surface to normal setting, if necessary. Raise the side rails. Place the bed in the lowest position.* | |
| —— | —— | —— | 16. Clean transfer aids per facility policy, if not indicated for single patient use. Remove gloves or other PPE, if used. Perform hand hygiene. | |

*Skill Checklists for Taylor's Clinical Nursing Skills:*
*A Nursing Process Approach, 3rd edition*

Name _____   Date _____

Unit _____   Position _____

Instructor/Evaluator: _____   Position _____

| Excellent | Satisfactory | Needs Practice | SKILL 9-3 **Transferring a Patient From the Bed to a Stretcher** | |
|:---:|:---:|:---:|---|---|
| | | | **Goal:** The patient is transferred without injury to patient or nurse. | **Comments** |
| ___ | ___ | ___ | 1. Review the medical record and nursing plan of care for conditions that may influence the patient's ability to move or to be positioned. Assess for tubes, IV lines, incisions, or equipment that may alter the positioning procedure. Identify any movement limitations. Consult patient handling algorithm, if available, to plan appropriate approach to moving the patient. | |
| ___ | ___ | ___ | 2. Perform hand hygiene and put on PPE, if indicated. | |
| ___ | ___ | ___ | 3. Identify the patient. Explain the procedure to the patient. | |
| ___ | ___ | ___ | 4. Close curtains around bed and close the door to the room, if possible. Adjust the head of the bed to a flat position or as low as the patient can tolerate. Raise the bed to a height that is even with the transport stretcher (VISN 8 Patient Safety Center, 2009). Lower the side rails, if in place. | |
| ___ | ___ | ___ | 5. Place the bath blanket over the patient and remove the top covers from underneath. | |
| ___ | ___ | ___ | 6. If a friction-reducing transfer sheet is not in place under the patient, place one under the patient's midsection. Have patient fold arms against chest and move chin to chest. Use the friction-reducing sheet to move the patient to the side of the bed where the stretcher will be placed. Alternately, place a lateral-assist device under the patient. Follow manufacturer's directions for use. | |
| ___ | ___ | ___ | 7. Position the stretcher next to (and parallel) to the bed. ***Lock the wheels on the stretcher and the bed.*** | |
| ___ | ___ | ___ | 8. Two nurses should stand on the stretcher side of the bed. A third nurse should stand on the side of the bed without the stretcher. | |
| ___ | ___ | ___ | 9. Use the friction-reducing sheet to roll the patient away from the stretcher. Place the transfer board across the space between the stretcher and the bed, partially under the patient. Roll the patient onto his or her back, so that the patient is partially on the transfer board. | |

# Transferring a Patient From the Bed to a Stretcher *(Continued)*

| Excellent | Satisfactory | Needs Practice | | Comments |
|---|---|---|---|---|
| —— | —— | —— | 10. The nurse on the side of the bed without the stretcher should grasp the friction-reducing sheet at the head and chest areas of the patient. One nurse on the stretcher side of the bed should grasp the friction-reducing sheet at the head and chest, and the other nurse at the chest and leg areas of the patient. | |
| —— | —— | —— | 11. *At a signal given by one of the nurses, have the nurses standing on the stretcher side of the bed pull the friction-reducing sheet. At the same time, the nurse (or nurses) on the other side push, transferring the patient's weight toward the transfer board, and pushing the patient from the bed to the stretcher.* | |
| —— | —— | —— | 12. Once the patient is transferred to the stretcher, remove the transfer board, and secure the patient until the side rails are raised. Raise the side rails. To ensure the patient's comfort, cover the patient with blanket and remove the bath blanket from underneath. Leave the friction-reducing sheet in place for the return transfer. | |
| —— | —— | —— | 13. Clean transfer aids per facility policy, if not indicated for single patient use. Remove gloves and any other PPE, if used. Perform hand hygiene. | |

*Skill Checklists for Taylor's Clinical Nursing Skills:*
*A Nursing Process Approach, 3rd edition*

Name _____  Date _____

Unit _____  Position _____

Instructor/Evaluator: _____  Position _____

SKILL 9-4

# Transferring a Patient From the Bed to a Chair

**Goal:** The transfer is accomplished without injury to patient or nurse and the patient remains free of any complications of immobility.

| Excellent | Satisfactory | Needs Practice | | Comments |
|---|---|---|---|---|
| —— | —— | —— | 1. Review the medical record and nursing plan of care for conditions that may influence the patient's ability to move or to be positioned. Assess for tubes, IV lines, incisions, or equipment that may alter the positioning procedure. Identify any movement limitations. Consult patient-handling algorithm, if available, to plan appropriate approach to moving the patient. | |
| —— | —— | —— | 2. Perform hand hygiene and put on PPE, as indicated. | |
| —— | —— | —— | 3. Identify the patient. Explain the procedure to the patient. | |
| —— | —— | —— | 4. If needed, move equipment to make room for the chair. Close curtains around bed and close the door to the room, if possible. | |
| —— | —— | —— | 5. Place the bed in the lowest position. Raise the head of the bed to a sitting position, or as high as the patient can tolerate. | |
| —— | —— | —— | 6. *Make sure the bed brakes are locked. Put the chair next to the bed. If available, lock the brakes of the chair. If the chair does not have brakes, brace the chair against a secure object.* | |
| —— | —— | —— | 7. Encourage the patient to make use of a stand-assist aid, either freestanding or attached to the side of the bed, if available, to move to the side of the bed and to a side-lying position, facing the side of the bed on which the patient will sit. | |
| —— | —— | —— | 8. Lower the side rail, if necessary, and stand near the patient's hips. Stand with your legs shoulder width apart with one foot near the head of the bed, slightly in front of the other foot. | |
| —— | —— | —— | 9. Encourage the patient to make use of the stand-assist device. Assist the patient to sit up on the side of the bed; ask the patient to swing his or her legs over the side of the bed. At the same time, pivot on your back leg to lift the patient's trunk and shoulders. Keep your back straight; avoid twisting. | |

| Excellent | Satisfactory | Needs Practice | SKILL 9-4
**Transferring a Patient From the Bed to a Chair** (*Continued*) |
|---|---|---|---|
| | | | **Comments** |

| Excellent | Satisfactory | Needs Practice | | Comments |
|---|---|---|---|---|
| ___ | ___ | ___ | 10. *Stand in front of the patient, and assess for any balance problems or complaints of dizziness. Allow the patient's legs to dangle a few minutes before continuing.* | |
| ___ | ___ | ___ | 11. Assist the patient to put on a robe, as necessary, and nonskid footwear. | |
| ___ | ___ | ___ | 12. Wrap the gait belt around the patient's waist, based on assessed need and facility policy. | |
| ___ | ___ | ___ | 13. Stand facing the patient. Spread your feet about shoulder width apart and flex your hips and knees. | |
| ___ | ___ | ___ | 14. Ask the patient to slide his or her buttocks to the edge of the bed until the feet touch the floor. Position yourself as close as possible to the patient, with your foot positioned on the outside of the patient's foot. If a second staff person is assisting, have him or her assume a similar position. | |
| ___ | ___ | ___ | 15. Encourage the patient to make use of the stand-assist device. If necessary, have second staff person grasp gait belt on opposite side. Using the gait belt, assist the patient to stand. Rock back and forth while counting to three. ***On the count of three, use your legs (not your back) to help raise the patient to a standing position.*** If indicated, brace your front knee against the patient's weak extremity as he or she stands. Assess the patient's balance and leg strength. If the patient is weak or unsteady, return the patient to bed. | |
| ___ | ___ | ___ | 16. Pivot on your back foot and assist the patient to turn until the patient feels the chair against his or her legs. | |
| ___ | ___ | ___ | 17. Ask the patient to use an arm to steady him- or herself on the arm of the chair while slowly lowering to a sitting position. Continue to brace the patient's knees with your knees and hold the gait belt. Flex your hips and knees when helping the patient sit in the chair. | |
| ___ | ___ | ___ | 18. Assess the patient's alignment in the chair. Remove gait belt, if desired. Depending on patient comfort, it could be left in place to use when returning to bed. Cover with a blanket, if needed. Make sure call bell and other necessary items are within easy reach. | |
| ___ | ___ | ___ | 19. Clean transfer aids per facility policy, if not indicated for single patient use. Remove gloves and any other PPE, if used. Perform hand hygiene. | |

*Skill Checklists for Taylor's Clinical Nursing Skills:*
*A Nursing Process Approach, 3rd edition*

Name _____ Date _____

Unit _____ Position _____

Instructor/Evaluator: _____ Position _____

SKILL 9-5

# Transferring a Patient Using a Powered Full-Body Sling Lift

**Goal:** The transfer is accomplished without injury to patient or nurse and the patient is free of any complications of immobility.

| Excellent | Satisfactory | Needs Practice | | Comments |
|---|---|---|---|---|
| ___ | ___ | ___ | 1. Review the medical record and nursing plan of care for conditions that may influence the patient's ability to move or to be positioned. Assess for tubes, IV lines, incisions, or equipment that may alter the positioning procedure. Identify any movement limitations. | |
| ___ | ___ | ___ | 2. Perform hand hygiene and put on PPE, if indicated. | |
| ___ | ___ | ___ | 3. Identify the patient. Explain the procedure to the patient. | |
| ___ | ___ | ___ | 4. If needed, move the equipment to make room for the chair. Close curtains around bed and close the door to the room, if possible. | |
| ___ | ___ | ___ | 5. Adjust the bed to a comfortable working height, usually elbow height of the caregiver (VISN 8 Patient Safety Center, 2009). *Lock the bed brakes.* | |
| ___ | ___ | ___ | 6. Lower the side rail, if in use, on the side of the bed you are working. If the sling is for use with more than one patient, place a cover or pad on the sling. Place the sling evenly under the patient. Roll the patient to one side and place half of the sling with the sheet or pad on it under the patient from shoulders to mid-thigh. Raise the rail and move to the other side. Lower the rail, if necessary. Roll the patient to the other side and pull the sling under the patient. Raise the side rail. | |
| ___ | ___ | ___ | 7. Bring the chair to the side of the bed. *Lock the wheels, if present.* | |
| ___ | ___ | ___ | 8. Lower the side rail on the chair side of the bed. Roll the base of the lift under the side of the bed nearest to the chair. *Center the frame over the patient. Lock the wheels of the lift.* | |
| ___ | ___ | ___ | 9. *Using the base-adjustment lever, widen the stance of the base.* | |
| ___ | ___ | ___ | 10. Lower the arms close enough to attach the sling to the frame. | |

## SKILL 9-5
# Transferring a Patient Using a Powered Full-Body Sling Lift (Continued)

| Excellent | Satisfactory | Needs Practice | | Comments |
|---|---|---|---|---|
| —— | —— | —— | 11. Place the strap or chain hooks through the holes of the sling. Short straps attach behind the patient's back and long straps attach at the other end of the sling. Check the patient to make sure the hooks are not pressing into the skin. Some lifts have straps on the sling that attach to hooks on the frame. Check the manufacturer's instructions for each lift. | |
| —— | —— | —— | 12. Check all equipment, lines, and drains attached to the patient so that they are not interfering with the device. Have the patient fold his or her arms across the chest. | |
| —— | —— | —— | 13. With a person standing on each side of the lift, tell the patient that he or she will be lifted from the bed. Support injured limbs as necessary. Engage the pump to raise the patient about 6 inches above the bed. | |
| —— | —— | —— | 14. Unlock the wheels of the lift. *Carefully wheel the patient straight back and away from the bed. Support the patient's limbs, as needed.* | |
| —— | —— | —— | 15. Position the patient over the chair with the base of the lift straddling the chair. Lock the wheels of the lift. | |
| —— | —— | —— | 16. Gently lower the patient to the chair until the hooks or straps are slightly loosened from the sling or frame. Guide the patient into the chair with your hands as the sling lowers. | |
| —— | —— | —— | 17. Disconnect the hooks or strap from the frame. Keep the sling in place under the patient. | |
| —— | —— | —— | 18. Adjust the patient's position, using pillows, if necessary. Check the patient's alignment in the chair. Cover the patient with a blanket, if necessary. Make sure call bell and other necessary items are within easy reach. When it is time for the patient to return to bed, reattach the hooks or straps and reverse the steps. | |
| —— | —— | —— | 19. Clean transfer aids per facility policy, if not indicated for single patient use. Remove gloves and any other PPE, if used. Perform hand hygiene. | |

*Skill Checklists for Taylor's Clinical Nursing Skills:*
*A Nursing Process Approach, 3rd edition*

Name _____     Date _____

Unit _____     Position _____

Instructor/Evaluator: _____     Position _____

SKILL 9-6

# Providing Range-of-Motion Exercises

| Excellent | Satisfactory | Needs Practice | **Goal:** The patient maintains joint mobility. | **Comments** |
|---|---|---|---|---|
| ____ | ____ | ____ | 1. Review the physician's orders and nursing plan of care for patient activity. Identify any movement limitations. | |
| ____ | ____ | ____ | 2. Perform hand hygiene and put on PPE, if indicated. | |
| ____ | ____ | ____ | 3. Identify the patient. Explain the procedure to the patient. | |
| ____ | ____ | ____ | 4. Close curtains around bed and close the door to the room, if possible. Place the bed at an appropriate and comfortable working height, usually elbow height of the caregiver (VISN 8 Patient Safety Center, 2009). Adjust the head of the bed to a flat position or as low as the patient can tolerate. | |
| ____ | ____ | ____ | 5. Stand on the side of the bed where the joints are to be exercised. Lower side rail on that side, if in place. Uncover only the limb to be used during the exercise. | |
| ____ | ____ | ____ | 6. Perform the exercises slowly and gently, providing support by holding the areas proximal and distal to the joint. Repeat each exercise two to five times, moving each joint in a smooth and rhythmic manner. *Stop movement if the patient complains of pain or if you meet resistance.* | |
| ____ | ____ | ____ | 7. While performing the exercises, begin at the head and move down one side of the body at a time. *Encourage the patient to do as many of these exercises by him- or herself as possible.* | |
| ____ | ____ | ____ | 8. Move the chin down to rest on the chest. Return the head to a normal upright position. Tilt the head as far as possible toward each shoulder. | |
| ____ | ____ | ____ | 9. Move the head from side to side, bringing the chin toward each shoulder. | |
| ____ | ____ | ____ | 10. Start with the arm at the patient's side and lift the arm forward to above the head. Return the arm to the starting position at the side of the body. | |
| ____ | ____ | ____ | 11. With the arm back at the patient's side, move the arm laterally to an upright position above the head, and then return it to the original position. Move the arm across the body as far as possible. | |

## SKILL 9-6

# Providing Range-of-Motion Exercises *(Continued)*

| Excellent | Satisfactory | Needs Practice | | Comments |
|---|---|---|---|---|
| ___ | ___ | ___ | 12. Raise the arm at the side until the upper arm is in line with the shoulder. Bend the elbow at a 90-degree angle and move the forearm upward and downward, then return the arm to the side. | |
| ___ | ___ | ___ | 13. Bend the elbow and move the lower arm and hand upward toward the shoulder. Return the lower arm and hand to the original position while straightening the elbow. | |
| ___ | ___ | ___ | 14. Rotate the lower arm and hand so the palm is up. Rotate the lower arm and hand so the palm of the hand is down. | |
| ___ | ___ | ___ | 15. Move the hand downward toward the inner aspect of the forearm. Return the hand to a neutral position even with the forearm. Then move the dorsal portion of the hand backward as far as possible. | |
| ___ | ___ | ___ | 16. Bend the fingers to make a fist, and then straighten them out. Spread the fingers apart and return them back together. Touch the thumb to each finger on the hand. | |
| ___ | ___ | ___ | 17. Extend the leg and lift it upward. Return the leg to the original position beside the other leg. | |
| ___ | ___ | ___ | 18. Lift the leg laterally away from the patient's body. Return the leg back toward the other leg and try to extend it beyond the midline. | |
| ___ | ___ | ___ | 19. Turn the foot and leg toward the other leg to rotate it internally. Turn the foot and leg outward away from the other leg to rotate it externally. | |
| ___ | ___ | ___ | 20. Bend the leg and bring the heel toward the back of the leg. Return the leg to a straight position. | |
| ___ | ___ | ___ | 21. At the ankle, move the foot up and back until the toes are upright. Move the foot with the toes pointing downward. | |
| ___ | ___ | ___ | 22. Turn the sole of the foot toward the midline. Turn the sole of the foot outward. | |
| ___ | ___ | ___ | 23. Curl the toes downward, and then straighten them out. Spread the toes apart and bring them together. | |
| ___ | ___ | ___ | 24. Repeat these exercises on the other side of the body. Encourage the patient to do as many of these exercises by him- or herself as possible. | |
| ___ | ___ | ___ | 25. *When finished, make sure the patient is comfortable, with the side rails up and the bed in the lowest position.* | |
| ___ | ___ | ___ | 26. Remove gloves and any other PPE, if used. Perform hand hygiene. | |

*Skill Checklists for Taylor's Clinical Nursing Skills:*
*A Nursing Process Approach, 3rd edition*

Name _____     Date _____

Unit _____     Position _____

Instructor/Evaluator: _____     Position _____

## SKILL 9-7
## Assisting a Patient With Ambulation

| Excellent | Satisfactory | Needs Practice | | Comments |
|---|---|---|---|---|
| | | | **Goal:** The patient ambulates safely, without falls or injury. | |
| ___ | ___ | ___ | 1. Review the medical record and nursing plan of care for conditions that may influence the patient's ability to move and ambulate. Assess for tubes, IV lines, incisions, or equipment that may alter the procedure for ambulation. Identify any movement limitations. | |
| ___ | ___ | ___ | 2. Perform hand hygiene. Put on PPE, as indicated. | |
| ___ | ___ | ___ | 3. Identify the patient. Explain the procedure to the patient. Ask the patient to report any feelings of dizziness, weakness, or shortness of breath while walking. Decide how far to walk. | |
| ___ | ___ | ___ | 4. Place the bed in the lowest position. | |
| ___ | ___ | ___ | 5. *Encourage the patient to make use of a stand-assist aid, either freestanding or attached to the side of the bed, if available, to move to the side of the bed.* Assist the patient to the side of the bed, if necessary. | |
| ___ | ___ | ___ | 6. Have the patient sit on the side of the bed for several minutes and assess for dizziness or lightheadedness. Have the patient stay sitting until he or she feels secure. | |
| ___ | ___ | ___ | 7. Assist the patient to put on footwear and a robe, if desired. | |
| ___ | ___ | ___ | 8. Wrap the gait belt around the patient's waist, based on assessed need and facility policy. | |
| ___ | ___ | ___ | 9. Encourage the patient to make use of the stand-assist device. Assist the patient to stand, using the gait belt, if necessary. Assess the patient's balance and leg strength. If the patient is weak or unsteady, return the patient to the bed or assist to a chair. | |

## SKILL 9-7

# Assisting a Patient With Ambulation *(Continued)*

| Excellent | Satisfactory | Needs Practice | | Comments |
|---|---|---|---|---|
| —— | —— | —— | 10. If you are the only nurse assisting, position yourself to the side and slightly behind the patient. Support the patient by the waist or transfer belt. | |
| —— | —— | —— | When two nurses assist, position yourself to the side and slightly behind the patient, supporting the patient by the waist or gait belt. Have the other nurse carry or manage equipment or provide additional support from the other side. | |
| —— | —— | —— | Alternatively, when two nurses assist, stand at the patient's sides (one nurse on each side) with near hands grasping the gait belt and far hands holding the patient's lower arm or hand. | |
| —— | —— | —— | 11. Take several steps forward with the patient. Continue to assess the patient's strength and balance. Remind the patient to stand erect. | |
| —— | —— | —— | 12. Continue with ambulation for the planned distance and time. Return the patient to the bed or chair based on the patient's tolerance and condition. | |
| —— | —— | —— | 13. Remove gait belts. Clean transfer aids per facility policy, if not indicated for single patient use. Remove gloves and any other PPE, if used. Perform hand hygiene. | |

*Skill Checklists for Taylor's Clinical Nursing Skills:*
*A Nursing Process Approach, 3rd edition*

Name _____     Date _____

Unit _____     Position _____

Instructor/Evaluator: _____     Position _____

| Excellent | Satisfactory | Needs Practice | SKILL 9-8<br><br>**Assisting a Patient With Ambulation Using a Walker**<br><br>**Goal:** The patient ambulates safely with the walker and is free from falls or injury. | Comments |
|---|---|---|---|---|
| —— | —— | —— | 1. Review the medical record and nursing plan of care for conditions that may influence the patient's ability to move and ambulate, and for specific instructions for ambulation such as distance. Assess for tubes, IV lines, incisions, or equipment that may alter the procedure for ambulation. Assess the patient's knowledge and previous experience regarding the use of a walker. Identify any movement limitations. | |
| —— | —— | —— | 2. Perform hand hygiene. Put on PPE, if indicated. | |
| —— | —— | —— | 3. Identify the patient. Explain the procedure to the patient. Tell the patient to report any feelings of dizziness, weakness, or shortness of breath while walking. Decide how far to walk. | |
| —— | —— | —— | 4. Place the bed in the lowest position, if the patient is in bed. | |
| —— | —— | —— | 5. *Encourage the patient to make use of a stand-assist aid, either free-standing or attached to the side of the bed, if available, to move to the side of the bed.* | |
| —— | —— | —— | 6. Assist the patient to the side of the bed, if necessary. Have the patient sit on the side of the bed. Assess for dizziness or lightheadedness. Have the patient stay seated until he or she feels secure. | |
| —— | —— | —— | 7. Assist the patient to put on footwear and a robe, if desired. | |
| —— | —— | —— | 8. Wrap the gait belt around the patient's waist, based on assessed need and facility policy. | |
| —— | —— | —— | 9. *Place the walker directly in front of the patient.* Ask the patient to push him- or herself off the bed or chair; make use of the stand-assist device, or assist the patient to stand. Once the patient is standing, have him or her hold the walker's hand grips firmly and equally. Stand slightly behind the patient, on one side. | |
| —— | —— | —— | 10. Have the patient move the walker forward 6 to 8 inches and set it down, making sure all four feet of the walker stay on the floor. Then, tell the patient to step forward with either foot into the walker, supporting him- or herself on his or her arms. Follow through with the other leg. | |

SKILL 9-8

# Assisting a Patient With Ambulation Using a Walker (Continued)

| Excellent | Satisfactory | Needs Practice | | Comments |
|---|---|---|---|---|
| — | — | — | 11. Move the walker forward again, and continue the same pattern. Continue with ambulation for the planned distance and time. Return the patient to the bed or chair based on the patient's tolerance and condition, ensuring that the patient is comfortable. Make sure call bell and other necessary items are within easy reach. | |
| — | — | — | 12. Remove gait belts. Clean transfer aids per facility policy, if not indicated for single patient use. Remove gloves and any other PPE, if used. Perform hand hygiene. | |

*Skill Checklists for Taylor's Clinical Nursing Skills:*
*A Nursing Process Approach, 3rd edition*

Name _____     Date _____

Unit _____     Position _____

Instructor/Evaluator: _____     Position _____

| Excellent | Satisfactory | Needs Practice | SKILL 9-9<br>**Assisting a Patient With Ambulation Using Crutches** | Comments |
|---|---|---|---|---|
| | | | **Goal:** The patient ambulates safely without experiencing falls or injury. | |
| —— | —— | —— | 1. Review the medical record and nursing plan of care for conditions that may influence the patient's ability to move and ambulate. Assess for tubes, IV lines, incisions, or equipment that may alter the procedure for ambulation. Assess the patient's knowledge and previous experience regarding the use of crutches. Determine that the appropriate size crutch has been obtained. | |
| —— | —— | —— | 2. Perform hand hygiene. Put on PPE, if indicated. | |
| —— | —— | —— | 3. Identify the patient. Explain the procedure to the patient. Tell the patient to report any feelings of dizziness, weakness, or shortness of breath while walking. Decide how far to walk. | |
| —— | —— | —— | 4. ***Encourage the patient to make use of the stand-assist device, if available.*** Assist the patient to stand erect, face forward in the tripod position. This means the patient holds the crutches 12 inches in front of and 12 inches to the side of each foot. | |
| —— | —— | —— | 5. For the four-point gait: | |
| —— | —— | —— | a. Have the patient move the right crutch forward 12 inches and then move the left foot forward to the level of the right crutch. | |
| —— | —— | —— | b. Then have the patient move the left crutch forward 12 inches and then move the right foot forward to the level of the left crutch. | |
| —— | —— | —— | 6. For the three-point gait: | |
| —— | —— | —— | a. Have the patient move the affected leg and both crutches forward about 12 inches. | |
| —— | —— | —— | b. Have the patient move the stronger leg forward to the level of the crutches. | |
| —— | —— | —— | 7. For the two-point gait: | |
| —— | —— | —— | a. Have the patient move the left crutch and the right foot forward about 12 inches at the same time. | |
| —— | —— | —— | b. Have the patient move the right crutch and left leg forward to the level of the left crutch at the same time. | |

| Excellent | Satisfactory | Needs Practice | |
|---|---|---|---|

## Assisting a Patient With Ambulation
## Using Crutches *(Continued)*

Comments

—— —— ——  8. For the swing-to gait:

—— —— ——     a. Have the patient move both crutches forward about 12 inches.

—— —— ——     b. Have the patient lift the legs and swing them to the crutches, supporting his or her body weight on the crutches.

—— —— ——  9. Continue with ambulation for the planned distance and time. Return the patient to the bed or chair based on the patient's tolerance and condition, ensuring that the patient is comfortable. Make sure call bell and other necessary items are within easy reach.

—— —— ——  10. Remove PPE, if used. Perform hand hygiene.

*Skill Checklists for Taylor's Clinical Nursing Skills:*
*A Nursing Process Approach, 3rd edition*

Name _____  Date _____

Unit _____  Position _____

Instructor/Evaluator: _____  Position _____

| Excellent | Satisfactory | Needs Practice | SKILL 9-10<br><br>**Assisting a Patient With Ambulation Using a Cane** | |
|---|---|---|---|---|
| | | | **Goal:** The patient ambulates safely without falls or injury. | **Comments** |
| —— | —— | —— | 1. Review the medical record and nursing plan of care for conditions that may influence the patient's ability to move and ambulate. Assess for tubes, IV lines, incisions, or equipment that may alter the procedure for ambulation. | |
| —— | —— | —— | 2. Perform hand hygiene. Put on PPE, as indicated. | |
| —— | —— | —— | 3. Identify the patient. Explain the procedure to the patient. Tell the patient to report any feelings of dizziness, weakness, or shortness of breath while walking. Decide how far to walk. | |
| —— | —— | —— | 4. *Encourage the patient to make use of a stand-assist aid, either free-standing or attached to the side of the bed, if available, to move to and sit on the side of the bed.* | |
| —— | —— | —— | 5. Wrap the gait belt around the patient's waist, based on assessed need and facility policy. | |
| —— | —— | —— | 6. Encourage the patient to make use of the stand-assist device to stand with weight evenly distributed between the feet and the cane. | |
| —— | —— | —— | 7. Have the patient hold the cane on his or her stronger side, close to the body, while the nurse stands to the side and slightly behind the patient. | |
| —— | —— | —— | 8. Tell the patient to advance the cane 4 to 12 inches (10 to 30 cm) and then, while supporting his or her weight on the stronger leg and the cane, advance the weaker foot forward, parallel with the cane. | |
| —— | —— | —— | 9. While supporting his or her weight on the weaker leg and the cane, have the patient advance the stronger leg forward ahead of the cane (heel slightly beyond the tip of the cane). | |
| —— | —— | —— | 10. Tell the patient to move the weaker leg forward until it is even with the stronger leg, and then advance the cane again. | |
| —— | —— | —— | 11. Continue with ambulation for the planned distance and time. Return the patient to the bed or chair based on the patient's tolerance and condition, ensuring the patient's comfort. Make sure call bell and other necessary items are within easy reach. | |
| —— | —— | —— | 12. Clean transfer aids per facility policy, if not indicated for single patient use. Remove PPE, if used. Perform hand hygiene. | |

*Skill Checklists for Taylor's Clinical Nursing Skills:*
*A Nursing Process Approach, 3rd edition*

Name _____  Date _____

Unit _____  Position _____

Instructor/Evaluator: _____  Position _____

SKILL 9-11

# Applying and Removing Antiembolism Stockings

**Goal:** The stockings are applied and removed with minimal discomfort to the patient.

| Excellent | Satisfactory | Needs Practice | | Comments |
|---|---|---|---|---|
| —— | —— | —— | 1. Review the medical record and medical orders to determine the need for antiembolism stockings. | |
| —— | —— | —— | 2. Perform hand hygiene. Put on PPE, as indicated. | |
| —— | —— | —— | 3. Identify the patient. Explain what you are going to do and the rationale for use of elastic stockings. | |
| —— | —— | —— | 4. Close curtains around bed and close the door to the room, if possible. | |
| —— | —— | —— | 5. Adjust the bed to a comfortable working height, usually elbow height of the caregiver (VISN 8 Patient Safety Center, 2009). | |
| —— | —— | —— | 6. Assist patient to supine position. If patient has been sitting or walking, have him or her lie down with legs and feet well elevated for at least 15 minutes before applying stockings. | |
| —— | —— | —— | 7. Expose legs one at a time. Wash and dry legs, if necessary. Powder the leg lightly unless patient has a breathing problem, dry skin, or sensitivity to the powder. If the skin is dry, a lotion may be used. Powders and lotions are not recommended by some manufacturers; check the package material for manufacturer specifications. | |
| —— | —— | —— | 8. Stand at the foot of the bed. Place hand inside stocking and grasp heel area securely. Turn stocking inside-out to the heel area, leaving the foot inside the stocking leg. | |
| —— | —— | —— | 9. With the heel pocket down, ease the stocking foot over the foot and heel. Check that patient's heel is centered in heel pocket of stocking. | |
| —— | —— | —— | 10. Using your fingers and thumbs, carefully grasp edge of stocking and pull it up smoothly over ankle and calf, toward the knee. Make sure it is distributed evenly. | |
| —— | —— | —— | 11. Pull forward slightly on toe section. If the stocking has a toe window, make sure it is properly positioned. Adjust if necessary to ensure material is smooth. | |
| —— | —— | —— | 12. If the stockings are knee-length, make sure each stocking top is 1 to 2 inches below the patella. Make sure the stocking does not roll down. | |

## SKILL 9-11
## Applying and Removing Antiembolism Stockings *(Continued)*

| Excellent | Satisfactory | Needs Practice | | Comments |
|---|---|---|---|---|
| — | — | — | 13. If applying thigh-length stocking, continue the application. Flex the patient's leg. Stretch the stocking over the knee. | |
| — | — | — | 14. Pull the stocking over the thigh until the top is 1 to 3 inches below the gluteal fold. Adjust the stocking, as necessary, to distribute the fabric evenly. Make sure the stocking does not roll down. | |
| — | — | — | 15. Remove equipment and return patient to a position of comfort. Remove your gloves. Raise side rail and lower bed. | |
| — | — | — | 16. Remove any other PPE, if used. Perform hand hygiene. | |
| | | | **Removing Stockings** | |
| — | — | — | 17. To remove stocking, grasp top of stocking with your thumb and fingers and smoothly pull stocking off inside out to heel. Support foot and ease stocking over it. | |

*Skill Checklists for Taylor's Clinical Nursing Skills:*
*A Nursing Process Approach, 3rd edition*

Name _____  Date _____

Unit _____  Position _____

Instructor/Evaluator: _____  Position _____

| | | | SKILL 9-12 | |
|---|---|---|---|---|
| **Excellent** | **Satisfactory** | **Needs Practice** | **Applying Pneumatic Compression Devices** | **Comments** |
| | | | **Goal:** The patient maintains adequate circulation in extremities and is free from symptoms of neurovascular compromise. | |
| ___ | ___ | ___ | 1. Review the medical record and nursing plan of care for conditions that may contraindicate the use of the PCD. | |
| ___ | ___ | ___ | 2. Perform hand hygiene. Put on PPE, as indicated. | |
| ___ | ___ | ___ | 3. Identify the patient. Explain the procedure to the patient. | |
| ___ | ___ | ___ | 4. Close curtains around bed and close the door to the room, if possible. Place the bed at an appropriate and comfortable working height, usually elbow height of the caregiver (VISN 8 Patient Safety Center, 2009). | |
| ___ | ___ | ___ | 5. Hang the compression pump on the foot of the bed and plug it into an electrical outlet. Attach the connecting tubing to the pump. | |
| ___ | ___ | ___ | 6. Remove the compression sleeves from the package and unfold them. Lay the unfolded sleeves on the bed with the cotton lining facing up. *Note the markings indicating the correct placement for the ankle and popliteal areas.* | |
| ___ | ___ | ___ | 7. Apply antiembolism stockings, if ordered. Place a sleeve under the patient's leg with the tubing toward the heel. Each one fits either leg. *For total leg sleeves, place the behind-the-knee opening at the popliteal space to prevent pressure there. For knee-high sleeves, make sure the back of the ankle is over the ankle marking.* | |
| ___ | ___ | ___ | 8. Wrap the sleeve snugly around the patient's leg so that two fingers fit between the leg and the sleeve. Secure the sleeve with the Velcro fasteners. Repeat for the second leg, if bilateral therapy is ordered. Connect each sleeve to the tubing, following manufacturer's recommendations. | |
| ___ | ___ | ___ | 9. Set the pump to the prescribed maximal pressure (usually 35 to 55 mm Hg). Make sure the tubing is free from kinks. Check that the patient can move about without interrupting the airflow. Turn on the pump. Initiate cooling setting, if available. | |
| ___ | ___ | ___ | 10. *Observe the patient and the device during the first cycle. Check the audible alarms. Check the sleeves and pump at least once per shift or per facility policy.* | |

| Excellent | Satisfactory | Needs Practice | | Comments |
|---|---|---|---|---|

SKILL 9-12

## Applying Pneumatic Compression Devices *(Continued)*

| Excellent | Satisfactory | Needs Practice | | Comments |
|---|---|---|---|---|
| ___ | ___ | ___ | 11. Place the bed in the lowest position. Make sure the call bell and other necessary items are within easy reach. | |
| ___ | ___ | ___ | 12. Remove PPE, if used. Perform hand hygiene. | |
| ___ | ___ | ___ | 13. Assess the extremities for peripheral pulses, edema, changes in sensation, and movement. Remove the sleeves and assess and document skin integrity every 8 hours. | |

*Skill Checklists for Taylor's Clinical Nursing Skills:*
*A Nursing Process Approach, 3rd edition*

Name _____  Date _____

Unit _____  Position _____

Instructor/Evaluator: _____  Position _____

| Excellent | Satisfactory | Needs Practice | SKILL 9-13<br>**Applying a Continuous Passive Motion Device** | |
|---|---|---|---|---|
| | | | **Goal:** The patient experiences increased joint mobility. | **Comments** |
| —— | —— | —— | 1. Review the medical record and nursing plan of care for the appropriate degrees of flexion and extension, the cycle rate, and the length of time the CPM is to be used. | |
| —— | —— | —— | 2. Obtain equipment. Apply the soft goods to the CPM device. | |
| —— | —— | —— | 3. Perform hand hygiene. Put on PPE, as indicated. | |
| —— | —— | —— | 4. Identify the patient. Explain the procedure to the patient. | |
| —— | —— | —— | 5. Close curtains around bed and close the door to the room, if possible. Place the bed at an appropriate and comfortable working height, usually elbow height of the caregiver (VISN 8 Patient Safety Center, 2009). | |
| —— | —— | —— | 6. Using the tape measure, determine the distance between the gluteal crease and the popliteal space. | |
| —— | —— | —— | 7. Measure the leg from the knee to 14 inches beyond the bottom of the foot. | |
| —— | —— | —— | 8. Position the patient in the middle of the bed. The affected extremity should be in a slightly abducted position. | |
| —— | —— | —— | 9. Support the affected extremity and elevate it, placing it in the padded CPM device. | |
| —— | —— | —— | 10. *Make sure the knee is at the hinged joint of the CPM device.* | |
| —— | —— | —— | 11. *Adjust the footplate to maintain the patient's foot in a neutral position. Assess the patient's position to make sure the leg is not internally or externally rotated.* | |
| —— | —— | —— | 12. Apply the restraining straps under the CPM device and around the leg. *Check that two fingers fit between the strap and the leg.* | |
| —— | —— | —— | 13. Explain the use of the STOP/GO button to the patient. Set the controls to the prescribed levels of flexion and extension and cycles per minute. Turn on the power to the CPM. | |
| —— | —— | —— | 14. Set the device to ON and start the therapy by pressing the GO button. Observe the patient and the device during the first cycle. Determine the angle of flexion when the device reaches its greatest height using the goniometer. Compare with prescribed degree. | |

SKILL 9-13

# Applying a Continuous Passive Motion Device *(Continued)*

| Excellent | Satisfactory | Needs Practice | | Comments |
|---|---|---|---|---|
| —— | —— | —— | 15. Check the patient's level of comfort and perform skin and neurovascular assessments at least every 8 hours or per facility policy. | |
| —— | —— | —— | 16. Place the bed in the lowest position, with the side rails up. Make sure the call bell and other necessary items are within easy reach. | |
| —— | —— | —— | 17. Remove PPE, if used. Perform hand hygiene. | |

*Skill Checklists for Taylor's Clinical Nursing Skills:*
*A Nursing Process Approach, 3rd edition*

Name _____ Date _____

Unit _____ Position _____

Instructor/Evaluator: _____ Position _____

| Excellent | Satisfactory | Needs Practice | SKILL 9-14 **Applying a Sling** | Comments |
|---|---|---|---|---|
| | | | **Goal:** The arm is immobilized, and the patient maintains muscle strength and joint range of motion. | |
| ____ | ____ | ____ | 1. Review the medical record and nursing plan of care to determine the need for the use of a sling. | |
| ____ | ____ | ____ | 2. Perform hand hygiene. Put on PPE, as indicated. | |
| ____ | ____ | ____ | 3. Identify the patient. Explain the procedure to the patient. | |
| ____ | ____ | ____ | 4. Close curtains around bed and close the door to the room, if possible. Place the bed at an appropriate and comfortable working height, if necessary. | |
| ____ | ____ | ____ | 5. Assist the patient to a sitting position. Place the patient's forearm across the chest with the elbow flexed and the palm against the chest. Measure the sleeve length, if indicated. | |
| ____ | ____ | ____ | 6. Enclose the arm in the sling, making sure the elbow fits into the corner of the fabric. Run the strap up the patient's back and across the shoulder opposite the injury, then down the chest to the fastener on the end of the sling. | |
| ____ | ____ | ____ | 7. Place the ABD pad under the strap, between the strap and the patient's neck. *Ensure that the sling and forearm are slightly elevated and at a right angle to the body.* | |
| ____ | ____ | ____ | 8. Place the bed in the lowest position, with the side rails up. Make sure the call bell and other necessary items are within easy reach. | |
| ____ | ____ | ____ | 9. Remove PPE, if used. Perform hand hygiene. | |
| ____ | ____ | ____ | 10. Check the patient's level of comfort, arm positioning, and neurovascular status of the affected limb every 4 hours or according to facility policy. Assess the axillary and cervical skin frequently for irritation or breakdown. | |

*Skill Checklists for Taylor's Clinical Nursing Skills:*
*A Nursing Process Approach, 3rd edition*

Name _____  Date _____

Unit _____  Position _____

Instructor/Evaluator: _____  Position _____

SKILL 9-15

# Applying a Figure-Eight Bandage

| Excellent | Satisfactory | Needs Practice | **Goal:** The bandage is applied correctly without injury or complications. | Comments |
|-----------|--------------|----------------|------------------------------------------------------------------------------|----------|
| ____ | ____ | ____ | 1. Review the medical record and nursing plan of care to determine the need for a figure-eight bandage. | |
| ____ | ____ | ____ | 2. Perform hand hygiene. Put on PPE, as indicated. | |
| ____ | ____ | ____ | 3. Identify the patient. Explain the procedure to the patient. | |
| ____ | ____ | ____ | 4. Close curtains around bed and close the door to the room, if possible. Place the bed at an appropriate and comfortable working height, usually elbow height of the caregiver (VISN 8 Patient Safety Center, 2009). | |
| ____ | ____ | ____ | 5. Assist the patient to a comfortable position, with the affected body part in a normal functioning position. | |
| ____ | ____ | ____ | 6. Hold the bandage roll with the roll facing upward in one hand while holding the free end of the roll in the other hand. Make sure to hold the bandage roll so it is close to the affected body part. | |
| ____ | ____ | ____ | 7. Wrap the bandage around the limb twice, below the joint, to anchor it. | |
| ____ | ____ | ____ | 8. Use alternating ascending and descending turns to form a figure eight. Overlap each turn of the bandage by one-half to two-thirds the width of the strip. | |
| ____ | ____ | ____ | 9. *Unroll the bandage as you wrap, not before wrapping.* | |
| ____ | ____ | ____ | 10. *Wrap firmly, but not tightly. Assess the patient's comfort as you wrap. If the patient reports tingling, itching, numbness, or pain, loosen the bandage.* | |
| ____ | ____ | ____ | 11. After the area is covered, wrap the bandage around the limb twice, above the joint, to anchor it. Secure the end of the bandage with tape, pins, or self-closures. Avoid metal clips. | |
| ____ | ____ | ____ | 12. Place the bed in the lowest position, with the side rails up. Make sure the call bell and other necessary items are within easy reach. | |
| ____ | ____ | ____ | 13. Remove PPE, if used. Perform hand hygiene. | |
| ____ | ____ | ____ | 14. Elevate the wrapped extremity for 15 to 30 minutes after application of the bandage. | |

SKILL 9-15

# Applying a Figure-Eight Bandage *(Continued)*

| Excellent | Satisfactory | Needs Practice | | Comments |
|---|---|---|---|---|
| ―― | ―― | ―― | 15. Assess the distal circulation after the bandage is in place. | |
| ―― | ―― | ―― | 16. Lift the distal end of the bandage and assess the skin for color, temperature, and integrity. Assess for pain and perform a neurovascular assessment of the affected extremity after applying the bandage and at least every 4 hours, or per facility policy. | |
| ―― | ―― | ―― | 17. Perform hand hygiene. | |

*Skill Checklists for Taylor's Clinical Nursing Skills:*
*A Nursing Process Approach, 3rd edition*

Name _____  Date _____

Unit _____  Position _____

Instructor/Evaluator: _____  Position _____

## SKILL 9-16
# Assisting With Cast Application

| Excellent | Satisfactory | Needs Practice | **Goal:** The cast is applied without interfering with neurovascular function; and patient demonstrates signs of healing. | **Comments** |
|---|---|---|---|---|
| —— | —— | —— | 1. Review the medical record and medical orders to determine the need for the cast. | |
| —— | —— | —— | 2. Perform hand hygiene. Put on gloves and/or other PPE, as indicated. | |
| —— | —— | —— | 3. Identify the patient. Explain the procedure to the patient and verify area to be casted. | |
| —— | —— | —— | 4. Perform a pain assessment and assess for muscle spasm. Administer prescribed medications in sufficient time to allow for the full effect of the analgesic and/or muscle relaxant. | |
| —— | —— | —— | 5. Close curtains around bed and close the door to the room, if possible. Place the bed at an appropriate and comfortable working height, if necessary. | |
| —— | —— | —— | 6. Position the patient as needed, depending on the type of cast being applied and the location of the injury. Support the extremity or body part to be casted. | |
| —— | —— | —— | 7. Drape the patient with the waterproof pads. | |
| —— | —— | —— | 8. Cleanse and dry the affected body part. | |
| —— | —— | —— | 9. Position and maintain the affected body part in the position indicated by the physician as the stockinette, sheet wadding, and padding is applied. The stockinette should extend beyond the ends of the cast. As the wadding is applied, check for wrinkles. | |
| —— | —— | —— | 10. Continue to position and maintain the affected body part in the position indicated by the physician or advanced practice professional as the casting material is applied. Assist with finishing by folding the stockinette or other padding down over the outer edge of the cast. | |
| —— | —— | —— | 11. *Support the cast during hardening.* Handle hardening plaster casts with the palms of hands, not fingers. Support the cast on a firm, smooth surface. Do not rest it on a hard surface or sharp edges. Avoid placing pressure on the cast. | |
| —— | —— | —— | 12. *Elevate the injured limb above heart level with pillow or bath blankets, as ordered, making sure pressure is evenly distributed under the cast.* | |

SKILL 9-16

# Assisting With Cast Application *(Continued)*

| Excellent | Satisfactory | Needs Practice | | Comments |
|---|---|---|---|---|
| —— | —— | —— | 13. Place the bed in the lowest position, with the side rails up. Make sure the call bell and other necessary items are within easy reach. | |
| —— | —— | —— | 14. Remove gloves and any other PPE, if used. Perform hand hygiene. | |
| —— | —— | —— | 15. Obtain x-rays, as ordered. | |
| —— | —— | —— | 16. Instruct the patient to report pain, odor, drainage, changes in sensation, abnormal sensation, or the inability to move fingers or toes of the affected extremity. | |
| —— | —— | —— | 17. Leave the cast uncovered and exposed to the air. Reposition the patient every 2 hours. Depending on facility policy, a fan may be used to dry the cast. | |

*Skill Checklists for Taylor's Clinical Nursing Skills:*
*A Nursing Process Approach, 3rd edition*

Name _____ Date _____

Unit _____ Position _____

Instructor/Evaluator: _____ Position _____

SKILL 9-17

# Caring for a Cast

| Excellent | Satisfactory | Needs Practice | | Comments |
|---|---|---|---|---|

**Goal:** The cast remains intact, and the patient does not experience neurovascular compromise.

| | | | |
|---|---|---|---|
| —— —— —— | 1. Review the medical record and the nursing plan of care to determine the need for cast care and care for the affected body part. | |
| —— —— —— | 2. Perform hand hygiene. Put on PPE, as indicated. | |
| —— —— —— | 3. Identify the patient. Explain the procedure to the patient. | |
| —— —— —— | 4. Close curtains around bed and close the door to the room, if possible. Place the bed at an appropriate and comfortable working height, if necessary. | |
| —— —— —— | 5. If a plaster cast was applied, handle the casted extremity or body area with the palms of your hands for the first 24 to 36 hours, until the cast is fully dry. | |
| —— —— —— | 6. If the cast is on an extremity, elevate the affected area on pillows covered with waterproof pads. *Maintain the normal curvatures and angles of the cast.* | |
| —— —— —— | 7. Keep cast (plaster) uncovered until fully dry. | |
| —— —— —— | 8. Assess the condition of the cast. Be alert for cracks, dents, or the presence of drainage from the cast. Perform skin and neurovascular assessments according to facility policy, as often as every 1 to 2 hours. *Check for pain, edema, inability to move body parts distal to the cast, pallor, pulses, and abnormal sensations. If the cast is on an extremity, compare it with the uncasted extremity.* | |
| —— —— —— | 9. If breakthrough bleeding or drainage is noted on the cast, mark the area on the cast, according to facility policy. Indicate the date and time next to the area. Follow physician orders or facility policy regarding the amount of drainage that needs to be reported to the physician. | |
| —— —— —— | 10. Assess for signs of infection. Monitor the patient's temperature. Assess for a foul odor from the cast, increased pain, or extreme warmth over an area of the cast. | |

# Caring for a Cast *(Continued)*

| Excellent | Satisfactory | Needs Practice | | Comments |
|---|---|---|---|---|
| —— | —— | —— | 11. Reposition the patient every 2 hours. Provide back and skin care frequently. Encourage range-of-motion exercises for unaffected joints. Encourage the patient to cough and deep breathe. | |
| —— | —— | —— | 12. Instruct the patient to report pain, odor, drainage, changes in sensation, abnormal sensation, or the inability to move fingers or toes of the affected extremity. | |
| —— | —— | —— | 13. Remove PPE, if used. Place bed in lowest position. Perform hand hygiene. | |

*Skill Checklists for Taylor's Clinical Nursing Skills:*
*A Nursing Process Approach, 3rd edition*

Name _____     Date _____

Unit _____     Position _____

Instructor/Evaluator: _____     Position _____

## SKILL 9-18
# Applying Skin Traction and Caring for a Patient in Skin Traction

**Goal:** The traction is maintained with the appropriate counterbalance and the patient is free from complications of immobility.

| Excellent | Satisfactory | Needs Practice | | Comments |
|---|---|---|---|---|
| —— | —— | —— | 1. Review the medical record and the nursing plan of care to determine the type of traction being used and care for the affected body part. | |
| —— | —— | —— | 2. Perform hand hygiene. Put on PPE, as indicated. | |
| —— | —— | —— | 3. Identify the patient. Explain the procedure to the patient, emphasizing the importance of maintaining counterbalance, alignment, and position. | |
| —— | —— | —— | 4. Perform a pain assessment and assess for muscle spasm. Administer prescribed medications in sufficient time to allow for the full effect of the analgesic and/or muscle relaxant. | |
| —— | —— | —— | 5. Close curtains around bed and close the door to the room, if possible. Place the bed at an appropriate and comfortable working height. | |
| | | | **Applying Skin Traction** | |
| —— | —— | —— | 6. Ensure the traction apparatus is attached securely to the bed. Assess the traction setup. | |
| —— | —— | —— | 7. Check that the ropes move freely through the pulleys. Check that all knots are tight and are positioned away from the pulleys. Pulleys should be free from the linens. | |
| —— | —— | —— | 8. Place the patient in a supine position with the foot of the bed elevated slightly. The patient's head should be near the head of the bed and in alignment. | |
| —— | —— | —— | 9. Cleanse the affected area. Place the elastic stocking on the affected limb, as appropriate. | |
| —— | —— | —— | 10. Place the traction boot over the patient's leg. Be sure the patient's heel is in the heel of the boot. Secure the boot with the straps. | |
| —— | —— | —— | 11. Attach the traction cord to the footplate of the boot. Pass the rope over the pulley fastened at the end of the bed. Attach the weight to the hook on the rope, usually 5 to 10 pounds for an adult. Gently let go of the weight. *The weight should hang freely, not touching the bed or the floor.* | |
| —— | —— | —— | 12. *Check the patient's alignment with the traction.* | |

SKILL 9-18

# Applying Skin Traction and Caring for a Patient in Skin Traction *(Continued)*

| Excellent | Satisfactory | Needs Practice | | Comments |
|---|---|---|---|---|

| | | | | |
|---|---|---|---|---|
| ___ | ___ | ___ | 13. *Check the boot for placement and alignment. Make sure the line of pull is parallel to the bed and not angled downward.* | |
| ___ | ___ | ___ | 14. Place the bed in the lowest position that still allows the weight to hang freely. | |
| ___ | ___ | ___ | 15. Remove PPE, if used. Perform hand hygiene. | |

**Caring for a Patient With Skin Traction**

| | | | | |
|---|---|---|---|---|
| ___ | ___ | ___ | 16. Perform a skin-traction assessment per facility policy. This assessment includes checking the traction equipment, examining the affected body part, maintaining proper body alignment, and performing skin and neurovascular assessments. | |
| ___ | ___ | ___ | 17. Remove the straps every 4 hours per the physician's order or facility policy. Check bony prominences for skin breakdown, abrasions, and pressure areas. Remove the boot, per physician's order or facility policy, every 8 hours. Put on gloves and wash, rinse, and thoroughly dry the skin. | |
| ___ | ___ | ___ | 18. Assess the extremity distal to the traction for edema, and assess peripheral pulses. Assess the temperature, color, and capillary refill, and compare with the unaffected limb. Check for pain, inability to move body parts distal to the traction, pallor, and abnormal sensations. Assess for indicators of deep-vein thrombosis, including calf tenderness, and swelling. | |
| ___ | ___ | ___ | 19. Replace the traction and remove gloves and dispose of them appropriately. | |
| ___ | ___ | ___ | 20. Check the boot for placement and alignment. *Make sure the line of pull is parallel to the bed and not angled downward.* | |
| ___ | ___ | ___ | 21. *Ensure the patient is positioned in the center of the bed, with the affected leg aligned with the trunk of the patient's body.* | |
| ___ | ___ | ___ | 22. Examine the weights and pulley system. *Weights should hang freely, off the floor and bed. Knots should be secure. Ropes should move freely through the pulleys. The pulleys should not be constrained by knots.* | |
| ___ | ___ | ___ | 23. Perform range-of-motion exercises on all unaffected joint areas, unless contraindicated. Encourage the patient to cough and deep breathe every 2 hours. | |
| ___ | ___ | ___ | 24. Raise the side rails. Place the bed in the lowest position that still allows the weight to hang freely. | |
| ___ | ___ | ___ | 25. Remove PPE, if used. Perform hand hygiene. | |

*Skill Checklists for Taylor's Clinical Nursing Skills:*
*A Nursing Process Approach, 3rd edition*

Name _____   Date _____

Unit _____   Position _____

Instructor/Evaluator: _____   Position _____

| Excellent | Satisfactory | Needs Practice | SKILL 9-19<br>**Caring for a Patient in Skeletal Traction** | Comments |
|---|---|---|---|---|
| | | | **Goal:** The traction is maintained with the appropriate counterbalance and the patient is free from complications of immobility. | |
| —— | —— | —— | 1. Review the medical record and the nursing plan of care to determine the type of traction being used and the prescribed care. | |
| —— | —— | —— | 2. Perform hand hygiene. Put on PPE, as indicated. | |
| —— | —— | —— | 3. Identify the patient. Explain the procedure to the patient, emphasizing the importance of maintaining counterbalance, alignment, and position. | |
| —— | —— | —— | 4. Perform a pain assessment and assess for muscle spasm. Administer prescribed medications in sufficient time to allow for the full effect of the analgesic and/or muscle relaxant. | |
| —— | —— | —— | 5. Close curtains around bed and close the door to the room, if possible. Place the bed at an appropriate and comfortable working height. | |
| —— | —— | —— | 6. Ensure the traction apparatus is attached securely to the bed. Assess the traction setup, including application of the ordered amount of weight. *Be sure that the weights hang freely, not touching the bed or the floor.* | |
| —— | —— | —— | 7. *Check that the ropes move freely through the pulleys. Check that all knots are tight and are positioned away from the pulleys. Pulleys should be free from the linens.* | |
| —— | —— | —— | 8. Check the alignment of the patient's body, as prescribed. | |
| —— | —— | —— | 9. Perform a skin assessment. Pay attention to pressure points, including the ischial tuberosity, popliteal space, Achilles' tendon, sacrum, and heel. | |
| —— | —— | —— | 10. Perform a neurovascular assessment. Assess the extremity distal to the traction for edema and peripheral pulses. Assess the temperature and color and compare with the unaffected limb. Check for pain, inability to move body parts distal to the traction, pallor, and abnormal sensations. Assess for indicators of deep-vein thrombosis, including calf tenderness, and swelling. | |
| —— | —— | —— | 11. Assess the site at and around the pins for redness, edema, and odor. Assess for skin tenting, prolonged or purulent drainage, elevated body temperature, elevated pin site temperature, and bowing or bending of the pins. | |

# Caring for a Patient in Skeletal Traction *(Continued)*

| Excellent | Satisfactory | Needs Practice | | Comments |
|---|---|---|---|---|
| —— | —— | —— | 12. Provide pin site care. | |
| —— | —— | —— |    a. Using sterile technique, open the applicator package and pour the cleansing agent into the sterile container. | |
| —— | —— | —— |    b. Put on the sterile gloves. | |
| —— | —— | —— |    c. Place the applicators into the solution. | |
| —— | —— | —— |    d. *Clean the pin site starting at the insertion area and working outward, away from the pin site.* | |
| —— | —— | —— |    e. *Use each applicator once. Use a new applicator for each pin site.* | |
| —— | —— | —— | 13. Depending on physician order and facility policy, apply the antimicrobial ointment to pin sites and apply a dressing. | |
| —— | —— | —— | 14. Remove gloves and any other PPE, if used. Perform hand hygiene. | |
| —— | —— | —— | 15. Perform range-of-motion exercises on all joint areas, unless contraindicated. Encourage the patient to cough and deep breathe every 2 hours. | |

*Skill Checklists for Taylor's Clinical Nursing Skills:*
*A Nursing Process Approach, 3rd edition*

Name _____  Date _____

Unit _____  Position _____

Instructor/Evaluator: _____  Position _____

## SKILL 9-20
# Caring for a Patient With an External Fixation Device

**Goal:** The patient shows no evidence of complication, such as infection, contractures, venous stasis, thrombus formation, or skin breakdown.

| Excellent | Satisfactory | Needs Practice | | Comments |
|---|---|---|---|---|
| ___ | ___ | ___ | 1. Review the medical record and the nursing plan of care to determine the type of device being used and prescribed care. | |
| ___ | ___ | ___ | 2. Perform hand hygiene. Put on PPE, as indicated. | |
| ___ | ___ | ___ | 3. Identify the patient. Explain the procedure to the patient. Assure the patient that there will be little pain after the fixation device is in place. Reinforce that the patient will be able to adjust to the device and will be able to move about with the device, allowing him or her to resume normal activities more quickly. | |
| ___ | ___ | ___ | 4. *After the fixation device is in place, apply ice to the surgical site, as ordered or per facility policy. Elevate the affected body part, if appropriate.* | |
| ___ | ___ | ___ | 5. Perform a pain assessment and assess for muscle spasm. Administer prescribed medications in sufficient time to allow for the full effect of the analgesic and/or muscle relaxant. | |
| ___ | ___ | ___ | 6. Administer analgesics, as ordered, before exercising or mobilizing the affected body part. | |
| ___ | ___ | ___ | 7. Perform neurovascular assessments, per facility policy or physician's order, usually every 2 to 4 hours for 24 hours, then every 4 to 8 hours. Assess the affected body part for color, motion, sensation, edema, capillary refill, and pulses. If appropriate, compare with the unaffected side. Assess for pain not relieved by analgesics, and for burning, tingling, and numbness. | |
| ___ | ___ | ___ | 8. Close curtains around bed and close the door to the room, if possible. Place the bed at an appropriate and comfortable working height, usually elbow height of the caregiver (VISN 8 Patient Safety Center, 2009). | |
| ___ | ___ | ___ | 9. Assess the pin site for redness, tenting of the skin, prolonged or purulent drainage, swelling, and bowing, bending, or loosening of the pins. Monitor body temperature. | |

# Caring for a Patient With an External Fixation Device *(Continued)*

| Excellent | Satisfactory | Needs Practice | | Comments |
|---|---|---|---|---|
| —— | —— | —— | 10. Perform pin site care. | |
| —— | —— | —— |    a. Using sterile technique, open the applicator package and pour the cleansing agent into the sterile container. | |
| —— | —— | —— |    b. Put on the sterile gloves. | |
| —— | —— | —— |    c. Place the applicators into the solution. | |
| —— | —— | —— |    d. *Clean the pin site starting at the insertion area and working outward, away from the pin site.* | |
| —— | —— | —— |    e. *Use each applicator once. Use a new applicator for each pin site.* | |
| —— | —— | —— | 11. Depending on physician order and facility policy, apply the antimicrobial ointment to pin sites and apply a dressing. | |
| —— | —— | —— | 12. Place the bed in the lowest position, with the side rails up. Make sure the call bell and other necessary items are within easy reach. | |
| —— | —— | —— | 13. Remove gloves and any other PPE, if used. Perform hand hygiene. | |

*Skill Checklists for Taylor's Clinical Nursing Skills:*
*A Nursing Process Approach, 3rd edition*

Name _____   Date _____

Unit _____   Position _____

Instructor/Evaluator: _____   Position _____

SKILL 10-1

# Promoting Patient Comfort

| Excellent | Satisfactory | Needs Practice | **Goal:** The patient experiences relief from discomfort and/or pain without adverse effect. | Comments |
|---|---|---|---|---|
| —— | —— | —— | 1. Perform hand hygiene and put on PPE, if indicated. | |
| —— | —— | —— | 2. Identify the patient. | |
| —— | —— | —— | 3. Discuss pain with the patient, acknowledging that the patient's pain exists. Explain how pain medications and other pain management therapies work together to provide pain relief. Allow the patient to help choose interventions for pain relief. | |
| | | | 4. Assess the patient's pain, using an appropriate assessment tool and measurement scale (see Fundamentals Review 10-1 through 10-5). | |
| —— | —— | —— | 5. Provide pharmacologic interventions, if indicated and ordered. | |
| —— | —— | —— | 6. Adjust the patient's environment to promote comfort. | |
| —— | —— | —— |    a. Adjust and maintain the room temperature per the patient's preference. | |
| —— | —— | —— |    b. Reduce harsh lighting, but provide adequate lighting per the patient's preference. | |
| —— | —— | —— |    c. Reduce harsh and unnecessary noise. Avoid having conversations immediately outside the patient's room. | |
| —— | —— | —— |    d. Close room door and/or curtain whenever possible. | |
| | | |    e. Provide good ventilation in the patient's room. Reduce unpleasant odors by promptly emptying bedpans, urinals, and emesis basins after use. Remove trash and laundry promptly. | |
| —— | —— | —— | 7. Prevent unnecessary interruptions and coordinate patient activities to group activities together. Allow for and plan rest periods without disturbance. | |
| —— | —— | —— | 8. Assist the patient to change position frequently. Assist the patient to a comfortable position, maintaining good alignment and supporting extremities as needed. Raise the head of the bed as appropriate. (See Chapter 9, Activity, for more information on positioning.) | |

# Promoting Patient Comfort *(Continued)*

| Excellent | Satisfactory | Needs Practice | | Comments |
|---|---|---|---|---|

—— —— ——  9. Provide oral hygiene as often as necessary to keep the mouth and mucous membranes clean and moist, as often as every 1 or 2 hours if necessary. This is especially important for patients who cannot drink or are not permitted fluids by mouth. (See Chapter 7, Hygiene, for additional information about mouth care.)

—— —— —— 10. Ensure the availability of appropriate fluids for drinking, unless contraindicated. Make sure the patient's water pitcher is filled and within reach. Make other fluids of the patient's choice available.

—— —— —— 11. Remove physical situations that might cause discomfort.

—— —— ——      a. Change soiled and/or wet dressings; replace soiled and/or wet bed linens.

—— —— ——      b. Smooth wrinkles in bed linens.

—— —— ——      c. Ensure patient is not lying or sitting on tubes, tubing, wires, or other equipment.

—— —— —— 12. Assist the patient as necessary with ambulation, and active or passive range-of-motion exercises, as appropriate. (See Chapter 9, Activity, for more information about activity.)

—— —— —— 13. Assess the patient's spirituality needs related to the pain experience. Ask the patient if he/she would like a spiritual counselor to visit.

—— —— —— 14. Consider the use of distraction. Distraction requires the patient to focus on something other than the pain.

—— —— ——      a. Have the patient recall a pleasant experience or focus attention on an enjoyable experience.

—— —— ——      b. Offer age or developmentally appropriate games, toys, books, audiobooks, access to television, and/or videos, or other items of interest to the patient.

—— —— ——      c. Encourage the patient to hold or stroke a loved person, pet, or toy.

—— —— ——      d. Offer access to music the patient prefers. Turn on the music when pain begins, or before anticipated painful stimuli. The patient can close his or her eyes and concentrate on listening. Raising or lowering the volume as pain increases or decreases can be helpful.

—— —— —— 15. Consider the use of guided imagery.

—— —— ——      a. Help the patient to identify a scene or experience that the patient describes as happy, pleasant, or peaceful.

| Excellent | Satisfactory | Needs Practice | SKILL 10-1 **Promoting Patient Comfort** *(Continued)* | Comments |
|---|---|---|---|---|
| —— | —— | —— | b. Encourage the patient to begin with several minutes of focused breathing, relaxation, or meditation. (Refer to specific information in steps 15 and 16.) | |
| —— | —— | —— | c. Help the patient concentrate on the peaceful, pleasant image. | |
| —— | —— | —— | d. If indicated, read a description of the identified scene or experience, using a soothing, soft voice. | |
| —— | —— | —— | e. Encourage the patient to concentrate on the details of the image, such as its sight, sounds, smells, tastes, and touch. | |
| —— | —— | —— | 16. Consider the use of relaxation activities, such as deep breathing. | |
| —— | —— | —— | a. Have the patient sit or recline comfortably and place hands on stomach. Close the eyes. | |
| —— | —— | —— | b. Ask the patient to mentally count to maintain a comfortable rate and rhythm. Have the patient inhale slowly and deeply while letting the abdomen expand as much as possible. Have the patient hold his or her breath for a few seconds. | |
| —— | —— | —— | c. Tell the patient to exhale slowly through mouth, blowing through puckered lips. Have the patient continue to count to maintain comfortable rate and rhythm, concentrating on the rise and fall of abdomen. | |
| —— | —— | —— | d. When the patient's abdomen feels empty, have the patient begin again with a deep inhalation. | |
| —— | —— | —— | e. Encourage patient to practice at least twice a day, for 10 minutes, and then use as needed to assist with pain management (Schaffer & Yucha, 2004). | |
| —— | —— | —— | 17. Consider the use of relaxation activities, such as progressive muscle relaxation. | |
| —— | —— | —— | a. Assist the patient to a comfortable position. | |
| —— | —— | —— | b. Direct the patient to focus on a particular muscle group. Start with the muscles of the jaw, then repeat with the muscles of the neck, shoulder, upper and lower arm, hand, abdomin, buttocks, thigh, lower leg, and foot. | |
| —— | —— | —— | c. Ask the patient to tighten the muscle group and note the sensation that the tightened muscles produce. After 5 to 7 seconds, tell the patient to relax the muscles all at once and concentrate on the sensation of the relaxed state, noting the difference in feeling in the muscles when contracted and relaxed. | |

SKILL 10-1

# Promoting Patient Comfort *(Continued)*

| Excellent | Satisfactory | Needs Practice | | Comments |
|---|---|---|---|---|
| —— | —— | —— | d. Have the patient continue to tighten-hold-relax each muscle group until the entire body has been covered. | |
| —— | —— | —— | e. Encourage patient to practice at least twice a day, for 10 minutes, and then use as needed to assist with pain management (Schaffer & Yucha, 2004). | |
| —— | —— | —— | 18. Consider the use of cutaneous stimulation, such as the intermittent application of heat or cold, or both. (See Chapter 8, Skin Integrity and Wound Care, for additional information on heat and cold therapy.) | |
| —— | —— | —— | 19. Consider the use of cutaneous stimulation, such as massage (see Skill 10-2). | |
| —— | —— | —— | 20. Discuss the potential for use of cutaneous stimulation, such as TENS, with the patient and primary care provider. (See Skill 10-3.) | |
| —— | —— | —— | 21. Remove equipment and return patient to a position of comfort. Remove gloves, if used. Raise side rail and lower bed. | |
| —— | —— | —— | 22. Remove additional PPE, if used. Perform hand hygiene. | |
| —— | —— | —— | 23. Evaluate the patient's response to interventions. Reassess level of discomfort or pain using original assessment tools. Reassess and alter plan of care as appropriate. | |

*Skill Checklists for Taylor's Clinical Nursing Skills:*
*A Nursing Process Approach, 3rd edition*

Name _____  Date _____

Unit _____  Position _____

Instructor/Evaluator: _____  Position _____

## SKILL 10-2

# Giving a Back Massage

**Goal:** The patient reports increased comfort and decreased pain and exhibits a relaxed state.

| Excellent | Satisfactory | Needs Practice | | Comments |
|---|---|---|---|---|
| ___ | ___ | ___ | 1. Perform hand hygiene and put on PPE, if indicated. | |
| ___ | ___ | ___ | 2. Identify the patient. | |
| ___ | ___ | ___ | 3. Offer a back massage to the patient and explain the procedure. | |
| ___ | ___ | ___ | 4. Put on gloves, if indicated. | |
| ___ | ___ | ___ | 5. Close room door and/or curtain. | |
| ___ | ___ | ___ | 6. Assess the patient's pain, using an appropriate assessment tool and measurement scale. (See Fundamentals Review 10-1 through 10-6.) | |
| ___ | ___ | ___ | 7. Raise the bed to a comfortable working position, usually elbow height of the caregiver (VISN 8 Patient Safety Center, 2009), and lower the side rail. | |
| ___ | ___ | ___ | 8. Assist the patient to a comfortable position, preferably the prone or side-lying position. Remove the covers and move the patient's gown just enough to expose the patient's back from the shoulders to sacral area. Drape the patient, as needed, with the bath blanket. | |
| ___ | ___ | ___ | 9. Warm the lubricant or lotion in the palm of your hand, or place the container in small basin of warm water. *During massage, observe the patient's skin for reddened or open areas. Pay particular attention to the skin over bony prominences.* (See Chapter 8, Skin Integrity and Wound Care, for detailed information regarding skin assessment.) | |
| ___ | ___ | ___ | 10. Using light, gliding strokes (*effleurage*), apply lotion to patient's shoulders, back, and sacral area. | |
| ___ | ___ | ___ | 11. Place your hands beside each other at the base of the patient's spine and stroke upward to the shoulders and back downward to the buttocks in slow, continuous strokes. Continue for several minutes. | |
| ___ | ___ | ___ | 12. Massage the patient's shoulder, entire back, areas over iliac crests, and sacrum with circular stroking motions. *Keep your hands in contact with the patient's skin.* Continue for several minutes, applying additional lotion, as necessary. | |

# Giving a Back Massage *(Continued)*

| Excellent | Satisfactory | Needs Practice | | Comments |
|-----------|--------------|----------------|---|---------|
| —— | —— | —— | 13. Knead the patient's skin by gently alternating grasping and compression motions (*pétrissage*). | |
| —— | —— | —— | 14. Complete the massage with additional long, stroking movements that eventually become lighter in pressure. | |
| —— | —— | —— | 15. Use the towel to pat the patient dry and to remove excess lotion. | |
| —— | —— | —— | 16. Remove gloves, if worn. Reposition patient's gown and covers. Raise side rail and lower bed. Assist patient to a position of comfort. | |
| —— | —— | —— | 17. Remove additional PPE, if used. Perform hand hygiene. | |
| —— | —— | —— | 18. Evaluate the patient's response to interventions. Reassess level of discomfort or pain using original assessment tools. Reassess and alter plan of care, as appropriate. | |

*Skill Checklists for Taylor's Clinical Nursing Skills:*
*A Nursing Process Approach, 3rd edition*

Name _____  Date _____

Unit _____  Position _____

Instructor/Evaluator: _____  Position _____

SKILL 10-3

# Applying and Caring for a Patient Using a TENS Unit

**Goal:** The patient reports increased comfort and decreased pain; and is free from injury, skin irritation or breakdown.

| Excellent | Satisfactory | Needs Practice | | Comments |
|---|---|---|---|---|
| ___ | ___ | ___ | 1. Perform hand hygiene and put on PPE, if indicated. | |
| ___ | ___ | ___ | 2. Identify the patient. | |
| ___ | ___ | ___ | 3. Show the patient the device, and explain its function and the reason for its use. | |
| ___ | ___ | ___ | 4. Assess the patient's pain, using an appropriate assessment tool and measurement scale. (See Fundamentals Review 10-1 through 10-6.) | |
| ___ | ___ | ___ | 5. Inspect the area where the electrodes are to be placed. Clean the patient's skin, using skin cleanser and water. Dry the area thoroughly. | |
| ___ | ___ | ___ | 6. Remove the adhesive backing from the electrodes and apply them to the specified location. *If the electrodes are not pregelled, apply a small amount of electrode gel to the bottom of each electrode.* If the electrodes are not self-adhering, tape them in place. | |
| ___ | ___ | ___ | 7. *Check the placement of the electrodes; leave at least a 2" (5 cm) space (about the width of one electrode) between them.* | |
| ___ | ___ | ___ | 8. *Check the controls on the TENS unit to make sure that they are off.* Connect the wires to the electrodes (if not already attached) and plug them into the unit. | |
| ___ | ___ | ___ | 9. Turn on the unit and adjust the intensity setting to the lowest intensity and determine if the patient can feel a tingling, burning, or buzzing sensation. Then adjust the intensity to the prescribed amount or the setting most comfortable for the patient. Secure the unit to the patient. | |
| ___ | ___ | ___ | 10. Set the pulse width (duration of the each pulsation) as indicated or recommended. | |
| ___ | ___ | ___ | 11. Assess the patient's pain level during therapy. | |
| ___ | ___ | ___ |    a. If intermittent use is ordered, turn the unit off after the specified duration of treatment and remove the electrodes. Provide skin care to the area. | |

| Excellent | Satisfactory | Needs Practice | | Comments |
|---|---|---|---|---|
| | | | **SKILL 10-3** <br> **Applying and Caring for a Patient Using a** <br> **TENS Unit** *(Continued)* | |
| ___ | ___ | ___ | b. If continuous therapy is ordered, periodically remove the electrodes from the skin (after turning the unit off) to inspect the area and clean the skin, according to facility policy. Reapply the electrodes and continue therapy. Change the electrodes according to manufacturer's directions. | |
| ___ | ___ | ___ | 12. When therapy is discontinued, turn the unit off and remove the electrodes. Clean the patient's skin. Clean the unit and replace the batteries. | |
| ___ | ___ | ___ | 13. Remove PPE, if used. Perform hand hygiene. | |

*Skill Checklists for Taylor's Clinical Nursing Skills:*
*A Nursing Process Approach, 3rd edition*

Name _____  Date _____

Unit _____  Position _____

Instructor/Evaluator: _____  Position _____

### SKILL 10-4

# Caring for a Patient Receiving Patient-Controlled Analgesia

**Goal:** The patient reports increased comfort and decreased pain; and shows no signs of adverse effects, oversedation, or respiratory depression.

| Excellent | Satisfactory | Needs Practice | | Comments |
|---|---|---|---|---|
| —— | —— | —— | 1. Gather equipment. Check the medication order against the original physician's order according to agency policy. Clarify any inconsistencies. Check the patient's chart for allergies. | |
| —— | —— | —— | 2. Know the actions, special nursing considerations, safe dose ranges, purpose of administration, and adverse effects of the medications to be administered. Consider the appropriateness of the medication for this patient. | |
| —— | —— | —— | 3. Prepare the medication syringe or other container, based on facility policy, for administration. (See Chapter 5, Medications, for additional information.) | |
| —— | —— | —— | 4. Perform hand hygiene and put on PPE, if indicated. | |
| —— | —— | —— | 5. Identify the patient. | |
| —— | —— | —— | 6. Show the patient the device, and explain its function and the reason for use. Explain the purpose and action of the medication to the patient. | |
| —— | —— | —— | 7. Plug the PCA device into the electrical outlet, if necessary. Check status of battery power, if appropriate. | |
| —— | —— | —— | 8. Close the door to the room or pull the bedside curtain. | |
| —— | —— | —— | 9. Complete necessary assessments before administering medication. Check allergy bracelet or ask patient about allergies. Assess the patient's pain, using an appropriate assessment tool and measurement scale. (See Fundamentals Review 10-1 through 10-6.) | |
| —— | —— | —— | 10. ***Check the label on the prefilled drug syringe with the medication record and patient identification.*** Obtain verification of information from a second nurse, according to facility policy. If using a barcode administration system, scan the barcode on the medication label, if required. | |
| —— | —— | —— | 11. If using a barcode administration system, scan the patient's barcode on the identification band, if required. | |
| —— | —— | —— | 12. Connect tubing to prefilled syringe and place the syringe into the PCA device. ***Prime the tubing.*** | |

# Caring for a Patient Receiving
## Patient-Controlled Analgesia *(Continued)*

| Excellent | Satisfactory | Needs Practice | | Comments |
|---|---|---|---|---|
| —— | —— | —— | 13. Set the PCA device to administer the loading dose, if ordered, and then program the device based on the medical order for medication dosage, dose interval, and lockout interval. Obtain verification of information from a second nurse, according to facility policy. | |
| —— | —— | —— | 14. Put on gloves. Using antimicrobial swab, clean connection port on IV infusion line or other site access, based on route of administration. Connect the PCA tubing to the patient's IV infusion line or appropriate access site, based on the specific site used. Secure the site per facility policy and procedure. Remove gloves. Initiate the therapy by activating the appropriate button on the pump. Lock the PCA device, per facility policy. | |
| —— | —— | —— | 15. Remind the patient to press the button each time he or she needs relief from pain. | |
| —— | —— | —— | 16. Assess the patient's pain at least every 4 hours or more often, as needed. Monitor vital signs, especially respiratory status, including oxygen saturation at least every 4 hours or more often as needed. | |
| —— | —— | —— | 17. Assess the patient's sedation score and end-tidal carbon dioxide level (capnography) at least every 4 hours or more often as needed. | |
| —— | —— | —— | 18. Assess the infusion site periodically, according to facility policy and nursing judgment. Assess the patient's use of the medication, noting number of attempts and number of doses delivered. Replace the drug syringe when it is empty. | |
| —— | —— | —— | 19. Make sure the patient control (dosing button) is within the patient's reach. | |
| —— | —— | —— | 20. Remove gloves and additional PPE, if used. Perform hand hygiene. | |

*Skill Checklists for Taylor's Clinical Nursing Skills:*
*A Nursing Process Approach, 3rd edition*

Name _____  Date _____

Unit _____  Position _____

Instructor/Evaluator: _____  Position _____

SKILL 10-5

# Caring for a Patient Receiving Epidural Analgesia

**Goal:** The patient reports increased comfort and decreased pain; and shows no signs of adverse effects, oversedation, or respiratory depression.

| Excellent | Satisfactory | Needs Practice | | Comments |
|---|---|---|---|---|
| —— | —— | —— | 1. Check the medication order against the original medical order according to agency policy. Clarify any inconsistencies. Check the patient's chart for allergies. | |
| —— | —— | —— | 2. Know the actions, special nursing considerations, safe dose ranges, purpose of administration, and adverse effects of the medications to be administered. Consider the appropriateness of the medication for this patient. | |
| —— | —— | —— | 3. Prepare the medication syringe or other container, based on facility policy, for administration. (See Chapter 5, Medications, for additional information.) | |
| —— | —— | —— | 4. Perform hand hygiene and put on PPE, if indicated. | |
| —— | —— | —— | 5. Identify the patient. | |
| —— | —— | —— | 6. Show the patient the device, and explain the function of the device and reason for use. Explain the purpose and action of the medication to the patient. | |
| —— | —— | —— | 7. Close the door to the room or pull the bedside curtain. | |
| —— | —— | —— | 8. Complete necessary assessments before administering medication. Check allergy bracelet or ask patient about allergies. Assess the patient's pain, using an appropriate assessment tool and measurement scale. (See Fundamentals Review 10-1 through 10-6.) Put on gloves. | |
| —— | —— | —— | 9. *Have an ampule of 0.4 mg naloxone (Narcan) and a syringe at the bedside.* | |
| —— | —— | —— | 10. After the catheter has been inserted and the infusion initiated by the anesthesiologist or radiologist, *check the label on the medication container and rate of infusion with the medication record and patient identification.* Obtain verification of information from a second nurse, according to facility policy. If using a barcode administration system, scan the barcode on the medication label, if required. | |
| —— | —— | —— | 11. Tape all connection sites. Label the bag, tubing, and pump apparatus "For Epidural Infusion Only." *Do not administer any other narcotics or adjuvant drugs without the approval of the clinician responsible for the epidural injection.* | |

# Caring for a Patient Receiving
# Epidural Analgesia *(Continued)*

| Excellent | Satisfactory | Needs Practice | | Comments |
|---|---|---|---|---|
| — | — | — | 12. Assess the catheter exit site and apply a transparent dressing over the catheter insertion site, if not already in place. Remove gloves and additional PPE, if used. Perform hand hygiene. | |
| — | — | — | 13. Monitor the infusion rate according to facility policy. Assess and record sedation level and respiratory status every hour for the first 24 hours, then at 4-hour intervals (or according to agency policy). ***Notify the physician if the sedation rating is 3 or 4, the respiratory depth decreases, or the respiratory rate falls below 10 breaths per minute.*** | |
| — | — | — | 14. Keep the head of bed elevated 30 degrees unless contraindicated. | |
| — | — | — | 15. Assess the patient's level of pain and the effectiveness of pain relief. | |
| — | — | — | 16. Monitor urinary output and assess for bladder distention. | |
| — | — | — | 17. Assess motor strength and sensation every 4 hours. | |
| — | — | — | 18. Monitor for adverse effects (pruritus, nausea, and vomiting). | |
| — | — | — | 19. Assess for signs of infection at the insertion site. | |
| — | — | — | 20. Change the dressing over the catheter exit site every 24 to 48 hours or as needed per agency policy using aseptic technique. Change the infusion tubing every 48 hours or as specified by agency policy. | |

*Skill Checklists for Taylor's Clinical Nursing Skills:*
*A Nursing Process Approach, 3rd edition*

Name _____  Date _____

Unit _____  Position _____

Instructor/Evaluator: _____  Position _____

| Excellent | Satisfactory | Needs Practice | SKILL 10-6<br>**Caring for a Patient Receiving Continuous Wound Perfusion Pain Management** | Comments |
|---|---|---|---|---|
| | | | **Goal:** The patient reports increased comfort and/or decreased pain, without adverse effects. | |
| ___ | ___ | ___ | 1. Check the medication order against the original medical order, according to agency policy. Clarify any inconsistencies. Check the patient's chart for allergies. | |
| ___ | ___ | ___ | 2. Know the actions, special nursing considerations, safe dose ranges, purpose of administration, and adverse effects of the medications to be administered. Consider the appropriateness of the medication for this patient. | |
| ___ | ___ | ___ | 3. Perform hand hygiene and put on PPE, if indicated. | |
| ___ | ___ | ___ | 4. Identify the patient. | |
| ___ | ___ | ___ | 5. Close the door to the room or pull the bedside curtain. | |
| ___ | ___ | ___ | 6. Assess the patient's pain. Administer postoperative analgesic, as ordered. | |
| ___ | ___ | ___ | 7. Check the medication label attached to the balloon. Compare with the medical order and MAR, per facility policy. Assess the patient for perioral numbness or tingling, numbness or tingling of fingers or toes, blurred vision, ringing in the ears, metallic taste in the mouth, confusion, seizures, drowsiness, nausea and/or vomiting. Assess the patient's vital signs. | |
| ___ | ___ | ___ | 8. Put on gloves. Assess the wound perfusion system. Inspect tubing for kinks; check that the white tubing clamps are open. If tubing appears crimped, massage area on tubing to facilitate flow. Check filter in tubing, which should be unrestricted and free from tape. | |
| ___ | ___ | ___ | 9. Check the flow restrictor to ensure it is in contact with the patient's skin. Tape in place, as necessary. | |
| ___ | ___ | ___ | 10. Check the insertion site dressing. Ensure that it is intact. Assess for leakage and dislodgement. Assess for redness, warmth, swelling, pain at site, and drainage. | |
| ___ | ___ | ___ | 11. Review the device with the patient. Review the function of the device and reason for use. Reinforce the purpose and action of the medication to the patient. | |

SKILL 10-6

# Caring for a Patient Receiving Continuous Wound Perfusion Pain Management *(Continued)*

| Excellent | Satisfactory | Needs Practice | | Comments |
|---|---|---|---|---|

**To Remove the Catheter**

12. Check to ensure that infusion is complete. Infusion is complete when the delivery time has passed and the balloon is no longer inflated.

13. Perform hand hygiene. Identify the patient. Put on gloves. Remove the catheter site dressing. Loosen adhesive skin closure strips at catheter site.

14. Grasp the catheter close to the patient's skin at the insertion site. Gently pull catheter to remove. Catheter should be easy to remove and not painful. Do not tug or quickly pull on the catheter during removal. Check the distal end of the catheter for the black marking.

15. Cover puncture site with a dry dressing, according to facility policy.

16. Dispose of the balloon, tubing, and catheter according to facility policy.

17. Remove gloves and additional PPE, if used. Perform hand hygiene.

*Skill Checklists for Taylor's Clinical Nursing Skills:*
*A Nursing Process Approach, 3rd edition*

Name _____     Date _____

Unit _____     Position _____

Instructor/Evaluator: _____     Position _____

| Excellent | Satisfactory | Needs Practice | SKILL 11-1 **Assisting a Patient With Eating** | Comments |
|---|---|---|---|---|
| | | | **Goal:** The patient consumes 50% to 60% of the contents of the meal tray. | |
| ___ | ___ | ___ | 1. Check the medical order for the type of diet prescribed for the patient. | |
| ___ | ___ | ___ | 2. Perform hand hygiene and put on PPE, if indicated. | |
| ___ | ___ | ___ | 3. Identify the patient. | |
| ___ | ___ | ___ | 4. Explain procedure to patient. | |
| ___ | ___ | ___ | 5. *Assess level of consciousness, for any physical limitations, decreased hearing or visual acuity. If patient uses a hearing aid or wears glasses or dentures, provide as needed. Ask if the patient has any cultural or religious preferences and food likes and dislikes, if possible.* | |
| ___ | ___ | ___ | 6. Pull the patient's bedside curtain. Assess the abdomen. Ask the patient if he/she has any nausea. Ask the patient if he/she has any difficulty swallowing. Assess the patient for nausea or pain and administer an antiemetic or analgesic as needed. | |
| ___ | ___ | ___ | 7. Offer to assist the patient with any elimination needs. | |
| ___ | ___ | ___ | 8. Provide hand hygiene and mouth care as needed. | |
| ___ | ___ | ___ | 9. Remove any bedpans or undesirable equipment and odors if possible from the vicinity where meal will be eaten. | |
| ___ | ___ | ___ | 10. Open the patient's bedside curtain. Assist to or position the patient in a high Fowler's or sitting position in the bed or chair. Position the bed in the low position, if the patient remains in bed. | |
| ___ | ___ | ___ | 11. Place protective covering or towel over the patient if desired. | |
| ___ | ___ | ___ | 12. Check tray to make sure that it is the correct tray before serving. Place tray on the overbed table so patient can see food if able. Ensure that hot foods are hot and cold foods are cold. Use caution with hot beverages, allowing sufficient time for cooling if needed. Ask the patient for his/her preference related to what foods are desired first. Cut food into small pieces as needed. Observe swallowing ability throughout the meal. | |

## SKILL 11-1

# Assisting a Patient With Eating *(Continued)*

| Excellent | Satisfactory | Needs Practice | | Comments |
|---|---|---|---|---|
| —— | —— | —— | 13. If possible, sit facing the patient while feeding is taking place. If patient is able, encourage him or her to hold finger foods and feed self as much as possible. Converse with patient during the meal as appropriate. If, however, the patient has **dysphagia,** limit questioning or conversation that would require patient response during eating. Play relaxation music if patient desires. | |
| —— | —— | —— | 14. Allow enough time for the patient to adequately chew and swallow the food. The patient may need to rest for short periods during eating. | |
| —— | —— | —— | 15. When the meal is completed or the patient is unable to eat any more, remove the tray from the room. *Note the amount and types of food consumed. Note the volume of liquid consumed.* | |
| —— | —— | —— | 16. Reposition the overbed table, remove the protective covering, offer hand hygiene as needed, and offer the bedpan. Assist the patient to a position of comfort and relaxation. | |
| —— | —— | —— | 17. Remove PPE, if used. Perform hand hygiene. | |

*Skill Checklists for Taylor's Clinical Nursing Skills:*
*A Nursing Process Approach, 3rd edition*

Name _____    Date _____

Unit _____    Position _____

Instructor/Evaluator: _____    Position _____

## SKILL 11-2

# Inserting a Nasogastric (NG) Tube

**Goal:** The tube is passed into the patient's stomach without any complications.

| Excellent | Satisfactory | Needs Practice | | Comments |
|---|---|---|---|---|
| —— | —— | —— | 1. Verify the medical order for insertion of an NG tube. | |
| —— | —— | —— | 2. Perform hand hygiene and put on PPE, if indicated. | |
| —— | —— | —— | 3. Identify the patient. | |
| —— | —— | —— | 4. Explain the procedure to the patient and provide the rationale as to why the tube is needed. Discuss the associated discomforts that may be experienced and possible interventions that may allay this discomfort. Answer any questions as needed. | |
| —— | —— | —— | 5. Gather equipment, including selection of the appropriate NG tube. | |
| —— | —— | —— | 6. Close the patient's bedside curtain or door. Raise bed to a comfortable working position; usually elbow height of the caregiver (VISN 8, 2009). Assist the patient to high Fowler's position or elevate the head of the bed 45 degrees if the patient is unable to maintain upright position. Drape chest with bath towel or disposable pad. Have emesis basin and tissues handy. | |
| —— | —— | —— | 7. *Measure the distance to insert tube by placing tip of tube at patient's nostril and extending to tip of earlobe and then to tip of xiphoid process.* Mark tube with an indelible marker. | |
| —— | —— | —— | 8. Put on gloves. Lubricate tip of tube (at least 2″–4″) with water-soluble lubricant. Apply topical anesthetic to nostril and oropharynx, as appropriate. | |
| —— | —— | —— | 9. After selecting the appropriate nostril, ask patient to slightly flex head back against the pillow. Gently insert the tube into the nostril while directing the tube upward and backward along the floor of the nose. Patient may gag when tube reaches pharynx. Provide tissues for tearing or watering of eyes. Offer comfort and reassurance to the patient. | |

| | | | |
|---|---|---|---|

# Inserting a Nasogastric (NG) Tube *(Continued)*

**Excellent**    **Satisfactory**    **Needs Practice**                          **Comments**

10. When pharynx is reached, instruct patient to touch chin to chest. Encourage patient to sip water through a straw or swallow even if no fluids are permitted. Advance tube in downward and backward direction when patient swallows. Stop when patient breathes. *If gagging and coughing persist, stop advancing the tube and check placement of tube with tongue blade and flashlight.* If tube is curled, straighten the tube and attempt to advance again. Keep advancing tube until pen marking is reached. *Do not use force. Rotate tube if it meets resistance.*

11. *Discontinue procedure and remove tube if there are signs of distress, such as gasping, coughing, cyanosis, and inability to speak or hum.*

12. Secure the tube loosely to the nose or cheek until it is determined that the tube is in the patient's stomach:

    a. Attach syringe to end of tube and aspirate a small amount of stomach contents.

    b. Measure the pH of aspirated fluid using pH paper or a meter. Place a drop of gastric secretions onto pH paper or place small amount in plastic cup and dip the pH paper into it. Within 30 seconds, compare the color on the paper with the chart supplied by the manufacturer.

    c. Visualize aspirated contents, checking for color and consistency.

    d. Obtain radiograph (x-ray) of placement of tube, based on facility policy (and ordered by physician).

13. Apply skin barrier to tip and end of nose and allow to dry. Remove gloves and secure tube with a commercially prepared device (follow manufacturer's directions) or tape to patient's nose. To secure with tape:

    a. Cut a 4″ piece of tape and split bottom 2″ or use packaged nose tape for NG tubes.

    b. Place unsplit end over bridge of patient's nose.

    c. Wrap split ends under tubing and up and over onto nose. *Be careful not to pull tube too tightly against nose.*

14. Put on gloves. Clamp tube and remove the syringe. Cap the tube or attach tube to suction according to the medical orders (see Chapter 13).

| Excellent | Satisfactory | Needs Practice | SKILL 11-2 **Inserting a Nasogastric (NG) Tube** *(Continued)* | |
|---|---|---|---|---|
| | | | | **Comments** |
| —— | —— | —— | 15. Measure length of exposed tube. Reinforce marking on tube at nostril with indelible ink. Ask the patient to turn their head to the side opposite the nostril the tube is inserted. Secure tube to patient's gown by using rubber band or tape and safety pin. For additional support, tube can be taped onto patient's cheek using a piece of tape. ***If a double-lumen tube (e.g., Salem sump) is used, secure vent above stomach level.*** Attach at shoulder level. | |
| —— | —— | —— | 16. Assist with or provide oral hygiene at 2- to 4-hour intervals. Lubricate the lips generously and clean nares and lubricate as needed. Offer analgesic throat lozenges or anesthetic spray for throat irritation if needed. | |
| —— | —— | —— | 17. Remove equipment and return patient to a position of comfort. Remove gloves. Raise side rail and lower bed. | |
| —— | —— | —— | 18. Remove additional PPE, if used. Perform hand hygiene. | |

*Skill Checklists for Taylor's Clinical Nursing Skills:*
*A Nursing Process Approach, 3rd edition*

Name _____ Date _____

Unit _____ Position _____

Instructor/Evaluator: _____ Position _____

| Excellent | Satisfactory | Needs Practice | SKILL 11-3<br>**Administering a Tube Feeding** | |
|---|---|---|---|---|
| | | | **Goal:** The patient receives the tube feeding without complaints of nausea or episodes of vomiting. | **Comments** |
| ‒‒ | ‒‒ | ‒‒ | 1. Assemble equipment. Check amount, concentration, type, and frequency of tube feeding on patient's chart. Check expiration date of formula. | |
| ‒‒ | ‒‒ | ‒‒ | 2. Perform hand hygiene and put on PPE, if indicated. | |
| ‒‒ | ‒‒ | ‒‒ | 3. Identify the patient. | |
| ‒‒ | ‒‒ | ‒‒ | 4. Explain the procedure to the patient and why this intervention is needed. Answer any questions as needed. | |
| ‒‒ | ‒‒ | ‒‒ | 5. Assemble equipment on overbed table within reach. | |
| ‒‒ | ‒‒ | ‒‒ | 6. Close the patient's bedside curtain or door. Raise bed to a comfortable working position, usually elbow height of the caregiver (VISN 8, 2009). Perform key abdominal assessments as described above. | |
| ‒‒ | ‒‒ | ‒‒ | 7. *Position patient with head of bed elevated at least 30 to 45 degrees or as near normal position for eating as possible.* | |
| ‒‒ | ‒‒ | ‒‒ | 8. Put on gloves. Unpin tube from patient's gown. Verify the position of the marking on the tube at the nostril. Measure length of exposed tube and compare with the documented length. | |
| ‒‒ | ‒‒ | ‒‒ | 9. Attach syringe to end of tube and aspirate a small amount of stomach contents, as described in Skill 11-2. | |
| ‒‒ | ‒‒ | ‒‒ | 10. Check the pH as described in Skill 11-2. | |
| ‒‒ | ‒‒ | ‒‒ | 11. Visualize aspirated contents, checking for color and consistency. | |
| ‒‒ | ‒‒ | ‒‒ | 12. If it is not possible to aspirate contents; assessments to check placement are inconclusive; the exposed tube length has changed; or there are any other indications that the tube is not in place, check placement by x-ray. | |
| ‒‒ | ‒‒ | ‒‒ | 13. After multiple steps have been taken to ensure that the feeding tube is located in the stomach or small intestine, *aspirate all gastric contents with the syringe and measure to check for the residual amount of feeding in the stomach.* Return the **residual** based on facility policy. Proceed with feeding if amount of residual does not exceed agency policy or the limit indicated in the medical record. | |

# Administering a Tube Feeding (Continued)

| Excellent | Satisfactory | Needs Practice | | Comments |
|---|---|---|---|---|
| ___ | ___ | ___ | 14. Flush tube with 30 mL of water for irrigation. Disconnect syringe from tubing and cap end of tubing while preparing the formula feeding equipment. Remove gloves. | |
| ___ | ___ | ___ | 15. Put on gloves before preparing, assembling and handling any part of the feeding system. | |
| ___ | ___ | ___ | 16. Administer feeding. | |
| | | | **When Using a Feeding Bag (Open System)** | |
| ___ | ___ | ___ | a. Label bag and/or tubing with date and time. Hang bag on IV pole and adjust to about 12″ above the stomach. Clamp tubing. | |
| ___ | ___ | ___ | b. Check the expiration date of the formula. Cleanse top of feeding container with a disinfectant before opening it. Pour formula into feeding bag and allow solution to run through tubing. Close clamp. | |
| ___ | ___ | ___ | c. Attach feeding setup to feeding tube, open clamp, and regulate drip according to the medical order, or allow feeding to run in over 30 minutes. | |
| ___ | ___ | ___ | d. *Add 30 to 60 mL (1–2 oz) of water for irrigation to feeding bag when feeding is almost completed and allow it to run through the tube.* | |
| ___ | ___ | ___ | e. Clamp tubing immediately after water has been instilled. Disconnect **feeding setup** from feeding tube. Clamp tube and cover end with cap. | |
| | | | **When Using a Large Syringe (Open System)** | |
| ___ | ___ | ___ | a. Remove plunger from 30- or 60-mL syringe. | |
| ___ | ___ | ___ | b. Attach syringe to feeding tube, pour premeasured amount of tube feeding formula into syringe, open clamp, and allow food to enter tube. *Regulate rate, fast or slow, by height of the syringe. Do not push formula with syringe plunger.* | |
| ___ | ___ | ___ | c. *Add 30 to 60 mL (1–2 oz) of water for irrigation to syringe when feeding is almost completed, and allow it to run through the tube.* | |
| ___ | ___ | ___ | d. When syringe has emptied, hold syringe high and disconnect from tube. Clamp tube and cover end with cap. | |
| | | | **When Using an Enteral Feeding Pump** | |
| ___ | ___ | ___ | a. Close flow-regulator clamp on tubing and fill feeding bag with prescribed formula. Amount used depends on agency policy. Place label on container with patient's name, date, and time the feeding was hung. | |

# Administering a Tube Feeding *(Continued)*

| Excellent | Satisfactory | Needs Practice | | Comments |
|---|---|---|---|---|
| — — — | | | b. Hang feeding container on IV pole. *Allow solution to flow through tubing.* | |
| — — — | | | c. Connect to feeding pump following manufacturer's directions. Set rate. Maintain the patient in the upright position throughout the feeding. If the patient needs to temporarily lie flat, the feeding should be paused. The feeding may be resumed after the patient's position has been changed back to at least 30 to 45 degrees. | |
| — — — | | | d. *Check placement of tube and gastric residual every 4 to 6 hours.* | |
| — — — | | | 17. Observe the patient's response during and after tube feeding and assess the abdomen at least once a shift. | |
| — — — | | | 18. *Have patient remain in upright position for at least 1 hour after feeding.* | |
| — — — | | | 19. Remove equipment and return patient to a position of comfort. Remove gloves. Raise side rail and lower bed. | |
| — — — | | | 20. Put on gloves. Wash and clean equipment or replace according to agency policy. Remove gloves. | |
| — — — | | | 21. Remove additional PPE, if used. Perform hand hygiene. | |

*Skill Checklists for Taylor's Clinical Nursing Skills:*
*A Nursing Process Approach, 3rd edition*

Name _____  Date _____

Unit _____  Position _____

Instructor/Evaluator: _____  Position _____

| | | | |
|---|---|---|---|

SKILL 11-4

# Removing a Nasogastric Tube

**Excellent** | **Satisfactory** | **Needs Practice**

**Goal:** The tube is removed with minimal discomfort to the patient, and the patient maintains an adequate nutritional intake.

**Comments**

| Excellent | Satisfactory | Needs Practice | | Comments |
|---|---|---|---|---|
| —— | —— | —— | 1. Check medical order for removal of NG tube. | |
| —— | —— | —— | 2. Perform hand hygiene and put on PPE, if indicated. | |
| —— | —— | —— | 3. Identify the patient. | |
| —— | —— | —— | 4. Explain the procedure to the patient and why this intervention is warranted. Describe that it will entail a quick few moments of discomfort. Perform key abdominal assessments as described above. | |
| —— | —— | —— | 5. Pull the patient's bedside curtain. Raise bed to a comfortable working position, usually elbow height of the caregiver (VISN 8, 2009). Assist the patient into a 30- to 45-degree position. Place towel or disposable pad across patient's chest. Give tissues and emesis basin to patient. | |
| —— | —— | —— | 6. Put on gloves. Discontinue suction and separate tube from suction. Unpin tube from patient's gown and carefully remove adhesive tape from patient's nose. | |
| —— | —— | —— | 7. Check placement (as outlined in Skill 11-2) and *attach syringe and flush with 10 mL of water or normal saline solution (optional) or clear with 30 to 50 mL of air.* | |
| —— | —— | —— | 8. *Clamp tube with fingers by doubling tube on itself. Instruct patient to take a deep breath and hold it. Quickly and carefully remove tube while patient holds breath.* Coil the tube in the disposable pad as you remove from the patient. | |
| —— | —— | —— | 9. Dispose of tube per agency policy. Remove gloves and place in bag. Perform hand hygiene. | |
| —— | —— | —— | 10. Offer mouth care to patient and facial tissue to blow nose. Lower the bed and assist the patient to a position of comfort as needed. | |
| —— | —— | —— | 11. Remove equipment and raise side rail and lower bed. | |
| —— | —— | —— | 12. Put on gloves and measure the amount of nasogastric drainage in the collection device and record on output flow record, subtracting irrigant fluids if necessary. Add solidifying agent to nasogastric drainage according to hospital policy. | |
| —— | —— | —— | 13. Remove additional PPE, if used. Perform hand hygiene. | |

*Skill Checklists for Taylor's Clinical Nursing Skills:*
*A Nursing Process Approach, 3rd edition*

Name _____   Date _____

Unit _____   Position _____

Instructor/Evaluator: _____   Position _____

| Excellent | Satisfactory | Needs Practice | SKILL 11-5<br>**Caring for a Gastrostomy Tube**<br><br>**Goal:** The patient ingests an adequate diet and exhibits no signs and symptoms of irritation, excoriation, or infection at the tube insertion site. | Comments |
|---|---|---|---|---|
| ___ | ___ | ___ | 1. Assemble equipment. Verify the medical order or facility policy and procedure regarding site care. | |
| ___ | ___ | ___ | 2. Perform hand hygiene and put on PPE, if indicated. | |
| ___ | ___ | ___ | 3. Identify the patient. | |
| ___ | ___ | ___ | 4. Explain the procedure to the patient and why this intervention is needed. Answer any questions as needed. | |
| ___ | ___ | ___ | 5. Assess patient for presence of pain at the tube insertion site. If pain is present, offer patient analgesic medication per physician's order and wait for medication absorption before beginning insertion site care. | |
| ___ | ___ | ___ | 6. Pull the patient's bedside curtain. Raise bed to a comfortable working position, usually elbow height of the caregiver (VISN 8, 2009). | |
| ___ | ___ | ___ | 7. Put on gloves. If gastrostomy tube is new and still has sutures holding it in place, dip cotton-tipped applicator into sterile saline solution and gently clean around the insertion site, removing any crust or drainage. Avoid adjusting or lifting the external disk for the first few days after placement except to clean the area. If the gastric tube insertion site has healed and the sutures are removed, wet a washcloth and apply a small amount of soap onto washcloth. Gently cleanse around the insertion, removing any crust or drainage. *Rinse site, removing all soap.* | |
| ___ | ___ | ___ | 8. Pat skin around insertion site dry. | |
| ___ | ___ | ___ | 9. If the sutures have been removed, *gently rotate the guard or external bumper 90 degrees at least once a day. Assess that the guard or external bumper is not digging into the surrounding skin. Avoid placing any tension on the feeding tube.* | |

# Caring for a Gastrostomy Tube *(Continued)*

| Excellent | Satisfactory | Needs Practice | | Comments |
|---|---|---|---|---|
| —— | —— | —— | 10. Leave the site open to air unless there is drainage. If drainage is present, place one thickness of precut gauze pad or drain sponge under the external bumper and change as needed to keep the area dry. Use a skin protectant or substance such as zinc oxide to prevent skin breakdown. | |
| —— | —— | —— | 11. Remove gloves. Lower the bed and assist the patient to a position of comfort as needed. | |
| —— | —— | —— | 12. Remove additional PPE, if used. Perform hand hygiene. | |

*Skill Checklists for Taylor's Clinical Nursing Skills:*
*A Nursing Process Approach, 3rd edition*

Name _____  Date _____

Unit _____  Position _____

Instructor/Evaluator: _____  Position _____

## SKILL 12-1

## Assisting With the Use of a Bedpan

**Goal:** The patient is able to void with assistance.

| Excellent | Satisfactory | Needs Practice | | Comments |
|---|---|---|---|---|
| ___ | ___ | ___ | 1. Review the patient's chart for any limitations in physical activity. (See Skill Variation: Assisting With Use of a Bedpan When the Patient Has Limited Movement.) | |
| ___ | ___ | ___ | 2. Bring bedpan and other necessary equipment to the bedside stand or overbed table. | |
| ___ | ___ | ___ | 3. Perform hand hygiene and put on PPE, if indicated. | |
| ___ | ___ | ___ | 4. Identify the patient. | |
| ___ | ___ | ___ | 5. Close curtains around bed and close the door to the room, if possible. Discuss the procedure with the patient and assess the patient's ability to assist with the procedure, as well as personal hygiene preferences. | |
| ___ | ___ | ___ | 6. Unless contraindicated, apply powder to the rim of the bedpan. Place bedpan and cover on chair next to bed. Put on gloves. | |
| ___ | ___ | ___ | 7. Adjust bed to comfortable working height, usually elbow height of the caregiver (VISN 8 Patient Safety Center, 2009). Place the patient in a supine position, with the head of the bed elevated about 30 degrees, unless contraindicated. | |
| ___ | ___ | ___ | 8. Fold top linen back just enough to allow placement of bedpan. If there is no waterproof pad on the bed and time allows, consider placing a waterproof pad under patient's buttocks before placing bedpan. | |
| ___ | ___ | ___ | 9. Ask the patient to bend the knees. Have the patient lift his or her hips upward. Assist patient, if necessary, by placing your hand that is closest to the patient palm up, under the lower back, and assist with lifting. Slip the bedpan into place with other hand. | |
| ___ | ___ | ___ | 10. *Ensure that bedpan is in proper position and patient's buttocks are resting on the rounded shelf of the regular bedpan or the shallow rim of the fracture bedpan.* | |
| ___ | ___ | ___ | 11. Raise head of bed as near to sitting position as tolerated, unless contraindicated. Cover the patient with bed linens. | |
| ___ | ___ | ___ | 12. *Place call bell and toilet tissue within easy reach. Place the bed in the lowest position.* Leave patient if it is safe to do so. Use side rails appropriately. | |

| Excellent | Satisfactory | Needs Practice | SKILL 12-1<br>**Assisting With the Use of a Bedpan** *(Continued)* | Comments |
|---|---|---|---|---|
| —— | —— | —— | 13. Remove gloves and additional PPE, if used. Perform hand hygiene. | |
| | | | **Removing the Bedpan** | |
| —— | —— | —— | 14. Perform hand hygiene and put on gloves and additional PPE, as indicated. Adjust bed to comfortable working height, usually elbow height of the caregiver (VISN 8 Patient Safety Center, 2009). Have a receptacle, such as plastic trash bag, handy for discarding tissue. | |
| —— | —— | —— | 15. Lower the head of the bed, if necessary, to about 30 degrees. Remove bedpan in the same manner in which it was offered, being careful to hold it steady. Ask the patient to bend the knees and lift the buttocks up from the bedpan. Assist patient, if necessary, by placing your hand that is closest to the patient palm up, under the lower back, and assist with lifting. Place the bedpan on the bedside chair and cover it. | |
| —— | —— | —— | 16. If patient needs assistance with hygiene, wrap tissue around the hand several times, and wipe patient clean, using one stroke from the pubic area toward the anal area. Discard tissue, and use more until patient is clean. Place patient on his or her side and spread buttocks to clean anal area. | |
| —— | —— | —— | 17. Do not place toilet tissue in the bedpan if a specimen is required or if output is being recorded. Place toilet tissue in appropriate receptacle. | |
| —— | —— | —— | 18. Return the patient to a comfortable position. Make sure the linens under the patient are dry. Replace or remove pad under the patient, as necessary. Remove your gloves and ensure that the patient is covered. | |
| —— | —— | —— | 19. Raise side rail. Lower bed height and adjust head of bed to a comfortable position. Reattach call bell. | |
| —— | —— | —— | 20. Offer patient supplies to wash and dry his or her hands, assisting as necessary. | |
| —— | —— | —— | 21. Put on clean gloves. Empty and clean the bedpan, measuring urine in graduated container, as necessary. Discard trash receptacle with used toilet paper per facility policy. | |
| —— | —— | —— | 22. Remove additional PPE, if used. Perform hand hygiene. | |

*Skill Checklists for Taylor's Clinical Nursing Skills:*
*A Nursing Process Approach, 3rd edition*

Name _____     Date _____

Unit _____     Position _____

Instructor/Evaluator: _____     Position _____

| Excellent | Satisfactory | Needs Practice | SKILL 12-2 **Assisting With the Use of a Urinal** | Comments |
|:---:|:---:|:---:|---|---|
| | | | **Goal:** The patient is able to void with assistance. | |
| ___ | ___ | ___ | 1. Review the patient's chart for any limitations in physical activity. | |
| ___ | ___ | ___ | 2. Bring urinal and other necessary equipment to the bedside stand or overbed table. | |
| ___ | ___ | ___ | 3. Perform hand hygiene and put on PPE, if indicated. | |
| ___ | ___ | ___ | 4. Identify the patient. | |
| ___ | ___ | ___ | 5. Close the curtains around the bed and close the door to the room, if possible. Discuss procedure with patient and assess the patient's ability to assist with the procedure, as well as personal hygiene preferences. | |
| ___ | ___ | ___ | 6. Put on gloves. | |
| ___ | ___ | ___ | 7. Assist the patient to an appropriate position, as necessary: standing at the bedside, lying on one side or back, sitting in bed with the head elevated, or sitting on the side of the bed. | |
| ___ | ___ | ___ | 8. If the patient remains in the bed, fold the linens just enough to allow for proper placement of the urinal. | |
| ___ | ___ | ___ | 9. If the patient is not standing, have him spread his legs slightly. *Hold the urinal close to the penis and position the penis completely within the urinal. Keep the bottom of the urinal lower than the penis. If necessary, assist the patient to hold the urinal in place.* | |
| ___ | ___ | ___ | 10. Cover the patient with the bed linens. | |
| ___ | ___ | ___ | 11. Place call bell and toilet tissue within easy reach. Have a receptacle, such as plastic trash bag, handy for discarding tissue. Ensure the bed is in the lowest position. Leave patient if it is safe to do so. Use side rails appropriately. | |
| ___ | ___ | ___ | 12. Remove gloves and additional PPE, if used. Perform hand hygiene. | |
| | | | **Removing the Urinal** | |
| ___ | ___ | ___ | 13. Perform hand hygiene. Put on gloves and additional PPE, as indicated. | |

# Assisting With the Use of a Urinal *(Continued)*

| Excellent | Satisfactory | Needs Practice | | Comments |
|---|---|---|---|---|
| —— | —— | —— | 14. Pull back the patient's bed linens just enough to remove the urinal. Remove the urinal. Cover the open end of the urinal. Place on the bedside chair. If patient needs assistance with hygiene, wrap tissue around the hand several times, and wipe patient clean. Place tissue in receptacle. | |
| —— | —— | —— | 15. Return the patient to a comfortable position. Make sure the linens under the patient are dry. Remove your gloves and ensure that the patient is covered. | |
| —— | —— | —— | 16. Ensure patient call bell is in reach. | |
| —— | —— | —— | 17. Offer patient supplies to wash and dry his hands, assisting as necessary. | |
| —— | —— | —— | 18. Put on clean gloves. Empty and clean the urinal, measuring urine in graduated container, as necessary. Discard trash receptacle with used toilet paper per facility policy. | |
| —— | —— | —— | 19. Remove gloves and additional PPE, if used, and perform hand hygiene. | |

*Skill Checklists for Taylor's Clinical Nursing Skills:*
*A Nursing Process Approach, 3rd edition*

Name _____   Date _____

Unit _____   Position _____

Instructor/Evaluator: _____   Position _____

| Excellent | Satisfactory | Needs Practice | SKILL 12-3<br>**Assisting With the Use of a Bedside Commode** | Comments |
|---|---|---|---|---|
| | | | **Goal:** The patient is able to void with assistance. | |
| ___ | ___ | ___ | 1. Review the patient's chart for any limitations in physical activity. | |
| ___ | ___ | ___ | 2. Bring the commode and other necessary equipment to the bedside. Obtain assistance for patient transfer from another staff member, if necessary. | |
| ___ | ___ | ___ | 3. Perform hand hygiene and put on PPE, if indicated. | |
| ___ | ___ | ___ | 4. Identify the patient. | |
| ___ | ___ | ___ | 5. Close the curtains around the bed and close the door to the room, if possible. Discuss procedure with the patient and assess the patient's ability to assist with the procedure, as well as personal hygiene preferences. | |
| ___ | ___ | ___ | 6. Place the commode close to, and parallel with, the bed. Raise or remove the seat cover. | |
| ___ | ___ | ___ | 7. Assist the patient to a standing position and then help the patient pivot to the commode. *While bracing one commode leg with your foot, ask the patient to place his or her hands one at a time on the armrests. Assist the patient to lower himself/herself slowly onto the commode seat.* | |
| ___ | ___ | ___ | 8. Cover the patient with a blanket. Place call bell and toilet tissue within easy reach. Leave patient if it is safe to do so. | |
| | | | **Assisting Patient Off Commode** | |
| ___ | ___ | ___ | 9. Perform hand hygiene. Put on gloves and additional PPE, as indicated. | |
| ___ | ___ | ___ | 10. Assist the patient to a standing position. If patient needs assistance with hygiene, wrap toilet tissue around your hand several times, and wipe patient clean, using one stroke from the pubic area toward the anal area. Discard tissue in an appropriate receptacle, according to facility policy, and continue with additional tissue until patient is clean. | |
| ___ | ___ | ___ | 11. Do not place toilet tissue in the commode if a specimen is required or if output is being recorded. Replace or lower the seat cover. | |

SKILL 12-3

# Assisting With the Use of a Bedside Commode *(Continued)*

| Excellent | Satisfactory | Needs Practice | | Comments |
|---|---|---|---|---|
| —— | —— | —— | 12. Remove your gloves. Return the patient to the bed or chair. If the patient returns to the bed, raise side rails, as appropriate. Ensure that the patient is covered and call bell is readily within reach. | |
| —— | —— | —— | 13. Offer patient supplies to wash and dry his or her hands, assisting as necessary. | |
| —— | —— | —— | 14. Put on clean gloves. Empty and clean the commode, measuring urine in graduated container, as necessary. | |
| —— | —— | —— | 15. Remove gloves and additional PPE, if used. Perform hand hygiene. | |

*Skill Checklists for Taylor's Clinical Nursing Skills:*
*A Nursing Process Approach, 3rd edition*

Name _____  Date _____

Unit _____  Position _____

Instructor/Evaluator: _____  Position _____

| Excellent | Satisfactory | Needs Practice | SKILL 12-4<br>**Assessing Bladder Volume Using an Ultrasound Bladder Scanner** | |
|---|---|---|---|---|
| | | | **Goal:** The volume of urine in the bladder is accurately measured. | **Comments** |
| —— | —— | —— | 1. Review the patient's chart for any limitations in physical activity. | |
| —— | —— | —— | 2. Bring the bladder scanner and other necessary equipment to the bedside. | |
| —— | —— | —— | 3. Perform hand hygiene and put on PPE, if indicated. | |
| —— | —— | —— | 4. Identify the patient. | |
| —— | —— | —— | 5. Close curtains around bed and close the door to the room, if possible. Discuss the procedure with the patient and assess the patient's ability to assist with the procedure, as well as personal hygiene preferences. | |
| —— | —— | —— | 6. Adjust the bed to a comfortable working height; usually elbow height of the caregiver (VISN 8 Patient Safety Center, 2009). Place the patient in a supine position. Drape patient. Stand on the patient's right side if you are right-handed, patient's left side if you are left-handed. | |
| —— | —— | —— | 7. Put on clean gloves. | |
| —— | —— | —— | 8. Press the ON button. Wait until the device warms up. Press the SCAN button to turn on the scanning screen. | |
| —— | —— | —— | 9. Press the appropriate gender button. The appropriate icon for male or female will appear on the screen. | |
| —— | —— | —— | 10. Clean the scanner head with the appropriate cleaner. | |
| —— | —— | —— | 11. *Gently palpate the patient's symphysis pubis. Place a generous amount of ultrasound gel or gel pad midline on the patient's abdomen, about 1 to 1.5 inches above the symphysis pubis (anterior midline junction of pubic bones).* | |
| —— | —— | —— | 12. *Place the scanner head on the gel or gel pad, with the directional icon on the scanner head toward the patient's head. Aim the scanner head toward the bladder (point the scanner head slightly downward toward the coccyx) (Patraca, 2005). Press and release the scan button.* | |
| —— | —— | —— | 13. Observe the image on the scanner screen. *Adjust the scanner head to center the bladder image on the crossbars.* | |
| —— | —— | —— | 14. Press and hold the DONE button until it beeps. Read the volume measurement on the screen. Print the results, if required, by pressing PRINT. | |

| Excellent | Satisfactory | Needs Practice | SKILL 12-4<br>**Assessing Bladder Volume Using an**<br>**Ultrasound Bladder Scanner** *(Continued)* | |
|---|---|---|---|---|
| | | | | **Comments** |
| —— | —— | —— | 15. Use a washcloth or paper towel to remove remaining gel from the patient's skin. Alternately, gently remove gel pad from patient's skin. Return the patient to a comfortable position. Remove your gloves and ensure that the patient is covered. | |
| —— | —— | —— | 16. Lower bed height and adjust head of bed to a comfortable position. Reattach call bell, if necessary. | |
| —— | —— | —— | 17. Remove additional PPE, if used. Perform hand hygiene. | |

*Skill Checklists for Taylor's Clinical Nursing Skills:*
*A Nursing Process Approach, 3rd edition*

Name _____  Date _____

Unit _____  Position _____

Instructor/Evaluator: _____  Position _____

SKILL 12-5

# Applying an External Condom Catheter

**Goal:** The patient's urinary elimination is maintained, with a urine output of at least 30 mL/hour, and the bladder is not distended.

| Excellent | Satisfactory | Needs Practice | | Comments |
|---|---|---|---|---|
| —— | —— | —— | 1. Bring necessary equipment to the bedside. | |
| —— | —— | —— | 2. Perform hand hygiene and put on PPE, if indicated. | |
| —— | —— | —— | 3. Identify the patient. | |
| —— | —— | —— | 4. Close curtains around bed and close the door to the room, if possible. Discuss the procedure with patient. Ask the patient if he has any allergies, especially to latex. | |
| —— | —— | —— | 5. Adjust bed to comfortable working height, usually elbow height of the caregiver (VISN 8 Patient Safety Center, 2009). Stand on the patient's right side if you are right-handed, or on patient's left side if you are left-handed. | |
| —— | —— | —— | 6. Prepare urinary drainage setup or reusable leg bag for attachment to condom sheath. | |
| —— | —— | —— | 7. Position patient on his back with thighs slightly apart. Drape patient so that only the area around the penis is exposed. Slide waterproof pad under patient. | |
| —— | —— | —— | 8. Put on disposable gloves. Trim any long pubic hair that is in contact with penis. | |
| —— | —— | —— | 9. Clean the genital area with washcloth, skin cleanser, and warm water. If patient is uncircumcised, retract foreskin and clean glans of penis. Replace foreskin. Clean the tip of the penis first, moving the washcloth in a circular motion from the meatus outward. Wash the shaft of the penis using downward strokes toward the pubic area. Rinse and dry. Remove gloves. Perform hand hygiene again. | |
| —— | —— | —— | 10. Apply skin protectant to penis and allow to dry. | |
| —— | —— | —— | 11. Roll condom sheath outward onto itself. Grasp penis firmly with nondominant hand. *Apply condom sheath by rolling it onto penis with dominant hand. Leave 1 to 2 inches (2.5 to 5 cm) of space between tip of penis and end of condom sheath.* | |
| —— | —— | —— | 12. *Apply pressure to sheath at the base of penis for 10 to 15 seconds.* | |
| —— | —— | —— | 13. Connect condom sheath to drainage setup. Avoid kinking or twisting drainage tubing. | |

SKILL 12-5

# Applying an External Condom Catheter *(Continued)*

| Excellent | Satisfactory | Needs Practice | | Comments |
|---|---|---|---|---|
| —— | —— | —— | 14. Remove gloves. Secure drainage tubing to the patient's inner thigh with Velcro leg strap or tape. Leave some slack in tubing for leg movement. | |
| —— | —— | —— | 15. Assist the patient to a comfortable position. Cover the patient with bed linens. Place the bed in the lowest position. | |
| —— | —— | —— | 16. Secure drainage bag below the level of the bladder. Check that drainage tubing is not kinked and that movement of side rails does not interfere with the drainage bag. | |
| —— | —— | —— | 17. Remove equipment. Remove gloves and additional PPE, if used. Perform hand hygiene. | |

*Skill Checklists for Taylor's Clinical Nursing Skills:*
*A Nursing Process Approach, 3rd edition*

Name _____ Date _____

Unit _____ Position _____

Instructor/Evaluator: _____ Position _____

SKILL 12-6

# Catheterizing the Female Urinary Bladder

**Goal:** The patient's urinary elimination is maintained, with a urine output of at least 30 mL/hour, and the patient's bladder is not distended.

| Excellent | Satisfactory | Needs Practice | | Comments |
|---|---|---|---|---|
| ___ | ___ | ___ | 1. Review the patient's chart for any limitations in physical activity. Confirm the medical order for indwelling catheter insertion. | |
| ___ | ___ | ___ | 2. Bring the catheter kit and other necessary equipment to the bedside. Obtain assistance from another staff member, if necessary. | |
| ___ | ___ | ___ | 3. Perform hand hygiene and put on PPE, if indicated. | |
| ___ | ___ | ___ | 4. Identify the patient. | |
| ___ | ___ | ___ | 5. Close curtains around bed and close the door to the room, if possible. Discuss the procedure with the patient and assess the patient's ability to assist with the procedure. Ask the patient if she has any allergies, especially to latex or iodine. | |
| ___ | ___ | ___ | 6. Provide good lighting. Artificial light is recommended (use of a flashlight requires an assistant to hold and position it). Place a trash receptacle within easy reach. | |
| ___ | ___ | ___ | 7. Adjust the bed to a comfortable working height, usually elbow height of the caregiver (VISN 8 Patient Safety Center, 2009). Stand on the patient's right side if you are right-handed, patient's left side if you are left-handed. | |
| ___ | ___ | ___ | 8. Assist the patient to a dorsal recumbent position with knees flexed, feet about 2 feet apart, with her legs abducted. Drape patient. Alternately, the Sims', or lateral, position can be used. Place the patient's buttocks near the edge of the bed with her shoulders at the opposite edge and her knees drawn toward her chest. Allow the patient to lie on either side, depending on which position is easiest for the nurse and best for the patient's comfort. Slide waterproof pad under patient. | |
| ___ | ___ | ___ | 9. Put on clean gloves. Clean the perineal area with washcloth, skin cleanser, and warm water, using a different corner of the washcloth with each stroke. Wipe from above orifice downward toward sacrum (front to back). Rinse and dry. Remove gloves. Perform hand hygiene again. | |

# Catheterizing the Female Urinary Bladder (Continued)

| Excellent | Satisfactory | Needs Practice | | Comments |
|---|---|---|---|---|
| —— | —— | —— | 10. Prepare urine drainage setup if a separate urine collection system is to be used. Secure to bed frame according to manufacturer's directions. | |
| —— | —— | —— | 11. Open sterile catheterization tray on a clean overbed table using sterile technique. | |
| —— | —— | —— | 12. Put on sterile gloves. Grasp upper corners of drape and unfold drape without touching unsterile areas. Fold back a corner on each side to make a cuff over gloved hands. Ask patient to lift her buttocks and slide sterile drape under her with gloves protected by cuff. | |
| —— | —— | —— | 13. Based on facility policy, position the fenestrated sterile drape. Place a fenestrated sterile drape over the perineal area, exposing the labia. | |
| —— | —— | —— | 14. Place sterile tray on drape between patient's thighs. | |
| —— | —— | —— | 15. Open all the supplies. Fluff cotton balls in tray before pouring antiseptic solution over them. Alternately, open package of antiseptic swabs. Open specimen container if specimen is to be obtained. | |
| —— | —— | —— | 16. Lubricate 1 to 2 inches of catheter tip. | |
| —— | —— | —— | 17. With thumb and one finger of nondominant hand, spread labia and identify meatus. ***Be prepared to maintain separation of labia with one hand until catheter is inserted and urine is flowing well and continuously.*** If the patient is in the side-lying position, lift the upper buttock and labia to expose the urinary meatus. | |
| —— | —— | —— | 18. Use the dominant hand to pick up a cotton ball or antiseptic swab. ***Clean one labial fold, top to bottom (from above the meatus down toward the rectum), then discard the cotton ball. Using a new cotton ball/swab for each stroke, continue to clean the other labial fold, then directly over the meatus.*** | |
| —— | —— | —— | 19. With your uncontaminated, dominant hand, place the drainage end of the catheter in receptacle. If the catheter is preattached to sterile tubing and drainage container (closed drainage system), position catheter and setup within easy reach on sterile field. Ensure that clamp on drainage bag is closed. | |

# Catheterizing the Female Urinary Bladder *(Continued)*

| Excellent | Satisfactory | Needs Practice | | Comments |
|---|---|---|---|---|
| ⎯ | ⎯ | ⎯ | 20. *Using your dominant hand, hold the catheter 2 to 3 inches from the tip and insert slowly into the urethra. Advance the catheter until there is a return of urine (approximately 2 to 3 inches [4.8 to 7.2 cm]). Once urine drains, advance catheter another 2 to 3 inches (4.8 to 7.2 cm). Do not force catheter through urethra into bladder.* Ask patient to breathe deeply, and rotate catheter gently if slight resistance is met as catheter reaches external sphincter. | |
| ⎯ | ⎯ | ⎯ | 21. Hold the catheter securely at the meatus with your nondominant hand. Use your dominant hand to inflate the catheter balloon. Inject entire volume of sterile water supplied in prefilled syringe. | |
| ⎯ | ⎯ | ⎯ | 22. Pull gently on catheter after balloon is inflated to feel resistance. | |
| ⎯ | ⎯ | ⎯ | 23. Attach catheter to drainage system if not already preattached. | |
| ⎯ | ⎯ | ⎯ | 24. Remove equipment and dispose of it according to facility policy. Discard syringe in sharps container. Wash and dry the perineal area, as needed. | |
| ⎯ | ⎯ | ⎯ | 25. Remove gloves. *Secure catheter tubing to the patient's inner thigh with Velcro leg strap or tape.* Leave some slack in catheter for leg movement. | |
| ⎯ | ⎯ | ⎯ | 26. Assist the patient to a comfortable position. Cover the patient with bed linens. Place the bed in the lowest position. | |
| ⎯ | ⎯ | ⎯ | 27. Secure drainage bag below the level of the bladder. Check that drainage tubing is not kinked and that movement of side rails does not interfere with catheter or drainage bag. | |
| ⎯ | ⎯ | ⎯ | 28. Put on clean gloves. Obtain urine specimen immediately, if needed, from drainage bag. Label specimen. Send urine specimen to the laboratory promptly or refrigerate it. | |
| ⎯ | ⎯ | ⎯ | 29. Remove gloves and additional PPE, if used. Perform hand hygiene. | |

*Skill Checklists for Taylor's Clinical Nursing Skills:*
*A Nursing Process Approach, 3rd edition*

Name _____  Date _____

Unit _____  Position _____

Instructor/Evaluator: _____  Position _____

## SKILL 12-7
# Catheterizing the Male Urinary Bladder

**Goal:** The patient's urinary elimination is maintained, with a urine output of at least 30 mL/hour, and the patient's bladder is not distended.

| Excellent | Satisfactory | Needs Practice | | Comments |
|---|---|---|---|---|
| —— | —— | —— | 1. Review chart for any limitations in physical activity. Confirm the medical order for indwelling catheter insertion. | |
| —— | —— | —— | 2. Bring catheter kit and other necessary equipment to the bedside. Obtain assistance from another staff member, if necessary. | |
| —— | —— | —— | 3. Perform hand hygiene and put on PPE, if indicated. | |
| —— | —— | —— | 4. Identify the patient. | |
| —— | —— | —— | 5. Close curtains around bed and close the door to the room, if possible. Discuss the procedure with the patient and assess patient's ability to assist with the procedure. Ask the patient if he has any allergies, especially to latex or iodine. | |
| —— | —— | —— | 6. Provide good lighting. Artificial light is recommended (use of a flashlight requires an assistant to hold and position it). Place a trash receptacle within easy reach. | |
| —— | —— | —— | 7. Adjust the bed to a comfortable working height, usually elbow height of the caregiver (VISN 8 Patient Safety Center, 2009). Stand on the patient's right side if you are right-handed, patient's left side if you are left-handed. | |
| —— | —— | —— | 8. Position the patient on his back with thighs slightly apart. Drape the patient so that only the area around the penis is exposed. Slide waterproof pad under patient. | |
| —— | —— | —— | 9. Put on clean gloves. Clean the genital area with washcloth, skin cleanser, and warm water. Clean the tip of the penis first, moving the washcloth in a circular motion from the meatus outward. Wash the shaft of the penis using downward strokes toward the pubic area. Rinse and dry. Remove gloves. Perform hand hygiene again. | |
| —— | —— | —— | 10. Prepare urine drainage setup if a separate urine collection system is to be used. Secure to bed frame according to manufacturer's directions. | |
| —— | —— | —— | 11. Open sterile catheterization tray on a clean overbed table, using sterile technique. | |
| —— | —— | —— | 12. Put on sterile gloves. Open sterile drape and place on patient's thighs. Place fenestrated drape with opening over penis. | |

SKILL 12-7

# Catheterizing the Male Urinary Bladder *(Continued)*

| Excellent | Satisfactory | Needs Practice | | Comments |
|---|---|---|---|---|
| ___ | ___ | ___ | 13. Place catheter set on or next to patient's legs on sterile drape. | |
| ___ | ___ | ___ | 14. Open all the supplies. Fluff cotton balls in tray before pouring antiseptic solution over them. Alternately, open package of antiseptic swabs. Open specimen container if specimen is to be obtained. Remove cap from syringe pre-filled with lubricant. | |
| ___ | ___ | ___ | 15. Place drainage end of catheter in receptacle. If the catheter is preattached to sterile tubing and drainage container (closed drainage system), position catheter and setup within easy reach on sterile field. Ensure that clamp on drainage bag is closed. | |
| ___ | ___ | ___ | 16. Lift penis with nondominant hand. Retract foreskin in uncircumcised patient. *Be prepared to keep this hand in this position until catheter is inserted and urine is flowing well and continuously. Using the dominant hand and the forceps, pick up a cotton ball or antiseptic swab. Using a circular motion, clean the penis, moving from the meatus down the glans of the penis. Repeat this cleansing motion two more times, using a new cotton ball/swab each time. Discard each cotton ball/swab after one use.* | |
| ___ | ___ | ___ | 17. Hold penis with slight upward tension and perpendicular to patient's body. Use the dominant hand to pick up the lubricant syringe. *Gently insert tip of syringe with lubricant into urethra and instill the 10 mL of lubricant (Society of Urologic Nurses and Associates, 2005c).* | |
| ___ | ___ | ___ | 18. Use the dominant hand to pick up the catheter and hold it an inch or two from the tip. Ask the patient to bear down as if voiding. *Insert catheter tip into meatus. Ask the patient to take deep breaths. Advance the catheter to the bifurcation or "Y" level of the ports. Do not use force to introduce the catheter.* If the catheter resists entry, ask patient to breathe deeply and rotate catheter slightly. | |
| ___ | ___ | ___ | 19. Hold the catheter securely at the meatus with your nondominant hand. Use your dominant hand to inflate the catheter balloon. *Inject the entire volume of sterile water supplied in the prefilled syringe. Once the balloon is inflated, the catheter may be gently pulled back into place. Replace foreskin over catheter.* Lower penis. | |
| ___ | ___ | ___ | 20. Pull gently on catheter after balloon is inflated to feel resistance. | |
| ___ | ___ | ___ | 21. Attach catheter to drainage system, if necessary. | |

SKILL 12-7

# Catheterizing the Male Urinary Bladder *(Continued)*

| Excellent | Satisfactory | Needs Practice | | Comments |
|---|---|---|---|---|
| —— | —— | —— | 22. Remove equipment and dispose of it according to facility policy. Discard syringe in sharps container. Wash and dry the perineal area as needed. | |
| —— | —— | —— | 23. Remove gloves. Secure catheter tubing to the patient's inner thigh or lower abdomen (with the penis directed toward the patient's chest) with Velcro leg strap or tape. Leave some slack in catheter for leg movement. | |
| —— | —— | —— | 24. Assist the patient to a comfortable position. Cover the patient with bed linens. Place the bed in the lowest position. | |
| —— | —— | —— | 25. Secure drainage bag below the level of the bladder. Check that drainage tubing is not kinked and that movement of side rails does not interfere with catheter or drainage bag. | |
| —— | —— | —— | 26. Put on clean gloves. Obtain urine specimen immediately, if needed, from drainage bag. Label specimen. Send urine specimen to the laboratory promptly or refrigerate it. | |
| —— | —— | —— | 27. Remove gloves and additional PPE, if used. Perform hand hygiene. | |

Name _____   Date _____

Unit _____   Position _____

Instructor/Evaluator: _____   Position _____

| Excellent | Satisfactory | Needs Practice | SKILL 12-8 **Removing an Indwelling Catheter** | Comments |
|---|---|---|---|---|
| | | | **Goal:** The catheter is removed without difficulty and with minimal patient discomfort. | |
| ____ | ____ | ____ | 1. Confirm the order for catheter removal in the medical record. | |
| ____ | ____ | ____ | 2. Bring necessary equipment to the bedside. | |
| ____ | ____ | ____ | 3. Perform hand hygiene and put on PPE, if indicated. | |
| ____ | ____ | ____ | 4. Identify the patient. | |
| ____ | ____ | ____ | 5. Close curtains around the bed and close the door to the room, if possible. Discuss the procedure with the patient and assess the patient's ability to assist with the procedure. | |
| ____ | ____ | ____ | 6. Adjust bed to comfortable working height, usually elbow height of the caregiver (VISN 8 Patient Safety Center, 2009). Stand on the patient's right side if you are right-handed, patient's left side if you are left-handed. | |
| ____ | ____ | ____ | 7. Position the patient as for catheter insertion. Drape the patient so that only the area around the catheter is exposed. Slide waterproof pad between the female patient's legs or over the male patient's thighs. | |
| ____ | ____ | ____ | 8. Remove the leg strap, tape, or other device used to secure the catheter to the patient's thigh or abdomen. | |
| ____ | ____ | ____ | 9. *Insert the syringe into the balloon inflation port. Allow water to come back by gravity (Mercer Smith, 2003). Alternately, aspirate the entire amount of sterile water used to inflate the balloon. Refer to manufacturer's instructions for deflation. Do not cut the inflation port.* | |
| ____ | ____ | ____ | 10. Ask the patient to take several slow deep breaths. *Slowly and gently remove the catheter.* Place it on the waterproof pad and wrap it in the pad. | |
| ____ | ____ | ____ | 11. Wash and dry the perineal area, as needed. | |
| ____ | ____ | ____ | 12. Remove gloves. Assist the patient to a comfortable position. Cover the patient with bed linens. Place the bed in the lowest position. | |
| ____ | ____ | ____ | 13. Put on clean gloves. Remove equipment and dispose of it according to facility policy. Note characteristics and amount of urine in drainage bag. | |
| ____ | ____ | ____ | 14. Remove gloves and additional PPE, if used. Perform hand hygiene. | |

*Skill Checklists for Taylor's Clinical Nursing Skills:*
*A Nursing Process Approach, 3rd edition*

Name _____  Date _____

Unit _____  Position _____

Instructor/Evaluator: _____  Position _____

SKILL 12-9

# Performing Intermittent Closed Catheter Irrigation

**Goal:** The patient exhibits the free flow of urine through the catheter.

| Excellent | Satisfactory | Needs Practice | | Comments |
|---|---|---|---|---|
| ___ | ___ | ___ | 1. Confirm the order for catheter irrigation in the medical record. | |
| ___ | ___ | ___ | 2. Bring necessary equipment to the bedside. | |
| ___ | ___ | ___ | 3. Perform hand hygiene and put on PPE, if indicated. | |
| ___ | ___ | ___ | 4. Identify the patient. | |
| ___ | ___ | ___ | 5. Close curtains around bed and close the door to the room, if possible. Discuss the procedure with patient. | |
| ___ | ___ | ___ | 6. Adjust bed to comfortable working height, usually elbow height of the caregiver (VISN 8 Patient Safety Center, 2009). | |
| ___ | ___ | ___ | 7. Put on gloves. Empty the catheter drainage bag and measure the amount of urine, noting the amount and characteristics of the urine. Remove gloves. | |
| ___ | ___ | ___ | 8. Assist patient to comfortable position and expose access port on catheter setup. Place waterproof pad under catheter and aspiration port. Remove catheter from device or tape anchoring catheter to the patient. | |
| ___ | ___ | ___ | 9. Open supplies, using aseptic technique. Pour sterile solution into sterile basin. Aspirate the prescribed amount of irrigant (usually 30 to 60 mL) into sterile syringe. Put on gloves. | |
| ___ | ___ | ___ | 10. *Cleanse the access port on catheter with antimicrobial swab.* | |
| ___ | ___ | ___ | 11. Clamp or fold catheter tubing below the access port. | |
| ___ | ___ | ___ | 12. Attach the syringe to the access port on the catheter using a twisting motion. *Gently instill solution into catheter.* | |
| ___ | ___ | ___ | 13. Remove syringe from access port. *Unclamp or unfold tubing and allow irrigant and urine to flow into the drainage bag.* Repeat procedure, as necessary. | |
| ___ | ___ | ___ | 14. Remove gloves. Secure catheter tubing to the patient's inner thigh or lower abdomen (if a male patient) with anchoring device or tape. Leave some slack in the catheter for leg movement. | |

| Excellent | Satisfactory | Needs Practice | | Comments |
|---|---|---|---|---|
| —— | —— | —— | 15. Assist the patient to a comfortable position. Cover the patient with bed linens. Place the bed in the lowest position. | |
| —— | —— | —— | 16. Secure drainage bag below the level of the bladder. Check that drainage tubing is not kinked and that movement of side rails does not interfere with catheter or drainage bag. | |
| —— | —— | —— | 17. Remove equipment and discard syringe in appropriate receptacle. Remove gloves and additional PPE, if used. Perform hand hygiene. | |
| —— | —— | —— | 18. Assess patient's response to the procedure and the quality and amount of drainage after the irrigation. | |

*Skill Checklists for Taylor's Clinical Nursing Skills:*
*A Nursing Process Approach, 3rd edition*

Name _____  Date _____

Unit _____  Position _____

Instructor/Evaluator: _____  Position _____

| Excellent | Satisfactory | Needs Practice | SKILL 12-10<br>**Administering a Continuous Closed Bladder Irrigation** | |
|---|---|---|---|---|
| | | | **Goal:** The patient exhibits free-flowing urine through the catheter. | **Comments** |
| —— | —— | —— | 1. Confirm the order for catheter irrigation in the medical record. Calculate the drip rate via gravity infusion for the prescribed infusion rate. | |
| —— | —— | —— | 2. Bring necessary equipment to the bedside. | |
| —— | —— | —— | 3. Perform hand hygiene and put on PPE, if indicated. | |
| —— | —— | —— | 4. Identify the patient. | |
| —— | —— | —— | 5. Close curtains around the bed and close the door to the room, if possible. Discuss the procedure with patient. | |
| —— | —— | —— | 6. Adjust bed to comfortable working height, usually elbow height of the caregiver (VISN 8 Patient Safety Center, 2009). | |
| —— | —— | —— | 7. Empty the catheter drainage bag and measure the amount of urine, noting the amount and characteristics of the urine. | |
| —— | —— | —— | 8. Assist patient to comfortable position and expose the irrigation port on the catheter setup. Place waterproof pad under the catheter and aspiration port. | |
| —— | —— | —— | 9. Prepare sterile irrigation bag for use as directed by manufacturer. Clearly label the solution as 'Bladder Irrigant.' Include the date and time on the label. Hang bag on IV pole 2.5 to 3 feet above the level of the patient's bladder. Secure tubing clamp and insert sterile tubing with drip chamber to container using aseptic technique. Release clamp and remove protective cover on end of tubing without contaminating it. Allow solution to flush tubing and remove air. Clamp tubing and replace end cover. | |
| —— | —— | —— | 10. Put on gloves. *Cleanse the irrigation port on the catheter with an alcohol swab. Using aseptic technique, attach irrigation tubing to irrigation port of three-way indwelling catheter.* | |
| —— | —— | —— | 11. Check the drainage tubing to make sure clamp, if present, is open. | |
| —— | —— | —— | 12. *Release clamp on irrigation tubing and regulate flow at determined drip rate, according to the ordered rate.* If the bladder irrigation is to be done with a medicated solution, use an electronic infusion device to regulate the flow. | |

| Excellent | Satisfactory | Needs Practice | | |
|---|---|---|---|---|
| | | | SKILL 12-10 **Administering a Continuous Closed Bladder Irrigation** *(Continued)* | |
| | | | | **Comments** |
| —— | —— | —— | 13. Remove gloves. Assist the patient to a comfortable position. Cover the patient with bed linens. Place the bed in the lowest position. | |
| —— | —— | —— | 14. Assess patient's response to the procedure, and quality and amount of drainage. | |
| —— | —— | —— | 15. Remove equipment. Remove gloves and additional PPE, if used. Perform hand hygiene. | |
| —— | —— | —— | 16. As irrigation fluid container nears empty, clamp the administration tubing. Do not allow drip chamber to empty. Disconnect empty bag and attach a new full irrigation solution bag. | |
| —— | —— | —— | 17. Put on gloves and empty drainage collection bag as each new container is hung and recorded. | |

*Skill Checklists for Taylor's Clinical Nursing Skills:*
*A Nursing Process Approach, 3rd edition*

Name _____ Date _____

Unit _____ Position _____

Instructor/Evaluator: _____ Position _____

| Excellent | Satisfactory | Needs Practice | SKILL 12-11 **Emptying and Changing a Stoma Appliance on an Ileal Conduit** | Comments |
|---|---|---|---|---|
| | | | **Goal:** The stoma appliance is applied correctly to the skin to allow urine to drain freely. | |
| —— | —— | —— | 1. Bring necessary equipment to the bedside stand or overbed table. | |
| —— | —— | —— | 2. Perform hand hygiene and put on PPE, if indicated. | |
| —— | —— | —— | 3. Identify the patient. | |
| —— | —— | —— | 4. Close curtains around bed and close the door to the room, if possible. Explain what you are going to do and why you are going to do it to the patient. Encourage patient to observe or participate, if possible. | |
| —— | —— | —— | 5. Assist patient to a comfortable sitting or lying position in bed or a standing or sitting position in the bathroom. If the patient is in bed, adjust the bed to a comfortable working height, usually elbow height of the caregiver (VISN 8 Patient Safety Center, 2009). Place waterproof pad under the patient at the stoma site. | |
| | | | **Emptying the Appliance** | |
| —— | —— | —— | 6. Put on gloves. Hold end of appliance over a bedpan, toilet, or measuring device. Remove the end cap from the spout. Open spout and empty contents into the bedpan, toilet, or measuring device. | |
| —— | —— | —— | 7. Close the spout. Wipe the spout with toilet tissue. Replace the cap. | |
| —— | —— | —— | 8. Remove equipment. Remove gloves. Assist patient to comfortable position. | |
| —— | —— | —— | 9. If appliance is not to be changed, place bed in lowest position. Remove additional PPE, if used. Perform hand hygiene. | |
| | | | **Changing the Appliance** | |
| —— | —— | —— | 10. Place a disposable waterproof pad on the overbed table or other work area. Set up the washbasin with warm water and the rest of the supplies. Place a trash bag within reach. | |
| —— | —— | —— | 11. Put on clean gloves. Place waterproof pad under the patient at the stoma site. Empty the appliance if necessary as described in steps 6–8. | |

# Emptying and Changing a Stoma Appliance on an Ileal Conduit *(Continued)*

| Excellent | Satisfactory | Needs Practice | | Comments |
|---|---|---|---|---|

| | | | | |
|---|---|---|---|---|
| —— | —— | —— | 12. Gently remove appliance faceplate from skin by pushing skin from appliance rather than pulling appliance from skin. Start at the top of the appliance, while keeping the skin taut. Apply a silicone-based adhesive remover by spraying or wiping with the remover wipe. | |
| —— | —— | —— | 13. Place the appliance in the trash bag, if disposable. If reusable, set aside to wash in lukewarm soap and water and allow to air dry after the new appliance is in place. | |
| —— | —— | —— | 14. Clean skin around stoma with mild soap and water or a cleansing agent and a washcloth. Remove all old adhesive from skin; additional adhesive remover may be used. Do not apply lotion to peristomal area. | |
| —— | —— | —— | 15. Gently pat area dry. *Make sure skin around stoma is thoroughly dry.* Assess stoma and condition of surrounding skin. | |
| —— | —— | —— | 16. Place one or two gauze squares over stoma opening. | |
| —— | —— | —— | 17. Apply skin protectant to a 2-inch (5-cm) radius around the stoma, and allow it to dry completely, which takes about 30 seconds. | |
| —— | —— | —— | 18. Lift the gauze squares for a moment and measure the stoma opening, using the measurement guide. Replace the gauze. Trace the same size opening on the back center of the appliance. Cut the opening 1/8 inch larger than the stoma size. Check that the spout is closed and the end cap is in place. | |
| —— | —— | —— | 19. Remove the backing from the appliance. Quickly remove the gauze squares and discard appropriately; ease the appliance over the stoma. *Gently press onto the skin while smoothing over the surface. Apply gentle pressure to the appliance for a few minutes.* | |
| —— | —— | —— | 20. Secure optional belt to appliance and around patient. | |
| —— | —— | —— | 21. Remove gloves. Assist the patient to a comfortable position. Cover the patient with bed linens. Place the bed in the lowest position. | |
| —— | —— | —— | 22. Put on clean gloves. Remove or discard any remaining equipment and assess patient's response to procedure. | |
| —— | —— | —— | 23. Remove gloves and additional PPE, if used. Perform hand hygiene. | |

*Skill Checklists for Taylor's Clinical Nursing Skills:*
*A Nursing Process Approach, 3rd edition*

Name _____    Date _____

Unit _____    Position _____

Instructor/Evaluator: _____    Position _____

## SKILL 12-12

# Caring for a Suprapubic Urinary Catheter

**Goal:** The patient's skin remains clean, dry, intact, and without evidence of irritation or breakdown; and the patient verbalizes an understanding of the purpose for, and care of the catheter, as appropriate.

| Excellent | Satisfactory | Needs Practice | | Comments |
|---|---|---|---|---|
| —— | —— | —— | 1. Bring necessary equipment to the bedside stand or overbed table. | |
| —— | —— | —— | 2. Perform hand hygiene and put on PPE, if indicated. | |
| —— | —— | —— | 3. Identify the patient. | |
| —— | —— | —— | 4. Close curtains around bed and close the door to the room, if possible. Explain what you are going to do, and why you are going to do it, to the patient. Encourage the patient to observe or participate, if possible. | |
| —— | —— | —— | 5. Adjust bed to comfortable working height, usually elbow height of the caregiver (VISN 8 Patient Safety Center, 2009). Assist patient to a supine position. Place waterproof pad under the patient at the stoma site. | |
| —— | —— | —— | 6. Put on clean gloves. Gently remove old dressing, if one is in place. Place dressing in trash bag. Remove gloves. Perform hand hygiene. | |
| —— | —— | —— | 7. Assess the insertion site and surrounding skin. | |
| —— | —— | —— | 8. Wet washcloth with warm water and apply skin cleanser. *Gently cleanse around suprapubic exit site.* Remove any encrustations. If this is a new suprapubic catheter, use sterile cotton-tipped applicators and sterile saline to clean the site until the incision has healed. *Moisten the applicators with the saline and clean in circular motion from the insertion site outward.* | |
| —— | —— | —— | 9. Rinse area of all cleanser. Pat dry. | |
| —— | —— | —— | 10. If the exit site has been draining, place small drain sponge around the catheter to absorb any drainage. Be prepared to change this sponge throughout the day, depending on the amount of drainage. Do not cut a 4 × 4 gauze to make a drain sponge. | |
| —— | —— | —— | 11. Remove gloves. Form a loop in tubing and anchor the tubing on the patient's abdomen. | |

# Caring for a Suprapubic Urinary Catheter *(Continued)*

| Excellent | Satisfactory | Needs Practice | | Comments |
|:---:|:---:|:---:|---|---|
| —— | —— | —— | 12. Assist the patient to a comfortable position. Cover the patient with bed linens. Place the bed in the lowest position. | |
| —— | —— | —— | 13. Put on clean gloves. Remove or discard equipment and assess the patient's response to the procedure. | |
| —— | —— | —— | 14. Remove gloves and additional PPE, if used. Perform hand hygiene. | |

*Skill Checklists for Taylor's Clinical Nursing Skills:*
*A Nursing Process Approach, 3rd edition*

Name _____   Date _____

Unit _____   Position _____

Instructor/Evaluator: _____   Position _____

SKILL 12-13

# Caring for a Peritoneal Dialysis Catheter

**Goal:** The peritoneal dialysis catheter dressing change is completed using aseptic technique without trauma to the site or patient; the site is clean, dry, and intact, without evidence of inflammation or infection.

| Excellent | Satisfactory | Needs Practice | | Comments |
|---|---|---|---|---|
| —— | —— | —— | 1. Bring necessary equipment to the bedside stand or overbed table. | |
| —— | —— | —— | 2. Perform hand hygiene and put on PPE, if indicated. | |
| —— | —— | —— | 3. Identify the patient. | |
| —— | —— | —— | 4. Close curtains around bed and close the door to the room, if possible. Explain what you are going to do and why you are going to do it to the patient. Encourage the patient to observe or participate if possible. | |
| —— | —— | —— | 5. Adjust bed to comfortable working height, usually elbow height of the caregiver (VISN 8 Patient Safety Center, 2009). Assist the patient to a supine position. Expose the abdomen, draping the patient's chest with the bath blanket, exposing only the catheter site. | |
| —— | —— | —— | 6. Put on unsterile gloves. Put on one of the facemasks; have patient put on the other mask. | |
| —— | —— | —— | 7. Gently remove old dressing, noting odor, amount and color of drainage, leakage, and condition of skin around the catheter. Discard dressing in appropriate container. | |
| —— | —— | —— | 8. Remove gloves and discard. Set up sterile field. Open packages. Using aseptic technique, place two sterile gauze squares in basin with antimicrobial agent. Leave two sterile gauze squares opened on sterile field. Alternately (based on facility's policy), place sterile antimicrobial swabs on the sterile field. Place sterile applicator on field. Squeeze a small amount of the topical antibiotic on one of the gauze squares on the sterile field. | |
| —— | —— | —— | 9. Put on sterile gloves. Pick up dialysis catheter with nondominant hand. *With the antimicrobial-soaked gauze/swab, cleanse the skin around the exit site using a circular motion, starting at the exit site and then slowly going outward 3 to 4 inches. Gently remove crusted scabs, if necessary.* | |

SKILL 12-13

# Caring for a Peritoneal Dialysis Catheter *(Continued)*

| Excellent | Satisfactory | Needs Practice | | Comments |
|---|---|---|---|---|
| —— | —— | —— | 10. *Continue to hold catheter with nondominant hand. After skin has dried, clean the catheter with an antimicrobial-soaked gauze, beginning at exit site, going around catheter, and then moving up to end of catheter. Gently remove crusted secretions on the tube, if necessary.* | |
| —— | —— | —— | 11. Using the sterile applicator, apply the topical antibiotic to the catheter exit site, if prescribed. | |
| —— | —— | —— | 12. Place sterile drain sponge around exit site. Then place a 4 × 4 gauze over exit site. Remove your gloves and secure edges of gauze pad with tape. Some institutions recommend placing a transparent dressing over the gauze pads instead of tape. Remove masks. | |
| —— | —— | —— | 13. Coil the exposed length of tubing and secure to the dressing or the patient's abdomen with tape. | |
| —— | —— | —— | 14. Assist the patient to a comfortable position. Cover the patient with bed linens. Place the bed in the lowest position. | |
| —— | —— | —— | 15. Put on clean gloves. Remove or discard equipment and assess the patient's response to the procedure. | |
| —— | —— | —— | 16. Remove gloves and additional PPE, if used. Perform hand hygiene. | |

*Skill Checklists for Taylor's Clinical Nursing Skills:*
*A Nursing Process Approach, 3rd edition*

Name _____     Date _____

Unit _____     Position _____

Instructor/Evaluator: _____     Position _____

## SKILL 12-14

# Caring for a Hemodialysis Access
# (Arteriovenous Fistula or Graft)

**Goal:** The graft or fistula remains patent; the patient verbalizes appropriate care measures and observations to be made, and demonstrates care measures.

| Excellent | Satisfactory | Needs Practice | | Comments |
|---|---|---|---|---|
| ___ | ___ | ___ | 1. Perform hand hygiene and put on PPE, if indicated. | |
| ___ | ___ | ___ | 2. Identify the patient. | |
| ___ | ___ | ___ | 3. Close curtains around bed and close the door to the room, if possible. Explain what you are going to do, and why you are going to do it, to the patient. | |
| ___ | ___ | ___ | 4. *Inspect area over access site for any redness, warmth, tenderness, or blemishes. Palpate over access site, feeling for a thrill or vibration. Palpate pulses distal to the site. Auscultate over access site with bell of stethoscope, listening for a bruit or vibration.* | |
| ___ | ___ | ___ | 5. Ensure that a sign is placed over head of bed informing the healthcare team which arm is affected. ***Do not measure blood pressure, perform a venipuncture, or start an IV on the access arm.*** | |
| ___ | ___ | ___ | 6. Instruct the patient not to sleep with the arm with the access site under head or body. | |
| ___ | ___ | ___ | 7. Instruct patient not to lift heavy objects with, or put pressure on, the arm with the access site. Advise the patient not to carry heavy bags (including purses) on the shoulder of that arm. | |
| ___ | ___ | ___ | 8. Remove PPE, if used. Perform hand hygiene. | |

*Skill Checklists for Taylor's Clinical Nursing Skills:*
*A Nursing Process Approach, 3rd edition*

Name _____     Date _____

Unit _____     Position _____

Instructor/Evaluator: _____     Position _____

## SKILL 13-1
# Administering a Large-Volume Cleansing Enema

**Goal**: The patient expels feces and is free from injury with minimal discomfort.

| Excellent | Satisfactory | Needs Practice | | Comments |
|---|---|---|---|---|
| ___ | ___ | ___ | 1. Verify the order for the enema. Bring necessary equipment to the bedside stand or overbed table. | |
| ___ | ___ | ___ | 2. Perform hand hygiene and put on PPE, if indicated. | |
| ___ | ___ | ___ | 3. Identify the patient. | |
| ___ | ___ | ___ | 4. Close curtains around the bed and close the door to the room, if possible. Explain what you are going to do and why you are going to do it to the patient. Discuss where the patient will defecate. Have a bedpan, commode, or nearby bathroom ready for use. | |
| ___ | ___ | ___ | 5. Warm solution in amount ordered, and check temperature with a bath thermometer, if available. If bath thermometer is not available, warm to room temperature or slightly higher, and test on inner wrist. If tap water is used, adjust temperature as it flows from faucet. | |
| ___ | ___ | ___ | 6. Add enema solution to container. Release clamp and allow fluid to progress through tube before reclamping. | |
| ___ | ___ | ___ | 7. Adjust bed to comfortable working height, usually elbow height of the caregiver (VISN 8 Patient Safety Center, 2009). Position the patient on the left side (Sims' position), as dictated by patient comfort and condition. Fold top linen back just enough to allow access to the patient's rectal area. Place a waterproof pad under the patient's hip. | |
| ___ | ___ | ___ | 8. Put on nonsterile gloves. | |
| ___ | ___ | ___ | 9. Elevate solution so that it is no higher than 18 inches (45 cm) above level of anus. Plan to give the solution slowly over a period of 5 to 10 minutes. Hang the container on an IV pole or hold it at the proper height. | |
| ___ | ___ | ___ | 10. Generously lubricate end of rectal tube 2 to 3 inches (5 to 7 cm). A disposable enema set may have a prelubricated rectal tube. | |
| ___ | ___ | ___ | 11. Lift buttock to expose anus. Slowly and gently insert the enema tube 3 to 4 inches (7 to 10 cm) for an adult. Direct it at an angle pointing toward the umbilicus, not bladder. Ask patient to take several deep breaths. | |

# Administering a Large-Volume Cleansing Enema *(Continued)*

| Excellent | Satisfactory | Needs Practice | | Comments |
|---|---|---|---|---|
| —— | —— | —— | 12. If resistance is met while inserting tube, permit a small amount of solution to enter, withdraw tube slightly, and then continue to insert it. ***Do not force entry of the tube.*** Ask patient to take several deep breaths. | |
| —— | —— | —— | 13. Introduce solution slowly over a period of 5 to 10 minutes. Hold tubing all the time that solution is being instilled. | |
| —— | —— | —— | 14. Clamp tubing or lower container if patient has desire to defecate or cramping occurs. Instruct the patient to take small, fast breaths or to pant. | |
| —— | —— | —— | 15. After solution has been given, clamp tubing and remove tube. Have paper towel ready to receive tube as it is withdrawn. | |
| —— | —— | —— | 16. Return the patient to a comfortable position. Encourage the patient to hold the solution until the urge to defecate is strong, usually in about 5 to 15 minutes. Make sure the linens under the patient are dry. Remove your gloves and ensure that the patient is covered. | |
| —— | —— | —— | 17. Raise side rail. Lower bed height and adjust head of bed to a comfortable position. | |
| —— | —— | —— | 18. Remove additional PPE, if used. Perform hand hygiene. | |
| —— | —— | —— | 19. When patient has a strong urge to defecate, place him or her in a sitting position on a bedpan or assist to commode or bathroom. Offer toilet tissues, if not in patient's reach. Stay with patient or have call bell readily accessible. | |
| —— | —— | —— | 20. Remind patient not to flush the commode before you inspect results of enema. | |
| —— | —— | —— | 21. Put on gloves and assist patient, if necessary, with cleaning of anal area. Offer washcloths, soap, and water for hand-washing. Remove gloves. | |
| —— | —— | —— | 22. Leave the patient clean and comfortable. Care for equipment properly. | |
| —— | —— | —— | 23. Perform hand hygiene. | |

*Skill Checklists for Taylor's Clinical Nursing Skills:*
*A Nursing Process Approach, 3rd edition*

Name _____  Date _____

Unit _____  Position _____

Instructor/Evaluator: _____  Position _____

## SKILL 13-2
# Administering a Small-Volume Cleansing Enema

**Goal:** The patient expels feces and reports a decrease in pain and discomfort.

| Excellent | Satisfactory | Needs Practice | | Comments |
|---|---|---|---|---|
| —— | —— | —— | 1. Verify the order for the enema. Bring necessary equipment to the bedside stand or overbed table. Warm the solution to body temperature in a bowl of warm water. | |
| —— | —— | —— | 2. Perform hand hygiene and put on PPE, if indicated. | |
| —— | —— | —— | 3. Identify the patient. | |
| —— | —— | —— | 4. Close curtains around bed and close the door to the room, if possible. Explain what you are going to do and why you are going to do it to the patient. Discuss where the patient will defecate. Have a bedpan, commode, or nearby bathroom ready for use. | |
| —— | —— | —— | 5. Adjust bed to comfortable working height, usually elbow height of the caregiver (VISN 8 Patient Safety Center, 2009). Position the patient on the left side (Sims' position), as dictated by patient comfort and condition. Fold top linen back just enough to allow access to the patient's rectal area. Place a waterproof pad under the patient's hip. | |
| —— | —— | —— | 6. Put on nonsterile gloves. | |
| —— | —— | —— | 7. Remove the cap and generously lubricate end of rectal tube 2 to 3 inches (5 to 7 cm). | |
| —— | —— | —— | 8. Lift buttock to expose anus. Slowly and gently insert the rectal tube 3 to 4 inches (7 to 10 cm) for an adult. Direct it at an angle pointing toward the umbilicus, not bladder. ***Do not force entry of the tube.*** Ask patient to take several deep breaths. | |
| —— | —— | —— | 9. Compress the container with your hands. Roll the end up on itself, toward the rectal tip. Administer all the solution in the container. | |
| —— | —— | —— | 10. After solution has been given, remove tube, keeping the container compressed. Have paper towel ready to receive tube as it is withdrawn. Encourage the patient to hold the solution until the urge to defecate is strong, usually in about 5 to 15 minutes. | |
| —— | —— | —— | 11. Remove gloves. Return the patient to a comfortable position. Make sure the linens under the patient are dry. Ensure that the patient is covered. | |

SKILL 13-2

# Administering a Small-Volume
# Cleansing Enema (Continued)

| Excellent | Satisfactory | Needs Practice | | Comments |
|---|---|---|---|---|
| —— | —— | —— | 12. Raise side rail. Lower bed height and adjust head of bed to a comfortable position. | |
| —— | —— | —— | 13. Remove additional PPE, if used. Perform hand hygiene. | |
| —— | —— | —— | 14. When patient has a strong urge to defecate, place him or her in a sitting position on a bedpan or assist to commode or bathroom. Stay with patient or have call bell readily accessible. | |
| —— | —— | —— | 15. Remind patient not to flush the commode before you inspect the results of the enema. | |
| —— | —— | —— | 16. Put on gloves and assist patient, if necessary, with cleaning of anal area. Offer washcloths, soap, and water for hand-washing. Remove gloves. | |
| —— | —— | —— | 17. Leave the patient clean and comfortable. Care for equipment properly. | |
| —— | —— | —— | 18. Perform hand hygiene. | |

*Skill Checklists for Taylor's Clinical Nursing Skills:*
*A Nursing Process Approach, 3rd edition*

Name _____  Date _____

Unit _____  Position _____

Instructor/Evaluator: _____  Position _____

| Excellent | Satisfactory | Needs Practice | SKILL 13-3<br>**Administering a Retention Enema**<br><br>**Goal:** The patient retains the solution for the prescribed, appropriate length of time and experiences the expected therapeutic effect of the solution. | Comments |
|---|---|---|---|---|
| ___ | ___ | ___ | 1. Verify the order for the enema. Bring necessary equipment to the bedside stand or overbed table. Warm the solution to body temperature in a bowl of warm water. | |
| ___ | ___ | ___ | 2. Perform hand hygiene and put on PPE, if indicated. | |
| ___ | ___ | ___ | 3. Identify the patient. | |
| ___ | ___ | ___ | 4. Close curtains around bed and close the door to the room, if possible. Explain what you are going to do and why you are going to do it to the patient. Have a bedpan, commode, or nearby bathroom ready for use. | |
| ___ | ___ | ___ | 5. Adjust bed to comfortable working height, usually elbow height of the caregiver (VISN 8 Patient Safety Center, 2009). Position the patient on the left side (Sims' position), as dictated by patient comfort and condition. Fold top linen back just enough to allow access to the patient's rectal area. Place a waterproof pad under the patient's hip. | |
| ___ | ___ | ___ | 6. Put on nonsterile gloves. | |
| ___ | ___ | ___ | 7. Remove cap of prepackaged enema solution. Apply a generous amount of lubricant to the tube. | |
| ___ | ___ | ___ | 8. Lift buttock to expose anus. Slowly and gently insert rectal tube 3 to 4 inches (7 to 10 cm) for an adult. Direct it at an angle pointing toward the umbilicus. Ask patient to take several deep breaths. | |
| ___ | ___ | ___ | 9. If resistance is met while inserting the tube, permit a small amount of solution to enter, withdraw tube slightly, and then continue to insert it. *Do not force entry of tube.* | |
| ___ | ___ | ___ | 10. Slowly squeeze enema container, emptying entire contents. | |
| ___ | ___ | ___ | 11. *Remove container while keeping it compressed.* Have paper towel ready to receive tube as it is withdrawn. | |
| ___ | ___ | ___ | 12. *Instruct patient to retain enema solution for at least 30 minutes or as indicated, per manufacturer's direction.* | |
| ___ | ___ | ___ | 13. Remove your gloves. Return the patient to a comfortable position. Make sure the linens under the patient are dry and ensure that the patient is covered. | |
| ___ | ___ | ___ | 14. Raise side rail. Lower bed height and adjust head of bed to a comfortable position. | |

| Excellent | Satisfactory | Needs Practice | | Comments |
|---|---|---|---|---|

**SKILL 13-3**

# Administering a Retention Enema *(Continued)*

| Excellent | Satisfactory | Needs Practice | | Comments |
|---|---|---|---|---|
| —— | —— | —— | 15. Remove additional PPE, if used. Perform hand hygiene. | |
| —— | —— | —— | 16. If the patient has a strong urge to dispel the solution, place him or her in a sitting position on bedpan or assist to commode or bathroom. Stay with patient or have call bell readily accessible. | |
| —— | —— | —— | 17. Remind patient not to flush commode before you inspect results of enema, if used for bowel evacuation. Record character of stool, as appropriate, and patient's reaction to enema. | |
| —— | —— | —— | 18. Put on gloves and assist patient, if necessary, with cleaning of anal area. Offer washcloths, soap, and water for handwashing. Remove gloves. | |
| —— | —— | —— | 19. Leave patient clean and comfortable. Care for equipment properly. | |
| —— | —— | —— | 20. Perform hand hygiene. | |

*Skill Checklists for Taylor's Clinical Nursing Skills:*
*A Nursing Process Approach, 3rd edition*

Name _____    Date _____

Unit _____    Position _____

Instructor/Evaluator: _____    Position _____

| Excellent | Satisfactory | Needs Practice | SKILL 13-4<br>**Digital Removal of Stool**<br><br>**Goal:** The patient expels feces with assistance and is free from trauma with minimal patient discomfort. | Comments |
|---|---|---|---|---|
| ___ | ___ | ___ | 1. Verify the order. Bring necessary equipment to the bedside stand or overbed table. | |
| ___ | ___ | ___ | 2. Perform hand hygiene and put on PPE, if indicated. | |
| ___ | ___ | ___ | 3. Identify the patient. | |
| ___ | ___ | ___ | 4. Close curtains around bed and close the door to the room, if possible. Explain what you are going to do and why you are going to do it to the patient. Discuss signs and symptoms of a slow heart rate. Instruct patient to alert you if any of these symptoms are felt during the procedure. Have a bedpan ready for use. | |
| ___ | ___ | ___ | 5. Adjust bed to comfortable working height, usually elbow height of the caregiver (VISN 8 Patient Safety Center, 2009). Position the patient on the left side (Sims' position), as dictated by patient comfort and condition. Fold top linen back just enough to allow access to the patient's rectal area. Place a waterproof pad under the patient's hip. | |
| ___ | ___ | ___ | 6. Put on nonsterile gloves. | |
| ___ | ___ | ___ | 7. Generously lubricate index finger with water-soluble lubricant and insert finger gently into anal canal, pointing toward the umbilicus. | |
| ___ | ___ | ___ | 8. Gently work the finger around and into the hardened mass to break it up and then remove pieces of it. Instruct patient to bear down, if possible, while extracting feces to ease in removal. Place extracted stool in bedpan. | |
| ___ | ___ | ___ | 9. Remove impaction at intervals if it is severe. ***Instruct patient to alert you if he or she begins to feel lightheaded or nauseated. If patient reports either symptom, stop removal and assess patient.*** | |
| ___ | ___ | ___ | 10. Put on clean gloves. Assist patient, if necessary, with cleaning of anal area. Offer washcloths, soap, and water for handwashing. If patient is able, offer sitz bath. | |

| Excellent | Satisfactory | Needs Practice | SKILL 13-4<br>**Digital Removal of Stool** *(Continued)* | |
|---|---|---|---|---|
| | | | | **Comments** |
| —— | —— | —— | 11. Remove gloves. Return the patient to a comfortable position. Make sure the linens under the patient are dry. Ensure that the patient is covered. | |
| —— | —— | —— | 12. Raise side rail. Lower bed height and adjust head of bed to a comfortable position. | |
| —— | —— | —— | 13. Remove additional PPE, if used. Perform hand hygiene. | |

*Skill Checklists for Taylor's Clinical Nursing Skills:*
*A Nursing Process Approach, 3rd edition*

Name _____   Date _____

Unit _____   Position _____

Instructor/Evaluator: _____   Position _____

## SKILL 13-5
## Applying a Fecal Incontinence Pouch

**Goal:** The patient expels feces into the pouch and maintains intact perianal skin.

| Excellent | Satisfactory | Needs Practice | | Comments |
|---|---|---|---|---|
| ___ | ___ | ___ | 1. Bring necessary equipment to the bedside stand or overbed table. | |
| ___ | ___ | ___ | 2. Perform hand hygiene and put on PPE, if indicated. | |
| ___ | ___ | ___ | 3. Identify the patient. | |
| ___ | ___ | ___ | 4. Close curtains around bed and close the door to the room, if possible. Explain what you are going to do and why you are going to do it to the patient. | |
| ___ | ___ | ___ | 5. Adjust bed to comfortable working height, usually elbow height of the caregiver (VISN 8 Patient Safety Center, 2009). Position the patient on the left side (Sims' position), as dictated by patient comfort and condition. Fold top linen back just enough to allow access to the patient's rectal area. Place a waterproof pad under the patient's hip. | |
| ___ | ___ | ___ | 6. Put on nonsterile gloves. Cleanse perianal area. Pat dry thoroughly. | |
| ___ | ___ | ___ | 7. Trim perianal hair with scissors, if needed. | |
| ___ | ___ | ___ | 8. Apply the skin protectant or barrier and allow it to dry. | |
| ___ | ___ | ___ | 9. Remove paper backing from adhesive of pouch. | |
| ___ | ___ | ___ | 10. With nondominant hand, separate buttocks. Apply fecal pouch to anal area with dominant hand, ensuring that opening of bag is over anus. | |
| ___ | ___ | ___ | 11. Release buttocks. Attach connector of fecal incontinence pouch to urinary drainage bag. Hang drainage bag below patient. | |
| ___ | ___ | ___ | 12. Remove gloves. Return the patient to a comfortable position. Make sure the linens under the patient are dry. Ensure that the patient is covered. | |
| ___ | ___ | ___ | 13. Raise side rail. Lower bed height and adjust head of bed to a comfortable position. | |
| ___ | ___ | ___ | 14. Remove additional PPE, if used. Perform hand hygiene. | |

*Skill Checklists for Taylor's Clinical Nursing Skills:*
*A Nursing Process Approach, 3rd edition*

Name _____   Date _____

Unit _____   Position _____

Instructor/Evaluator: _____   Position _____

SKILL 13-6

# Changing and Emptying an Ostomy Appliance

| Excellent | Satisfactory | Needs Practice | | Comments |
|---|---|---|---|---|
| | | | **Goal:** The stoma appliance is applied correctly to the skin to allow stool to drain freely. | |
| —— | —— | —— | 1. Bring necessary equipment to the bedside stand or overbed table. | |
| —— | —— | —— | 2. Perform hand hygiene and put on PPE, if indicated. | |
| —— | —— | —— | 3. Identify the patient. | |
| —— | —— | —— | 4. Close curtains around bed and close the door to the room, if possible. Explain what you are going to do and why you are going to do it to the patient. Encourage the patient to observe or participate, if possible. | |
| —— | —— | —— | 5. Assist patient to a comfortable sitting or lying position in bed or a standing or sitting position in the bathroom. | |
| | | | **Emptying an Appliance** | |
| —— | —— | —— | 6. Put on disposable gloves. Remove clamp and fold end of pouch upward like a cuff. | |
| —— | —— | —— | 7. Empty contents into bedpan, toilet, or measuring device. | |
| —— | —— | —— | 8. Wipe the lower 2 inches of the appliance or pouch with toilet tissue. | |
| —— | —— | —— | 9. Uncuff edge of appliance or pouch and apply clip or clamp, or secure Velcro closure. Ensure the curve of the clamp follows the curve of the patient's body. Remove gloves. Assist patient to a comfortable position. | |
| —— | —— | —— | 10. If appliance is not to be changed, remove additional PPE, if used. Perform hand hygiene. | |
| | | | **Changing an Appliance** | |
| —— | —— | —— | 11. Place a disposable pad on the work surface. Set up the wash basin with warm water and the rest of the supplies. Place a trash bag within reach. | |
| —— | —— | —— | 12. Put on clean gloves. Place waterproof pad under the patient at the stoma site. Empty the appliance as described previously. | |

SKILL 13-6

# Changing and Emptying an
# Ostomy Appliance *(Continued)*

| Excellent | Satisfactory | Needs Practice | | Comments |
|---|---|---|---|---|

| | | | |
|---|---|---|---|
| —— —— —— | 13. | Gently remove pouch faceplate from skin by pushing skin from appliance rather than pulling appliance from skin. Start at the top of the appliance, while keeping the abdominal skin taut. Apply a silicone-based adhesive remover by spraying or wiping with the remover wipe. | |
| —— —— —— | 14. | Place the appliance in the trash bag, if disposable. If reusable, set aside to wash in lukewarm soap and water and allow to air dry after the new appliance is in place. | |
| —— —— —— | 15. | Use toilet tissue to remove any excess stool from stoma. Cover stoma with gauze pad. Clean skin around stoma with mild soap and water or a cleansing agent and a washcloth. Remove all old adhesive from skin; use an adhesive remover, as necessary. Do not apply lotion to peristomal area. | |
| —— —— —— | 16. | Gently pat area dry. Make sure skin around stoma is thoroughly dry. Assess stoma and condition of surrounding skin. | |
| —— —— —— | 17. | Apply skin protectant to a 2-inch (5 cm) radius around the stoma, and allow it to dry completely, which takes about 30 seconds. | |
| —— —— —— | 18. | Lift the gauze squares for a moment and measure the stoma opening, using the measurement guide. Replace the gauze. Trace the same-size opening on the back center of the appliance. Cut the opening 1/8 inch larger than the stoma size. | |
| —— —— —— | 19. | Remove the backing from the appliance. Quickly remove the gauze squares and ease the appliance over the stoma. Gently press onto the skin while smoothing over the surface. Apply gentle pressure to appliance for 5 minutes. | |
| —— —— —— | 20. | Close bottom of appliance or pouch by folding the end upward and using the clamp or clip that comes with the product, or secure Velcro closure. Ensure the curve of the clamp follows the curve of the patient's body. | |
| —— —— —— | 21. | Remove gloves. Assist the patient to a comfortable position. Cover the patient with bed linens. Place the bed in the lowest position. | |
| —— —— —— | 22. | Put on clean gloves. Remove or discard equipment and assess patient's response to procedure. | |
| —— —— —— | 23. | Remove gloves and additional PPE, if used. Perform hand hygiene. | |

*Skill Checklists for Taylor's Clinical Nursing Skills:*
*A Nursing Process Approach, 3rd edition*

Name _____     Date _____

Unit _____     Position _____

Instructor/Evaluator: _____     Position _____

## SKILL 13-7
# Irrigating a Colostomy

| Excellent | Satisfactory | Needs Practice | **Goal:** The patient expels soft, formed stool. | **Comments** |
|---|---|---|---|---|
| ___ | ___ | ___ | 1. Verify the order for the irrigation. Bring necessary equipment to the bedside stand or overbed table. | |
| ___ | ___ | ___ | 2. Perform hand hygiene and put on PPE, if indicated. | |
| ___ | ___ | ___ | 3. Identify the patient. | |
| ___ | ___ | ___ | 4. Close curtains around bed and close the door to the room, if possible. Explain what you are going to do and why you are going to do it to the patient. Plan where the patient will receive irrigation. Assist patient onto bedside commode or into nearby bathroom. | |
| ___ | ___ | ___ | 5. Warm solution in amount ordered and check temperature with a bath thermometer, if available. If bath thermometer is not available, warm to room temperature or slightly higher, and test on inner wrist. If tap water is used, adjust temperature as it flows from faucet. | |
| ___ | ___ | ___ | 6. Add irrigation solution to container. Release clamp and allow fluid to progress through tube before reclamping. | |
| ___ | ___ | ___ | 7. Hang container so that bottom of bag will be at patient's shoulder level when seated. | |
| ___ | ___ | ___ | 8. Put on nonsterile gloves. | |
| ___ | ___ | ___ | 9. Remove ostomy appliance and attach irrigation sleeve. Place drainage end into toilet bowl or commode. | |
| ___ | ___ | ___ | 10. Lubricate end of cone with water-soluble lubricant. | |
| ___ | ___ | ___ | 11. Insert the cone into the stoma. Introduce solution slowly over a period of 5 to 6 minutes. Hold cone and tubing (or if patient is able, allow patient to hold) all the time that solution is being instilled. Control rate of flow by closing or opening the clamp. | |
| ___ | ___ | ___ | 12. *Hold cone in place for an additional 10 seconds after the fluid is infused.* | |
| ___ | ___ | ___ | 13. Remove cone. Patient should remain seated on toilet or bedside commode. | |
| ___ | ___ | ___ | 14. After majority of solution has returned, allow patient to clip (close) bottom of irrigating sleeve and continue with daily activities. | |

# Irrigating a Colostomy *(Continued)*

| Excellent | Satisfactory | Needs Practice | | Comments |
|---|---|---|---|---|
| ___ | ___ | ___ | 15. After solution has stopped flowing from stoma, put on clean gloves. Remove irrigating sleeve and cleanse skin around stoma opening with mild soap and water. Gently pat peristomal skin dry. | |
| ___ | ___ | ___ | 16. Attach new appliance to stoma or stoma cover (see Skill 13-6), as needed. | |
| ___ | ___ | ___ | 17. Remove gloves. Return the patient to a comfortable position. Make sure the linens under the patient are dry, if appropriate. Ensure that the patient is covered. | |
| ___ | ___ | ___ | 18. Raise side rail. Lower bed height and adjust head of bed to a comfortable position, as necessary. | |
| ___ | ___ | ___ | 19. Remove gloves and additional PPE, if used. Perform hand hygiene. | |

*Skill Checklists for Taylor's Clinical Nursing Skills:*
*A Nursing Process Approach, 3rd edition*

Name _____     Date _____

Unit _____     Position _____

Instructor/Evaluator: _____     Position _____

SKILL 13-8

# Irrigating a Nasogastric Tube Connected to Suction

| Excellent | Satisfactory | Needs Practice | | Comments |
|---|---|---|---|---|
| | | | **Goal:** The tube maintains patency with irrigation and patient remains free from injury. | |
| ___ | ___ | ___ | 1. Assemble equipment. Verify the medical order or facility policy and procedure regarding frequency of irrigation, solution type, and amount of irrigant. Check expiration dates on irrigating solution and irrigation set. | |
| ___ | ___ | ___ | 2. Perform hand hygiene and put on PPE, if indicated. | |
| ___ | ___ | ___ | 3. Identify the patient. | |
| ___ | ___ | ___ | 4. Explain the procedure to the patient and why this intervention is needed. Answer any questions as needed. Perform key abdominal assessments as described above. | |
| ___ | ___ | ___ | 5. Pull the patient's bedside curtain. Raise bed to a comfortable working position, usually elbow height of the caregiver (VISN 8 Patient Safety Center, 2009). Assist patient to 30- to 45-degree position, unless this is contraindicated. Pour the irrigating solution into container. | |
| ___ | ___ | ___ | 6. Put on gloves. *Check placement of NG tube.* (Refer to Skill 11-2.) | |
| ___ | ___ | ___ | 7. Draw up 30 mL of saline solution (or amount indicated in the order or policy) into syringe. | |
| ___ | ___ | ___ | 8. Clamp suction tubing near connection site. If needed, disconnect tube from suction apparatus and lay on disposable pad or towel, or hold both tubes upright in nondominant hand. | |
| ___ | ___ | ___ | 9. Place tip of syringe in tube. *If Salem sump or double-lumen tube is used, make sure that syringe tip is placed in drainage port and not in blue air vent.* Hold syringe upright and gently insert the irrigant (or allow solution to flow in by gravity if agency policy or physician indicates). *Do not force solution into tube.* | |
| ___ | ___ | ___ | 10. *If unable to irrigate tube, reposition patient and attempt irrigation again. Inject 10 to 20 mL of air and aspirate again. Check with physician or follow agency policy, if repeated attempts to irrigate tube fail.* | |

# Irrigating a Nasogastric Tube Connected to Suction *(Continued)*

| Excellent | Satisfactory | Needs Practice | | Comments |
|---|---|---|---|---|
| —— | —— | —— | 11. After irrigant has been instilled, hold end of NG tube over irrigation tray or emesis basin. Observe for return flow of NG drainage into available container. Alternately, you may reconnect the NG tube to suction and observe the return drainage as it drains into the suction container. | |
| —— | —— | —— | 12. *If not already done, reconnect drainage port to suction, if ordered.* | |
| —— | —— | —— | 13. *Inject air into blue air vent after irrigation is complete. Position the blue air vent above the patient's stomach.* | |
| —— | —— | —— | 14. Remove gloves. Lower the bed and raise side rails, as necessary. Assist the patient to a position of comfort. Perform hand hygiene. | |
| —— | —— | —— | 15. Put on gloves. Measure returned solution, if collected outside of suction apparatus. Rinse equipment if it will be reused. Label with the date, patient's name, room number, and purpose (for NG tube/irrigation). | |
| —— | —— | —— | 16. Remove gloves and additional PPE, if used. Perform hand hygiene. | |

*Skill Checklists for Taylor's Clinical Nursing Skills:*
*A Nursing Process Approach, 3rd edition*

Name _____  Date _____

Unit _____  Position _____

Instructor/Evaluator: _____  Position _____

## SKILL 14-1
# Using a Pulse Oximeter

**Goal:** The patient exhibits arterial blood oxygen saturation within acceptable parameters, or greater than 95%.

| Excellent | Satisfactory | Needs Practice | | Comments |
|---|---|---|---|---|
| —— | —— | —— | 1. Review chart for any health problems that would affect the patient's oxygenation status. | |
| —— | —— | —— | 2. Bring necessary equipment to the bedside stand or overbed table. | |
| —— | —— | —— | 3. Perform hand hygiene and put on PPE, if indicated. | |
| —— | —— | —— | 4. Identify the patient. | |
| —— | —— | —— | 5. Close curtains around bed and close the door to the room, if possible. Explain what you are going to do and why you are going to do it to the patient. | |
| —— | —— | —— | 6. Select an adequate site for application of the sensor. | |
| —— | —— | —— |    a. Use the patient's index, middle, or ring finger. | |
| —— | —— | —— |    b. Check the proximal pulse and capillary refill at the pulse closest to the site. | |
| —— | —— | —— |    c. If circulation at the site is inadequate, consider using the earlobe, forehead, or bridge of nose. | |
| —— | —— | —— |    d. Use a toe only if lower extremity circulation is not compromised. | |
| —— | —— | —— | 7. Select proper equipment: | |
| —— | —— | —— |    a. If one finger is too large for the probe, use a smaller one. A pediatric probe may be used for a small adult. | |
| —— | —— | —— |    b. Use probes appropriate for patient's age and size. | |
| —— | —— | —— |    c. Check if patient is allergic to adhesive. A nonadhesive finger clip or reflectance sensor is available. | |
| —— | —— | —— | 8. Prepare the monitoring site. Cleanse the selected area with the alcohol wipe or disposable cleansing cloth. Allow the area to dry. If necessary, remove nail polish and artificial nails after checking pulse oximeter's manufacturer instructions. | |
| —— | —— | —— | 9. *Apply probe securely to skin. Make sure that the light-emitting sensor and the light-receiving sensor are aligned opposite each other (not necessary to check if placed on forehead or bridge of nose).* | |

| Excellent | Satisfactory | Needs Practice | SKILL 14-1 **Using a Pulse Oximeter** *(Continued)* | Comments |
|---|---|---|---|---|
| —— | —— | —— | 10. Connect the sensor probe to the pulse oximeter, turn the oximeter on, and check operation of the equipment (audible beep, fluctuation of bar of light or waveform on face of oximeter). | |
| —— | —— | —— | 11. Set alarms on pulse oximeter. Check manufacturer's alarm limits for high and low pulse rate settings. | |
| —— | —— | —— | 12. Check oxygen saturation at regular intervals, as ordered by primary care provider, nursing assessment, and signaled by alarms. Monitor hemoglobin level. | |
| —— | —— | —— | 13. Remove sensor on a regular basis and check for skin irritation or signs of pressure (every 2 hours for spring-tension sensor or every 4 hours for adhesive finger or toe sensor). | |
| —— | —— | —— | 14. Clean nondisposable sensors according to the manufacturer's directions. Remove PPE, if used. Perform hand hygiene. | |

*Skill Checklists for Taylor's Clinical Nursing Skills:*
*A Nursing Process Approach, 3rd edition*

Name _____  Date _____

Unit _____  Position _____

Instructor/Evaluator: _____  Position _____

## SKILL 14-2
## Teaching Patient to Use an Incentive Spirometer

**Goal:** The patient accurately demonstrates the procedure for using the spirometer.

| Excellent | Satisfactory | Needs Practice | | Comments |
|---|---|---|---|---|
| —— | —— | —— | 1. Review chart for any health problems that would affect the patient's oxygenation status. | |
| —— | —— | —— | 2. Bring necessary equipment to the bedside stand or overbed table. | |
| —— | —— | —— | 3. Perform hand hygiene and put on PPE, if indicated. | |
| —— | —— | —— | 4. Identify the patient. | |
| —— | —— | —— | 5. Close curtains around bed and close the door to the room, if possible. Explain what you are going to do and why you are going to do it to the patient. | |
| —— | —— | —— | 6. Assist patient to an upright or semi-Fowler's position, if possible. Remove dentures if they fit poorly. Assess the patient's level of pain. Administer pain medication, as prescribed, if needed. Wait the appropriate amount of time for the medication to take effect. *If patient has recently undergone abdominal or chest surgery, place a pillow or folded blanket over a chest or abdominal incision for splinting.* | |
| —— | —— | —— | 7. Demonstrate how to steady the device with one hand and hold the mouthpiece with the other hand. If the patient cannot use hands, assist the patient with the incentive spirometer. | |
| —— | —— | —— | 8. Instruct the patient to exhale normally and then place lips securely around the mouthpiece. | |
| —— | —— | —— | 9. *Instruct patient to inhale slowly and as deeply as possible through the mouthpiece without using nose (if desired, a nose clip may be used).* | |
| —— | —— | —— | 10. When the patient cannot inhale anymore, *the patient should hold his or her breath and count to three.* Check position of gauge to determine progress and level attained. If patient begins to cough, splint an abdominal or chest incision. | |

| Excellent | Satisfactory | Needs Practice | SKILL 14-2<br>**Teaching Patient to Use an<br>Incentive Spirometer** *(Continued)* |
|---|---|---|---|
| | | | **Comments** |
| —— | —— | —— | 11. Instruct the patient to remove lips from mouthpiece and exhale normally. *If patient becomes light-headed during the process, tell him or her to stop and take a few normal breaths before resuming incentive spirometry.* |
| —— | —— | —— | 12. Encourage patient to perform incentive spirometry 5 to 10 times every 1 to 2 hours, if possible. |
| —— | —— | —— | 13. Clean the mouthpiece with water and shake to dry. Remove PPE, if used. Perform hand hygiene. |

*Skill Checklists for Taylor's Clinical Nursing Skills:*
*A Nursing Process Approach, 3rd edition*

Name _____  Date _____

Unit _____  Position _____

Instructor/Evaluator: _____  Position _____

| Excellent | Satisfactory | Needs Practice | SKILL 14-3<br>**Administering Oxygen by Nasal Cannula**<br><br>**Goal:** The patient exhibits an oxygen saturation level within acceptable parameters. | Comments |
|---|---|---|---|---|
| ⎯ | ⎯ | ⎯ | 1. Bring necessary equipment to the bedside stand or overbed table. | |
| ⎯ | ⎯ | ⎯ | 2. Perform hand hygiene and put on PPE, if indicated. | |
| ⎯ | ⎯ | ⎯ | 3. Identify the patient. | |
| ⎯ | ⎯ | ⎯ | 4. Close curtains around bed and close the door to the room, if possible. | |
| ⎯ | ⎯ | ⎯ | 5. Explain what you are going to do and the reason for doing it to the patient. Review safety precautions necessary when oxygen is in use. Place "No Smoking" signs in appropriate areas. | |
| ⎯ | ⎯ | ⎯ | 6. Connect nasal cannula to oxygen setup with humidification, if one is in use. Adjust flow rate as ordered. Check that oxygen is flowing out of prongs. | |
| ⎯ | ⎯ | ⎯ | 7. Place prongs in patient's nostrils. Place tubing over and behind each ear with adjuster comfortably under chin. Alternately, the tubing may be placed around the patient's head, with the adjuster at the back or base of the head. Place gauze pads at ear beneath the tubing, as necessary. | |
| ⎯ | ⎯ | ⎯ | 8. Adjust the fit of the cannula, as necessary. Tubing should be snug but not tight against the skin. | |
| ⎯ | ⎯ | ⎯ | 9. *Encourage patient to breathe through the nose, with the mouth closed.* | |
| ⎯ | ⎯ | ⎯ | 10. Reassess patient's respiratory status, including respiratory rate, effort, and lung sounds. Note any signs of respiratory distress, such as tachypnea, nasal flaring, use of accessory muscles, or dyspnea. | |
| ⎯ | ⎯ | ⎯ | 11. Remove PPE, if used. Perform hand hygiene. | |
| ⎯ | ⎯ | ⎯ | 12. Put on clean gloves. Remove and clean the cannula and assess nares at least every 8 hours, or according to agency recommendations. Check nares for evidence of irritation or bleeding. | |

*Skill Checklists for Taylor's Clinical Nursing Skills:*
*A Nursing Process Approach, 3rd edition*

Name _____     Date _____

Unit _____     Position _____

Instructor/Evaluator: _____     Position _____

| Excellent | Satisfactory | Needs Practice | SKILL 14-4<br>**Administering Oxygen by Mask**<br><br>**Goal:** The patient exhibits an oxygen saturation level within acceptable parameters. | Comments |
|---|---|---|---|---|
| ____ | ____ | ____ | 1. Bring necessary equipment to the bedside stand or overbed table. | |
| ____ | ____ | ____ | 2. Perform hand hygiene and put on PPE, if indicated. | |
| ____ | ____ | ____ | 3. Identify the patient. | |
| ____ | ____ | ____ | 4. Close curtains around bed and close the door to the room, if possible. | |
| ____ | ____ | ____ | 5. Explain what you are going to do and the reason for doing it to the patient. Review safety precautions necessary when oxygen is in use. Place "No Smoking" signs in appropriate areas. | |
| ____ | ____ | ____ | 6. Attach face mask to oxygen source (with humidification, if appropriate, for the specific mask). Start the flow of oxygen at the specified rate. For a mask with a reservoir, be sure to allow oxygen to fill the bag before proceeding to the next step. | |
| ____ | ____ | ____ | 7. Position face mask over the patient's nose and mouth. Adjust the elastic strap so that the mask fits snugly but comfortably on the face. Adjust the flow rate to the prescribed rate. | |
| ____ | ____ | ____ | 8. If the patient reports irritation or redness is noted, use gauze pads under the elastic strap at pressure points to reduce irritation to ears and scalp. | |
| ____ | ____ | ____ | 9. Reassess patient's respiratory status, including respiratory rate, effort, and lung sounds. Note any signs of respiratory distress, such as tachypnea, nasal flaring, use of accessory muscles, or dyspnea. | |
| ____ | ____ | ____ | 10. Remove PPE, if used. Perform hand hygiene. | |
| ____ | ____ | ____ | 11. *Remove the mask and dry the skin every 2 to 3 hours if the oxygen is running continuously. Do not use powder around the mask.* | |

*Skill Checklists for Taylor's Clinical Nursing Skills:*
*A Nursing Process Approach, 3rd edition*

Name _____  Date _____

Unit _____  Position _____

Instructor/Evaluator: _____  Position _____

| Excellent | Satisfactory | Needs Practice | SKILL 14-5 **Using an Oxygen Tent** | Comments |
|:---:|:---:|:---:|---|---|
| | | | **Goal:** The patient exhibits an oxygen saturation level within acceptable parameters. | |
| —— | —— | —— | 1. Bring necessary equipment to the bedside stand or overbed table. | |
| —— | —— | —— | 2. Perform hand hygiene and put on PPE, if indicated. | |
| —— | —— | —— | 3. Identify the patient. | |
| —— | —— | —— | 4. Close curtains around bed and close the door to the room, if possible. | |
| —— | —— | —— | 5. Explain what you are going to do and the reason for doing it to the patient and parents/guardians. Review safety precautions necessary when oxygen is in use. | |
| —— | —— | —— | 6. Calibrate the oxygen analyzer according to manufacturer's directions. | |
| —— | —— | —— | 7. Place tent over crib or bed. Connect the humidifier to the oxygen source in the wall and connect the tent tubing to the humidifier. Adjust flow rate as ordered by physician. Check that oxygen is flowing into tent. | |
| —— | —— | —— | 8. Turn analyzer on. Place oxygen analyzer probe in tent, out of patient's reach. | |
| —— | —— | —— | 9. Adjust oxygen as necessary, based on sensor readings. Once oxygen levels reach the prescribed amount, place patient in the tent. | |
| —— | —— | —— | 10. Roll small blankets like a jelly roll and tuck tent edges under blanket rolls, as necessary. | |
| —— | —— | —— | 11. *Encourage patient and family members to keep tent flap closed.* | |
| —— | —— | —— | 12. Reassess patient's respiratory status, including respiratory rate, effort, and lung sounds. Note any signs of respiratory distress, such as tachypnea, nasal flaring, use of accessory muscles, grunting, retractions, or dyspnea. | |
| —— | —— | —— | 13. Remove PPE, if used. Perform hand hygiene. | |
| —— | —— | —— | 14. Frequently check bedding and patient's pajamas for moisture. Change as needed to keep the patient dry. | |

*Skill Checklists for Taylor's Clinical Nursing Skills:*
*A Nursing Process Approach, 3rd edition*

Name _____    Date _____

Unit _____    Position _____

Instructor/Evaluator: _____    Position _____

| Excellent | Satisfactory | Needs Practice | SKILL 14-6<br>**Suctioning the Nasopharyngeal and**<br>**Oropharyngeal Airways**<br><br>**Goal:** The patient exhibits improved breath sounds and a clear, patent airway. | Comments |
|---|---|---|---|---|
| ___ | ___ | ___ | 1. Bring necessary equipment to the bedside stand or overbed table. | |
| ___ | ___ | ___ | 2. Perform hand hygiene and put on PPE, if indicated. | |
| ___ | ___ | ___ | 3. Identify the patient. | |
| ___ | ___ | ___ | 4. Close curtains around bed and close the door to the room, if possible. | |
| ___ | ___ | ___ | 5. Determine the need for suctioning. Verify the suction order in the patient's chart, if necessary. *For a postoperative patient, administer pain medication before suctioning.* | |
| ___ | ___ | ___ | 6. Explain what you are going to do and the reason for suctioning to the patient, even if the patient does not appear to be alert. Reassure the patient you will interrupt procedure if he or she indicates respiratory difficulty. | |
| ___ | ___ | ___ | 7. Adjust bed to comfortable working height, usually elbow height of the caregiver (VISN 8 Patient Safety Center, 2009). Lower side rail closest to you. *If patient is conscious, place him or her in a semi-Fowler's position. If patient is unconscious, place him or her in the lateral position, facing you.* Move the bedside table close to your work area and raise it to waist height. | |
| ___ | ___ | ___ | 8. Place towel or waterproof pad across the patient's chest. | |
| ___ | ___ | ___ | 9. *Adjust suction to appropriate pressure.* | |
| ___ | ___ | ___ | For a wall unit for an adult: 100–120 mm Hg (Roman, 2005); neonates: 60–80 mm Hg; infants: 80–100 mm Hg; children: 80–100 mm Hg; adolescents: 80–120 mm Hg (Ireton, 2007). | |
| ___ | ___ | ___ | For a portable unit for an adult: 10–15 cm Hg; neonates: 6–8 cm Hg; infants: 8–10 cm Hg; children: 8–10 cm Hg; adolescents: 8–10 cm Hg. | |
| ___ | ___ | ___ | *Put on a disposable, clean glove and occlude the end of the connecting tubing to check suction pressure.* Place the connecting tubing in a convenient location. | |

# Suctioning the Nasopharyngeal and Oropharyngeal Airways (Continued)

| Excellent | Satisfactory | Needs Practice | | Comments |
|---|---|---|---|---|
| —— | —— | —— | 10. Open sterile suction package using aseptic technique. The open wrapper or container becomes a sterile field to hold other supplies. Carefully remove the sterile container, touching only the outside surface. Set it up on the work surface and pour sterile saline into it. | |
| —— | —— | —— | 11. Place a small amount of water-soluble lubricant on the sterile field, taking care to avoid touching the sterile field with the lubricant package. | |
| —— | —— | —— | 12. Increase the patient's supplemental oxygen level or apply supplemental oxygen per facility policy or primary care provider order. | |
| —— | —— | —— | 13. Put on face shield or goggles and mask. Put on sterile gloves. *The dominant hand will manipulate the catheter and must remain sterile. The nondominant hand is considered clean rather than sterile and will control the suction valve (Y-port) on the catheter.* | |
| —— | —— | —— | 14. With dominant gloved hand, pick up sterile catheter. Pick up the connecting tubing with the nondominant hand and connect the tubing and suction catheter. | |
| —— | —— | —— | 15. Moisten the catheter by dipping it into the container of sterile saline. Occlude Y-tube to check suction. | |
| —— | —— | —— | 16. Encourage the patient to take several deep breaths. | |
| —— | —— | —— | 17. Apply lubricant to the first 2 to 3 inches of the catheter, using the lubricant that was placed on the sterile field. | |
| —— | —— | —— | 18. Remove the oxygen delivery device, if appropriate. Do not apply suction as the catheter is inserted. Hold the catheter between your thumb and forefinger. | |
| —— | —— | —— | 19. Insert the catheter: | |
| —— | —— | —— | a. **For nasopharyngeal suctioning,** gently insert catheter through the naris and along the floor of the nostril toward the trachea. Roll the catheter between your fingers to help advance it. Advance the catheter approximately 5″ to 6″ to reach the pharynx. | |
| —— | —— | —— | b. **For oropharyngeal suctioning,** insert catheter through the mouth, along the side of the mouth toward the trachea. Advance the catheter 3″ to 4″ to reach the pharynx. (See the Skill Variation in your skills book for nasotracheal suctioning.) | |
| —— | —— | —— | 20. *Apply suction by intermittently occluding the Y-port on the catheter with the thumb of your nondominant hand and gently rotating the catheter as it is being withdrawn. Do not suction for more than 10 to 15 seconds at a time.* | |

| Excellent | Satisfactory | Needs Practice | SKILL 14-6<br>**Suctioning the Nasopharyngeal and Oropharyngeal Airways** *(Continued)* |
|---|---|---|---|
| | | | **Comments** |
| —— | —— | —— | 21. Replace the oxygen delivery device using your nondominant hand, if appropriate, and have the patient take several deep breaths. |
| —— | —— | —— | 22. Flush catheter with saline. Assess effectiveness of suctioning and repeat, as needed, and according to patient's tolerance. Wrap the suction catheter around your dominant hand between attempts. |
| —— | —— | —— | 23. *Allow at least a 30-second to 1-minute interval if additional suctioning is needed. No more than three suction passes should be made per suctioning episode. Alternate the nares, unless contraindicated, if repeated suctioning is required.* Do not force the catheter through the nares. Encourage the patient to cough and deep breathe between suctioning. Suction the oropharynx after suctioning the nasopharynx. |
| —— | —— | —— | 24. When suctioning is completed, remove gloves from dominant hand over the coiled catheter, pulling them off inside out. Remove glove from nondominant hand and dispose of gloves, catheter, and container with solution in the appropriate receptacle. Assist patient to a comfortable position. Raise bed rail and place bed in the lowest position. |
| —— | —— | —— | 25. Turn off suction. Remove supplemental oxygen placed for suctioning, if appropriate. Remove face shield or goggles and mask. Perform hand hygiene. |
| —— | —— | —— | 26. Offer oral hygiene after suctioning. |
| —— | —— | —— | 27. Reassess patient's respiratory status, including respiratory rate, effort, oxygen saturation, and lung sounds. |
| —— | —— | —— | 28. Remove additional PPE, if used. Perform hand hygiene. |

*Skill Checklists for Taylor's Clinical Nursing Skills:*
*A Nursing Process Approach, 3rd edition*

Name _____  Date _____

Unit _____  Position _____

Instructor/Evaluator: _____  Position _____

SKILL 14-7

# Inserting an Oropharyngeal Airway

| Excellent | Satisfactory | Needs Practice | **Goal:** The patient sustains a patent airway. | Comments |
|---|---|---|---|---|
| —— | —— | —— | 1. Bring necessary equipment to the bedside stand or overbed table. | |
| —— | —— | —— | 2. Perform hand hygiene and put on PPE, if indicated. | |
| —— | —— | —— | 3. Identify the patient. | |
| —— | —— | —— | 4. Close curtains around bed and close the door to the room, if possible. | |
| —— | —— | —— | 5. Explain to the patient what you are going to do and the reason for doing it, even though the patient does not appear to be alert. | |
| —— | —— | —— | 6. Put on disposable gloves; put on goggles or face shield, as indicated. | |
| —— | —— | —— | 7. Measure the oropharyngeal airway for correct size. Measure the oropharyngeal airway by holding the airway on the side of the patient's face. The airway should reach from the opening of the mouth to the back angle of the jaw. | |
| —— | —— | —— | 8. *Check mouth for any loose teeth, dentures, or other foreign material. Remove dentures or material if present.* | |
| —— | —— | —— | 9. Position patient in semi-Fowler's position. | |
| —— | —— | —— | 10. Suction patient, if necessary. | |
| —— | —— | —— | 11. Open patient's mouth by using your thumb and index finger to gently pry teeth apart. *Insert the airway with the curved tip pointing up toward the roof of the mouth.* | |
| —— | —— | —— | 12. Slide the airway across the tongue to the back of the mouth. Rotate the airway 180 degrees as it passes the uvula. The tip should point down and the curvature should follow the contour of the roof of the mouth. A flashlight can be used to confirm the position of the airway with the curve fitting over the tongue. | |
| —— | —— | —— | 13. Ensure accurate placement and adequate ventilation by auscultating breath sounds. | |

| | | | SKILL 14-7 |
|---|---|---|---|

| Excellent | Satisfactory | Needs Practice | | Comments |
|---|---|---|---|---|
| ___ | ___ | ___ | 14. Position patient on his or her side when airway is in place. | |
| ___ | ___ | ___ | 15. Remove gloves and additional PPE, if used. Perform hand hygiene. | |
| ___ | ___ | ___ | 16. Remove the airway for a brief period every 4 hours, or according to facility policy. Assess mouth, provide mouth care, and clean the airway according to facility policy before reinserting it. | |

*Skill Checklists for Taylor's Clinical Nursing Skills:*
*A Nursing Process Approach, 3rd edition*

Name _____   Date _____

Unit _____   Position _____

Instructor/Evaluator: _____   Position _____

## SKILL 14-8
# Suctioning an Endotracheal Tube: Open System

**Goal:** The patient exhibits improved breath sounds and a clear, patent airway.

| Excellent | Satisfactory | Needs Practice | | Comments |
|---|---|---|---|---|
| —— | —— | —— | 1. Bring necessary equipment to the bedside stand or overbed table. | |
| —— | —— | —— | 2. Perform hand hygiene and put on PPE, if indicated. | |
| —— | —— | —— | 3. Identify the patient. | |
| —— | —— | —— | 4. Close curtains around bed and close the door to the room, if possible. | |
| —— | —— | —— | 5. Determine the need for suctioning. Verify the suction order in the patient's chart. *Assess for pain or the potential to cause pain. Administer pain medication, as prescribed, before suctioning.* | |
| —— | —— | —— | 6. Explain what you are going to do and the reason for doing it to the patient, even if the patient does not appear to be alert. Reassure the patient you will interrupt the procedure if he or she indicates respiratory difficulty. | |
| —— | —— | —— | 7. Adjust bed to comfortable working position, usually elbow height of the caregiver (VISN 8 Patient Safety Center, 2009). Lower side rail closest to you. *If patient is conscious, place him or her in a semi-Fowler's position. If patient is unconscious, place him or her in the lateral position, facing you. Move the overbed table close to your work area and raise it to waist height.* | |
| —— | —— | —— | 8. Place towel or waterproof pad across patient's chest. | |
| —— | —— | —— | 9. *Turn suction to appropriate pressure.* <br><br> For a wall unit for an adult: 100–120 mm Hg (Roman, 2005); neonates: 60–80 mm Hg; infants: 80–100 mm Hg; children: 80–100 mm Hg; adolescents: 80–120 mm Hg (Ireton, 2007). | |
| —— | —— | —— | For a portable unit for an adult: 10–15 cm Hg; neonates: 6–8 cm Hg; infants 8–10 cm Hg; children 8–10 cm Hg; adolescents: 8–10 cm Hg. | |
| —— | —— | —— | 10. Put on a disposable, clean glove and occlude the end of the connecting tubing to check suction pressure. Place the connecting tubing in a convenient location. Place the resuscitation bag connected to oxygen within convenient reach, if using. | |

# SKILL 14-8
## Suctioning an Endotracheal Tube: Open System *(Continued)*

| Excellent | Satisfactory | Needs Practice | | Comments |
|---|---|---|---|---|
| —— | —— | —— | 11. Open sterile suction package using aseptic technique. The open wrapper becomes a sterile field to hold other supplies. Carefully remove the sterile container, touching only the outside surface. Set it up on the work surface and pour sterile saline into it. | |
| —— | —— | —— | 12. Put on face shield or goggles and mask. Put on sterile gloves. *The dominant hand will manipulate the catheter and must remain sterile. The nondominant hand is considered clean rather than sterile and will control the suction valve (Y-port) on the catheter.* | |
| —— | —— | —— | 13. With dominant gloved hand, pick up sterile catheter. Pick up the connecting tubing with the nondominant hand and connect the tubing and suction catheter. | |
| —— | —— | —— | 14. Moisten the catheter by dipping it into the container of sterile saline, unless it is a silicone catheter. Occlude Y-tube to check suction. | |
| —— | —— | —— | 15. Hyperventilate the patient using your nondominant hand and a manual resuscitation bag and delivering three to six breaths or use the sigh mechanism on a mechanical ventilator. | |
| —— | —— | —— | 16. Open the adapter on the mechanical ventilator tubing or remove the manual resuscitation bag with your nondominant hand. | |
| —— | —— | —— | 17. Using your dominant hand, gently and quickly insert the catheter into the trachea. *Advance the catheter to the predetermined length. Do not occlude Y-port when inserting the catheter.* | |
| —— | —— | —— | 18. Apply suction by intermittently occluding the Y-port on the catheter with the thumb of your nondominant hand, and gently rotate the catheter as it is being withdrawn. *Do not suction for more than 10 to 15 seconds at a time.* | |
| —— | —— | —— | 19. Hyperventilate the patient using your nondominant hand and a manual resuscitation bag and delivering three to six breaths. Replace the oxygen delivery device, if applicable, using your nondominant hand and have the patient take several deep breaths. If the patient is mechanically ventilated, close the adapter on the mechanical ventilator tubing or replace the ventilator tubing and use the sigh mechanism on a mechanical ventilator. | |

# Suctioning an Endotracheal Tube: Open System *(Continued)*

| Excellent | Satisfactory | Needs Practice | | Comments |
|---|---|---|---|---|
| — | — | — | 20. Flush catheter with saline. Assess the effectiveness of suctioning and repeat, as needed, and according to patient's tolerance. | |
| — | — | — | Wrap the suction catheter around your dominant hand between attempts. | |
| — | — | — | 21. *Allow at least a 30-second to 1-minute interval if additional suctioning is needed. No more than three suction passes should be made per suctioning episode.* Suction the oropharynx after suctioning the trachea. Do not reinsert in the endotracheal tube after suctioning the mouth. | |
| — | — | — | 22. When suctioning is completed, remove gloves from dominant hand over the coiled catheter, pulling it off inside-out. Remove glove from nondominant hand and dispose of gloves, catheter, and container with solution in the appropriate receptacle. Assist patient to a comfortable position. Raise bed rail and place bed in the lowest position. | |
| — | — | — | 23. Turn off suction. Remove face shield or goggles and mask. Perform hand hygiene. | |
| — | — | — | 24. Offer oral hygiene after suctioning. | |
| — | — | — | 25. Reassess patient's respiratory status, including respiratory rate, effort, oxygen saturation, and lung sounds. | |
| — | — | — | 26. Remove additional PPE, if used. Perform hand hygiene. | |

*Skill Checklists for Taylor's Clinical Nursing Skills:*
*A Nursing Process Approach, 3rd edition*

Name _____     Date _____

Unit _____     Position _____

Instructor/Evaluator: _____     Position _____

## SKILL 14-9

# Suctioning an Endotracheal Tube: Closed System

**Goal:** The patient exhibits improved breath sounds and a clear, patent airway.

| Excellent | Satisfactory | Needs Practice | | Comments |
|---|---|---|---|---|
| —— | —— | —— | 1. Bring necessary equipment to the bedside stand or overbed table. | |
| —— | —— | —— | 2. Perform hand hygiene and put on PPE, if indicated. | |
| —— | —— | —— | 3. Identify the patient. | |
| —— | —— | —— | 4. Close curtains around bed and close the door to the room, if possible. | |
| —— | —— | —— | 5. Determine the need for suctioning. Verify the suction order in the patient's chart. *Assess for pain or the potential to cause pain. Administer pain medication, as prescribed, before suctioning.* | |
| | | | 6. Explain what you are going to do and the reason for doing it to the patient, even if the patient does not appear to be alert. Reassure the patient you will interrupt the procedure if he or she indicates respiratory difficulty. | |
| —— | —— | —— | 7. Adjust bed to comfortable working position, usually elbow height of the caregiver (VISN 8 Patient Safety Center, 2009). Lower side rail closest to you. *If patient is conscious, place him or her in a semi-Fowler's position. If patient is unconscious, place him or her in the lateral position, facing you. Move the overbed table close to your work area and raise to waist height.* | |
| —— | —— | —— | 8. *Turn suction to appropriate pressure.* | |
| —— | —— | —— | For a wall unit for an adult: 100–120 mm Hg (Roman, 2005); neonates: 60–80 mm Hg; infants: 80–100 mm Hg; children: 80–100 mm Hg; adolescents: 80–120 mm Hg (Ireton, 2007). | |
| —— | —— | —— | For a portable unit for an adult: 10–15 cm Hg; neonates: 6–8 cm Hg; infants 8–10 cm Hg; children 8–10 cm Hg; adolescents: 8–10 cm Hg. | |
| —— | —— | —— | 9. *Open the package of the closed suction device using aseptic technique. Make sure that the device remains sterile.* | |
| —— | —— | —— | 10. Put on sterile gloves. | |

| Excellent | Satisfactory | Needs Practice | |
|---|---|---|---|

SKILL 14-9

# Suctioning an Endotracheal Tube: Closed System *(Continued)*

**Comments**

| | | | |
|---|---|---|---|
| —— | —— | —— | 11. Using nondominant hand, disconnect ventilator from endotracheal tube. *Place ventilator tubing in a convenient location so that the inside of the tubing remains sterile or continue to hold the tubing in your nondominant hand.* |
| —— | —— | —— | 12. *Using dominant hand and keeping device sterile, connect the closed suctioning device so that the suctioning catheter is in line with the endotracheal tube.* |
| —— | —— | —— | 13. *Keeping the inside of the ventilator tubing sterile, attach ventilator tubing to port perpendicular to the endotracheal tube.* Attach suction tubing to suction catheter. |
| —— | —— | —— | 14. Pop top off sterile normal saline dosette. Open plug to port by suction catheter and insert saline dosette or syringe. |
| —— | —— | —— | 15. *Hyperventilate the patient by using the sigh button on the ventilator before suctioning.* Turn safety cap on suction button of catheter so that button is depressed easily. |
| —— | —— | —— | 16. Grasp suction catheter through protective sheath, about 6 inches (15 cm) from the endotracheal tube. Gently insert the catheter into the endotracheal tube. Release the catheter while holding on to the protective sheath. Move hand farther back on catheter. *Grasp catheter through sheath and repeat movement, advancing the catheter to the predetermined length. Do not occlude Y-port when inserting the catheter.* |
| —— | —— | —— | 17. Apply intermittent suction by depressing the suction button with thumb of nondominant hand. Gently rotate the catheter with thumb and index finger of dominant hand as catheter is being withdrawn. *Do not suction for more than 10 to 15 seconds at a time.* Hyperoxygenate or hyperventilate with sigh button on ventilator, as ordered. |
| —— | —— | —— | 18. Once catheter is withdrawn back into sheath, depress the suction button while gently squeezing the normal saline dosette until the catheter is clean. *Allow at least a 30-second to 1-minute interval if additional suctioning is needed. No more than three suction passes should be made per suctioning episode.* |
| —— | —— | —— | 19. *When procedure is completed, ensure that the catheter is withdrawn into the sheath, and turn the safety button. Remove normal saline dosette and apply cap to port.* |

## SKILL 14-9

# Suctioning an Endotracheal Tube:
## Closed System *(Continued)*

| Excellent | Satisfactory | Needs Practice | | Comments |
|---|---|---|---|---|
| —— | —— | —— | 20. Suction the oral cavity with a separate single-use, disposable catheter and perform oral hygiene. Remove gloves. Turn off suction. | |
| —— | —— | —— | 21. Assist patient to a comfortable position. Raise the bed rail and place the bed in the lowest position. | |
| —— | —— | —— | 22. Reassess patient's respiratory status, including respiratory rate, effort, oxygen saturation, and lung sounds. | |
| —— | —— | —— | 23. Remove additional PPE, if used. Perform hand hygiene. | |

*Skill Checklists for Taylor's Clinical Nursing Skills:*
*A Nursing Process Approach, 3rd edition*

Name _____     Date _____

Unit _____     Position _____

Instructor/Evaluator: _____     Position _____

## SKILL 14-10
## Securing an Endotracheal Tube

**Goal:** The tube remains in place, and the patient maintains bilaterally equal and clear lung sounds.

| Excellent | Satisfactory | Needs Practice | | Comments |
|---|---|---|---|---|
| —— | —— | —— | 1. Bring necessary equipment to the bedside stand or overbed table. | |
| —— | —— | —— | 2. Perform hand hygiene and put on PPE, if indicated. | |
| —— | —— | —— | 3. Identify the patient. | |
| —— | —— | —— | 4. Close curtains around bed and close the door to the room, if possible. | |
| —— | —— | —— | 5. Assess the need for endotracheal tube retaping. ***Administer pain medication or sedation, as prescribed, before attempting to retape endotracheal tube.*** Explain the procedure to the patient. | |
| —— | —— | —— | 6. Obtain the assistance of a second individual to hold the endotracheal tube in place while the old tape is removed and the new tape is placed. | |
| —— | —— | —— | 7. Adjust the bed to a comfortable working position, usually elbow height of the caregiver (VISN 8 Patient Safety Center, 2009). Lower side rail closest to you. ***If the patient is conscious, place him or her in a semi-Fowler's position. If the patient is unconscious, place him or her in the lateral position, facing you. Move the overbed table close to your work area and raise to waist height.*** Place a trash receptacle within easy reach of work area. | |
| —— | —— | —— | 8. Put on face shield or goggles and mask. Suction patient as described in Skill 14-8 or 14-9. | |
| —— | —— | —— | 9. Measure a piece of tape for the length needed to reach around the patient's neck to the mouth plus 8 inches. Cut tape. Lay it adhesive-side up on the table. | |
| —— | —— | —— | 10. Cut another piece of tape long enough to reach from one jaw around the back of the neck to the other jaw. Lay this piece on the center of the longer piece on the table, matching the tapes' adhesive sides together. | |
| —— | —— | —— | 11. Take one 3-mL syringe or tongue blade and wrap the sticky tape around the syringe until the nonsticky area is reached. Do this for the other side as well. | |

| Excellent | Satisfactory | Needs Practice | SKILL 14-10<br>**Securing an Endotracheal Tube** *(Continued)* | |
|-----------|--------------|----------------|---------------------------------------------------------------|---|
| | | | | **Comments** |
| ⎯ | ⎯ | ⎯ | 12. Take one of the 3-mL syringes or tongue blades and pass it under the patient's neck so that there is a 3-mL syringe on either side of the patient's head. | |
| ⎯ | ⎯ | ⎯ | 13. Put on disposable gloves. Have the assistant put on gloves as well. | |
| ⎯ | ⎯ | ⎯ | 14. *Provide oral care, including suctioning the oral cavity.* | |
| ⎯ | ⎯ | ⎯ | 15. Take note of the 'cm' position markings on the tube. Begin to unwrap old tape from around the endotracheal tube. After one side is unwrapped, have assistant hold the endotracheal tube as close to the lips or nares as possible to offer stabilization. | |
| ⎯ | ⎯ | ⎯ | 16. Carefully remove the remaining tape from the endotracheal tube. *After tape is removed, have assistant gently and slowly move endotracheal tube (if orally intubated) to the other side of the mouth. Assess mouth for any skin breakdown. Before applying new tape, make sure that markings on endotracheal tube are at same spot as when retaping began.* | |
| ⎯ | ⎯ | ⎯ | 17. Remove old tape from cheeks and side of face. Use adhesive remover to remove excess adhesive from tape. Clean the face and neck with washcloth and cleanser. If patient has facial hair, consider shaving cheeks. Pat cheeks dry with the towel. | |
| ⎯ | ⎯ | ⎯ | 18. Apply the skin barrier to the patient's face (under nose, cheeks, and lower lip) where the tape will sit. Unroll one side of the tape. Ensure that nonstick part of tape remains behind patient's neck while pulling firmly on the tape. *Place adhesive portion of tape snugly against patient's cheek.* Split the tape in half from the end to the corner of the mouth. | |
| ⎯ | ⎯ | ⎯ | 19. Place the top-half piece of tape under the patient's nose. Wrap the lower half around the tube in one direction, such as over and around the tube. Fold over tab on end of tape. | |
| ⎯ | ⎯ | ⎯ | 20. Unwrap second side of tape. Split to corner of the mouth. Place the bottom-half piece of tape along the patient's lower lip. Wrap the top half around the tube in the opposite direction, such as below and around the tube. Fold over tab on end of tape. Ensure tape is secure. | |
| ⎯ | ⎯ | ⎯ | 21. *Auscultate lung sounds. Assess for cyanosis, oxygen saturation, chest symmetry, and stability of endotracheal tube. Again check to ensure that the tube is at the correct depth.* | |

| Excellent | Satisfactory | Needs Practice | SKILL 14-10 **Securing an Endotracheal Tube** *(Continued)* | Comments |
|-----------|--------------|----------------|--------------|----------|
| —— | —— | —— | 22. *If the endotracheal tube is cuffed, check pressure of the balloon by attaching a handheld pressure gauge to the pilot balloon of the endotracheal tube.* | |
| —— | —— | —— | 23. Assist patient to a comfortable position. Raise the bed rail and place the bed in the lowest position. | |
| —— | —— | —— | 24. Remove face shield or goggles and mask. Remove additional PPE, if used. Perform hand hygiene. | |

*Skill Checklists for Taylor's Clinical Nursing Skills:*
*A Nursing Process Approach, 3rd edition*

Name _____   Date _____

Unit _____   Position _____

Instructor/Evaluator: _____   Position _____

| Excellent | Satisfactory | Needs Practice | SKILL 14-11<br>**Suctioning the Tracheostomy: Open System** | |
|---|---|---|---|---|
| | | | **Goal:** The patient exhibits improved breath sounds and a clear, patent airway. | **Comments** |
| —— | —— | —— | 1. Bring necessary equipment to the bedside stand or overbed table. | |
| —— | —— | —— | 2. Perform hand hygiene and put on PPE, if indicated. | |
| —— | —— | —— | 3. Identify the patient. | |
| —— | —— | —— | 4. Close curtains around bed and close the door to the room, if possible. | |
| —— | —— | —— | 5. Determine the need for suctioning. Verify the suction order in the patient's chart. *Assess for pain or the potential to cause pain. Administer pain medication, as prescribed, before suctioning.* | |
| —— | —— | —— | 6. Explain to the patient what you are going to do and the reason or doing it, even if the patient does not appear to be alert. Reassure the patient you will interrupt the procedure if he or she indicates respiratory difficulty. | |
| —— | —— | —— | 7. Adjust bed to comfortable working position, usually elbow height of the caregiver (VISN 8 Patient Safety Center, 2009). Lower side rail closest to you. *If patient is conscious, place him or her in a semi-Fowler's position. If patient is unconscious, place him or her in the lateral position, facing you.* Move the overbed table close to your work area and raise to waist height. | |
| —— | —— | —— | 8. Place towel or waterproof pad across patient's chest. | |
| —— | —— | —— | 9. *Turn suction to appropriate pressure.* | |
| —— | —— | —— | For a wall unit for an adult: 100–120 mm Hg (Roman, 2005); neonates: 60–80 mm Hg; infants: 80–100 mm Hg; children: 80–100 mm Hg; adolescents: 80–120 mm Hg (Ireton, 2007). | |
| —— | —— | —— | For a portable unit for an adult: 10–15 cm Hg; neonates: 6–8 cm Hg; infants 8–10 cm Hg; children 8–10 cm Hg; adolescents: 8–10 cm Hg. | |
| —— | —— | —— | *Put on a disposable, clean glove and occlude the end of the connecting tubing to check suction pressure. Place the connecting tubing in a convenient location. If using, place resuscitation bag connected to oxygen within convenient reach.* | |

| Excellent | Satisfactory | Needs Practice | | Comments |
|---|---|---|---|---|

# Suctioning the Tracheostomy: Open System *(Continued)*

---

_____  _____  _____  10. Open sterile suction package using aseptic technique. The open wrapper or container becomes a sterile field to hold other supplies. Carefully remove the sterile container, touching only the outside surface. Set it up on the work surface and pour sterile saline into it.

_____  _____  _____  11. Put on face shield or goggles and mask. Put on sterile gloves. ***The dominant hand will manipulate the catheter and must remain sterile. The nondominant hand is considered clean rather than sterile and will control the suction valve (Y-port) on the catheter.***

_____  _____  _____  12. With dominant gloved hand, pick up sterile catheter. Pick up the connecting tubing with the nondominant hand and connect the tubing and suction catheter.

_____  _____  _____  13. Moisten the catheter by dipping it into the container of sterile saline, unless it is a silicone catheter. Occlude Y-tube to check suction.

_____  _____  _____  14. Using your nondominant hand and a manual resuscitation bag, hyperventilate the patient, delivering three to six breaths or use the sigh mechanism on a mechanical ventilator.

_____  _____  _____  15. Open the adapter on the mechanical ventilator tubing or remove oxygen delivery setup with your nondominant hand.

_____  _____  _____  16. Using your dominant hand, gently and quickly insert catheter into trachea. ***Advance the catheter to the predetermined length. Do not occlude Y-port when inserting catheter.***

_____  _____  _____  17. Apply suction by intermittently occluding the Y-port on the catheter with the thumb of your nondominant hand, and gently rotate the catheter as it is being withdrawn. ***Do not suction for more than 10 to 15 seconds at a time.***

_____  _____  _____  18. Hyperventilate the patient using your nondominant hand and a manual resuscitation bag, delivering three to six breaths. Replace the oxygen delivery device, if applicable, using your nondominant hand and have the patient take several deep breaths. If the patient is mechanically ventilated, close the adapter on the mechanical ventilator tubing and use the sigh mechanism on a mechanical ventilator.

_____  _____  _____  19. Flush catheter with saline. Assess the effectiveness of suctioning and repeat, as needed, and according to patient's tolerance. Wrap the suction catheter around your dominant hand between attempts.

---

SKILL 14-11

# Suctioning the Tracheostomy: Open System *(Continued)*

| Excellent | Satisfactory | Needs Practice | | Comments |
|---|---|---|---|---|

**20.** *Allow at least a 30-second to 1-minute interval if additional suctioning is needed. No more than three suction passes should be made per suctioning episode. Encourage the patient to cough and deep breathe between suctionings.* Suction the oropharynx after suctioning the trachea. Do not reinsert in the tracheostomy after suctioning the mouth.

**21.** When suctioning is completed, remove gloves from dominant hand over the coiled catheter, pulling it off inside out. Remove glove from nondominant hand and dispose of gloves, catheter, and container with solution in the appropriate receptacle. Assist patient to a comfortable position. Raise bed rail and place bed in the lowest position.

**22.** Turn off suction. Remove supplemental oxygen placed for suctioning, if appropriate. Remove face shield or goggles and mask. Perform hand hygiene.

**23.** Offer oral hygiene after suctioning.

**24.** Reassess patient's respiratory status, including respiratory rate, effort, oxygen saturation, and lung sounds.

**25.** Remove additional PPE, if used. Perform hand hygiene.

*Skill Checklists for Taylor's Clinical Nursing Skills:*
*A Nursing Process Approach, 3rd edition*

Name _____ Date _____

Unit _____ Position _____

Instructor/Evaluator: _____ Position _____

SKILL 14-12

# Providing Tracheostomy Care

| Excellent | Satisfactory | Needs Practice | **Goal:** The patient exhibits a tracheostomy tube and site free from drainage, secretions, and skin irritation or breakdown. | Comments |
|---|---|---|---|---|
| ⎯ | ⎯ | ⎯ | 1. Bring necessary equipment to the bedside stand or overbed table. | |
| ⎯ | ⎯ | ⎯ | 2. Perform hand hygiene and put on PPE, if indicated. | |
| ⎯ | ⎯ | ⎯ | 3. Identify the patient. | |
| ⎯ | ⎯ | ⎯ | 4. Close curtains around bed and close the door to the room, if possible. | |
| ⎯ | ⎯ | ⎯ | 5. Determine the need for tracheostomy care. *Assess patient's pain and administer pain medication, if indicated.* | |
| ⎯ | ⎯ | ⎯ | 6. Explain what you are going to do and the reason to the patient, even if the patient does not appear to be alert. Reassure the patient you will interrupt procedure if he or she indicates respiratory difficulty. | |
| ⎯ | ⎯ | ⎯ | 7. Adjust bed to comfortable working position, usually elbow height of the caregiver (VISN 8 Patient Safety Center, 2009). Lower side rail closest to you. *If the patient is conscious, place him or her in a semi-Fowler's position. If patient is unconscious, place him or her in the lateral position, facing you.* Move the overbed table close to your work area and raise to waist height. Place a trash receptacle within easy reach of work area. | |
| ⎯ | ⎯ | ⎯ | 8. Put on face shield or goggles and mask. Suction tracheostomy, if necessary. If tracheostomy has just been suctioned, remove soiled site dressing and discard before removal of gloves used to perform suctioning. | |
| | | | **Cleaning the Tracheostomy: Disposable Inner Cannula** (See the Skill Variation in your skills book for steps for cleaning a nondisposable inner cannula.) | |
| ⎯ | ⎯ | ⎯ | 9. Carefully open the package with the new disposable inner cannula, taking care not to contaminate the cannula or the inside of the package. Carefully open the package with the sterile cotton-tipped applicators, taking care not to contaminate them. Open sterile cup or basin and fill 0.5 inch deep with saline. Open the plastic disposable bag and place within reach on work surface. | |

## SKILL 14-12

# Providing Tracheostomy Care (Continued)

| Excellent | Satisfactory | Needs Practice | | Comments |
|---|---|---|---|---|

—— —— —— 10. Put on disposable gloves.

—— —— —— 11. Remove the oxygen source if one is present. Stabilize the outer cannula and faceplate of the tracheostomy with your nondominant hand. Grasp the locking mechanism of the inner cannula with your dominant hand. Press the tabs and release lock. Gently remove inner cannula and place in disposal bag. If not already removed, remove site dressing and dispose of it in the trash.

—— —— —— 12. Discard gloves and put on sterile gloves. Pick up the new inner cannula with your dominant hand, stabilize the faceplate with your nondominant hand, and gently insert the new inner cannula into the outer cannula. Press the tabs to allow the lock to grab the outer cannula. Reapply oxygen source, if needed.

**Applying Clean Dressing and Holder**

(See the Skill Variations in your skills book for steps for an alternate site dressing if a commercially prepared sponge is not available and to secure a tracheostomy with a tracheostomy ties/tape instead of a collar.)

—— —— —— 13. Remove oxygen source, if necessary. Dip cotton-tipped applicator or gauze sponge in cup or basin with sterile saline and clean stoma under faceplate. *Use each applicator or sponge only once, moving from stoma site outward.*

—— —— —— 14. Pat skin gently with dry 4 × 4 gauze sponge.

—— —— —— 15. Slide commercially prepared tracheostomy dressing or pre-folded non-cotton-filled 4 × 4-inch dressing under the faceplate.

—— —— —— 16. Change the tracheostomy holder:

—— —— ——     a. *Obtain the assistance of a second individual to hold the tracheostomy tube in place while the old collar is removed and the new collar is placed.*

—— —— ——     b. Open the package for the new tracheostomy collar.

—— —— ——     c. Both nurses should put on clean gloves.

—— —— ——     d. One nurse holds the faceplate while the other pulls up the Velcro tabs. Gently remove the collar.

—— —— ——     e. The first nurse continues to hold the tracheostomy faceplate.

—— —— ——     f. The other nurse places the collar around the patient's neck and inserts first one tab, then the other, into the openings on the faceplate and secures the Velcro tabs on the tracheostomy holder.

| Excellent | Satisfactory | Needs Practice | SKILL 14-12<br>**Providing Tracheostomy Care** *(Continued)* | |
|:---:|:---:|:---:|---|---|
| | | | | **Comments** |
| —— | —— | —— | g. Check the fit of the tracheostomy collar. You should be able to fit one finger between the neck and the collar. Check to make sure that the patient can flex neck comfortably. Reapply oxygen source, if necessary. | |
| —— | —— | —— | 17. Remove gloves. Assist patient to a comfortable position. Raise the bed rail and place the bed in the lowest position. | |
| —— | —— | —— | 18. Remove face shield or goggles and mask. Remove additional PPE, if used. Perform hand hygiene. | |
| —— | —— | —— | 19. Reassess patient's respiratory status, including respiratory rate, effort, oxygen saturation, and lung sounds. | |

*Skill Checklists for Taylor's Clinical Nursing Skills:*
*A Nursing Process Approach, 3rd edition*

Name _____   Date _____

Unit _____   Position _____

Instructor/Evaluator: _____   Position _____

SKILL 14-13

# Providing Care of a Chest Drainage System

**Goal:** The patient does not experience any complications related to the chest drainage system or respiratory distress.

| Excellent | Satisfactory | Needs Practice | | Comments |
|---|---|---|---|---|
| —— | —— | —— | 1. Bring necessary equipment to the bedside stand or overbed table. | |
| —— | —— | —— | 2. Perform hand hygiene and put on PPE, if indicated. | |
| —— | —— | —— | 3. Identify the patient. | |
| —— | —— | —— | 4. Close curtains around bed and close the door to the room, if possible. | |
| —— | —— | —— | 5. Explain what you are going to do and the reason for doing it to the patient. | |
| —— | —— | —— | 6. Assess the patient's level of pain. Administer prescribed medication, as needed. | |
| —— | —— | —— | 7. Put on clean gloves. | |
| | | | **Assessing the Drainage System** | |
| —— | —— | —— | 8. Move the patient's gown to expose the chest tube insertion site. Keep the patient covered as much as possible, using a bath blanket to drape the patient, if necessary. *Observe the dressing around the chest tube insertion site and ensure that it is dry, intact, and occlusive.* | |
| —— | —— | —— | 9. Check that all connections are securely taped. Gently palpate around the insertion site, feeling for subcutaneous emphysema, a collection of air or gas under the skin. This may feel crunchy or spongy, or like "popping" under your fingers. | |
| —— | —— | —— | 10. Check drainage tubing to ensure that there are no dependent loops or kinks. Position the drainage collection device below the tube insertion site. | |
| —— | —— | —— | 11. If the chest tube is ordered to be suctioned, note the fluid level in the suction chamber and check it with the amount of ordered suction. Look for bubbling in the suction chamber. Temporarily disconnect the suction to check the level of water in the chamber. Add sterile water or saline, if necessary, to maintain correct amount of suction. | |

SKILL 14-13

# Providing Care of a Chest Drainage System *(Continued)*

| Excellent | Satisfactory | Needs Practice | | Comments |
|---|---|---|---|---|
| —— | —— | —— | 12. Observe the water-seal chamber for fluctuations of the water level with the patient's inspiration and expiration (tidaling). If suction is used, temporarily disconnect the suction to observe for fluctuation. ***Assess for the presence of bubbling in the water-seal chamber.*** Add water, if necessary, to maintain the level at the 2-cm mark, or the mark recommended by the manufacturer. | |
| —— | —— | —— | 13. Assess the amount and type of fluid drainage. Measure drainage output at the end of each shift by marking the level on the container or placing a small piece of tape at the drainage level to indicate date and time. The amount should be a running total, because the drainage system is never emptied. If the drainage system fills, it is removed and replaced. | |
| —— | —— | —— | 14. Remove gloves. Assist patient to a comfortable position. Raise the bed rail and place the bed in the lowest position, as necessary. | |
| —— | —— | —— | 15. Remove additional PPE, if used. Perform hand hygiene. | |
| | | | **Changing the Drainage System** | |
| —— | —— | —— | 16. Obtain two padded Kelly clamps, a new drainage system, and a bottle of sterile water. Add water to the water-seal chamber in the new system until it reaches the 2-cm mark or the mark recommended by the manufacturer. Follow manufacturer's directions to add water to suction system if suction is ordered. | |
| —— | —— | —— | 17. Put on clean gloves and additional PPE, as indicated. | |
| —— | —— | —— | 18. ***Apply Kelly clamps 1.5 to 2.5 inches from insertion site and 1 inch apart, going in opposite directions.*** | |
| —— | —— | —— | 19. Remove the suction from the current drainage system. Unroll or use scissors to carefully cut away any foam tape on the connection of the chest tube and drainage system. Using a slight twisting motion, remove the drainage system. ***Do not pull on the chest tube.*** | |
| —— | —— | —— | 20. ***Keeping the end of the chest tube sterile, insert the end of the new drainage system into the chest tube.*** Remove Kelly clamps. Reconnect suction, if ordered. Apply plastic bands or foam tape to chest tube/drainage system connection site. | |
| —— | —— | —— | 21. Assess the patient and the drainage system as outlined (Steps 5–15). | |
| —— | —— | —— | 22. Remove additional PPE, if used. Perform hand hygiene. | |

*Skill Checklists for Taylor's Clinical Nursing Skills:*
*A Nursing Process Approach, 3rd edition*

Name _____  Date _____

Unit _____  Position _____

Instructor/Evaluator: _____  Position _____

| | | | SKILL 14-14 | |
|---|---|---|---|---|

## Assisting With Removal of a Chest Tube

| Excellent | Satisfactory | Needs Practice | **Goal:** The chest tube is removed with minimal discomfort to the patient and the patient remains free of respiratory distress. | Comments |
|---|---|---|---|---|
| ___ | ___ | ___ | 1. Bring necessary equipment to the bedside stand or overbed table. | |
| ___ | ___ | ___ | 2. Perform hand hygiene and put on PPE, if indicated. | |
| ___ | ___ | ___ | 3. Identify the patient. | |
| ___ | ___ | ___ | 4. Administer pain medication, as prescribed. *Premedicate patient before the chest tube removal, at a sufficient interval to allow for the medication to take effect, based on the medication prescribed.* | |
| ___ | ___ | ___ | 5. Close curtains around bed and close the door to the room, if possible. | |
| ___ | ___ | ___ | 6. Explain what you are going to do and the reason for doing it to the patient. Explain any nonpharmacologic pain interventions the patient may use to decrease discomfort during tube removal. | |
| ___ | ___ | ___ | 7. Put on clean gloves. | |
| ___ | ___ | ___ | 8. Provide reassurance to the patient while the physician removes the dressing and then the tube. | |
| ___ | ___ | ___ | 9. *After physician has removed chest tube and secured the occlusive dressing, assess patient's lung sounds, respiratory rate, oxygen saturation, and pain level.* | |
| ___ | ___ | ___ | 10. Anticipate the physician ordering a chest x-ray. | |
| ___ | ___ | ___ | 11. Dispose of equipment appropriately. | |
| ___ | ___ | ___ | 12. Remove gloves and additional PPE, if used. Perform hand hygiene. | |

*Skill Checklists for Taylor's Clinical Nursing Skills:*
*A Nursing Process Approach, 3rd edition*

Name _____  Date _____

Unit _____  Position _____

Instructor/Evaluator: _____  Position _____

SKILL 14-15

# Using a Handheld Resuscitation Bag and Mask

| Excellent | Satisfactory | Needs Practice | | Comments |
|---|---|---|---|---|
| | | | **Goal:** The patient exhibits signs and symptoms of adequate oxygen saturation. | |
| —— | —— | —— | 1. If not a crisis situation, perform hand hygiene. | |
| —— | —— | —— | 2. Put on PPE, as indicated. | |
| —— | —— | —— | 3. If not an emergency, identify the patient. | |
| —— | —— | —— | 4. Explain what you are going to do and the reason for doing it to the patient, even if the patient does not appear to be alert. | |
| —— | —— | —— | 5. Put on disposable gloves. Put on face shield or goggles and mask. | |
| —— | —— | —— | 6. *Ensure that the mask is connected to the bag device, the oxygen tubing is connected to the oxygen source, and the oxygen is turned on, at a flow rate of 10 to 15 L per minute.* This may be done through visualization or by listening to the open end of the reservoir or tail: if air is heard flowing, the oxygen is attached and on. | |
| —— | —— | —— | 7. If possible, get behind head of bed and remove headboard. *Slightly hyperextend patient's neck (unless contraindicated). If unable to hyperextend, use jaw thrust maneuver to open airway.* | |
| —— | —— | —— | 8. Place mask over patient's face with opening over oral cavity. If mask is teardrop-shaped, the narrow portion should be placed over the bridge of the nose. | |
| —— | —— | —— | 9. *With dominant hand, place three fingers on the mandible, keeping head slightly hyperextended. Place thumb and one finger in C position around the mask, pressing hard enough to form a seal around the patient's face.* | |
| —— | —— | —— | 10. *Using nondominant hand, gently and slowly (over 2 to 3 seconds) squeeze the bag, watching chest for symmetric rise.* If two people are available, one person should maintain a seal on the mask with two hands while the other squeezes the bag to deliver the ventilation and oxygenation. | |

SKILL 14-15

# Using a Handheld Resuscitation Bag and Mask *(Continued)*

| Excellent | Satisfactory | Needs Practice | | Comments |
|---|---|---|---|---|
| —— | —— | —— | 11. Deliver the breaths with the patient's own inspiratory effort, if present. Avoid delivering breaths when the patient exhales. Deliver one breath every 5 seconds, if patient's own respiratory drive is absent. Continue delivering breaths until patient's drive returns or until patient is intubated and attached to mechanical ventilation. | |
| —— | —— | —— | 12. Dispose of equipment appropriately. | |
| —— | —— | —— | 13. Remove face shield or goggles and mask. Remove gloves and additional PPE, if used. Perform hand hygiene. | |

*Skill Checklists for Taylor's Clinical Nursing Skills:*
*A Nursing Process Approach, 3rd edition*

Name _____    Date _____

Unit _____    Position _____

Instructor/Evaluator: _____    Position _____

SKILL 15-1

# Initiating a Peripheral Venous Access IV Infusion

| Excellent | Satisfactory | Needs Practice | **Goal:** The access device is inserted on the first attempt, using sterile technique. | Comments |
|---|---|---|---|---|
| —— | —— | —— | 1. Verify the IV solution order on the MAR/CMAR with the medical order. Clarify any inconsistencies. Check the patient's chart for allergies. Check for color, leaking, and expiration date. Know techniques for IV insertion, precautions, purpose of the IV administration, and medications if ordered. | |
| —— | —— | —— | 2. Gather all equipment and bring to the bedside. | |
| —— | —— | —— | 3. Perform hand hygiene and put on PPE, if indicated. | |
| —— | —— | —— | 4. Identify the patient. | |
| —— | —— | —— | 5. Close curtains around bed and close the door to the room, if possible. Explain what you are going to do and why you are going to do it to the patient. Ask the patient about allergies to medications, tape, or skin antiseptics, as appropriate. If considering using a local anesthetic, inquire about allergies for these substances as well. | |
| —— | —— | —— | 6. If using a local anesthetic, explain the rationale and procedure to the patient. Apply the anesthetic to a few potential insertion sites. Allow sufficient time for the anesthetic to take effect. | |
| | | | **Prepare the IV Solution and Administration Set** | |
| —— | —— | —— | 7. Compare the IV container label with the MAR/CMAR. Remove IV bag from outer wrapper, if indicated. Check expiration dates. Scan bar code on container, if necessary. Compare on patient identification band with the MAR/CMAR. Alternately, label the solution container with the patient's name, solution type, additives, date, and time. Complete a time strip for the infusion and apply to IV container. | |
| —— | —— | —— | 8. Maintain aseptic technique when opening sterile packages and IV solution. Remove administration set from package. Apply label to tubing reflecting the day/date for next set change, per facility guidelines. | |

## SKILL 15-1
# Initiating a Peripheral Venous Access IV Infusion (Continued)

| Excellent | Satisfactory | Needs Practice | | Comments |
|---|---|---|---|---|
| —— | —— | —— | 9. Close the roller clamp or slide clamp on the IV administration set. Invert the IV solution container and remove the cap on the entry site, taking care not to touch the exposed entry site. Remove the cap from the spike on the administration set. Using a twisting and pushing motion, insert the administration set spike into the entry site of the IV container. Alternately, follow the manufacturer's directions for insertion. | |
| —— | —— | —— | 10. Hang the IV container on the IV pole. Squeeze the drip chamber and fill at least halfway. | |
| —— | —— | —— | 11. Open the IV tubing clamp, and allow fluid to move through tubing. Follow additional manufacturer's instructions for specific electronic infusion pump, as indicated. *Allow fluid to flow until all air bubbles have disappeared and the entire length of the tubing is primed (filled) with IV solution.* Close the clamp. Alternately, some brands of tubing may require removal of the cap at the end of the IV tubing to allow fluid to flow. Maintain its sterility. After fluid has filled the tubing, recap the end of the tubing. | |
| —— | —— | —— | 12. If an electronic device is to be used, follow manufacturer's instructions for inserting tubing into the device. | |
| | | | **Initiate Peripheral Venous Access** | |
| —— | —— | —— | 13. Place patient in low Fowler's position in bed. Place protective towel or pad under patient's arm. | |
| —— | —— | —— | 14. Provide emotional support, as needed. | |
| —— | —— | —— | 15. Open the short extension tubing package. Attach end cap, if not in place. Clean end cap with alcohol wipe. Insert syringe with normal saline into extension tubing. Fill extension tubing with normal saline and apply slide clamp. Remove the syringe and place extension tubing and syringe back on package, within easy reach. | |
| —— | —— | —— | 16. Select and palpate for an appropriate vein. Refer to guidelines in previous Assessment section. | |
| —— | —— | —— | 17. If the site is hairy and agency policy permits, clip a 2-inch area around the intended entry site. | |
| —— | —— | —— | 18. Put on gloves. | |
| —— | —— | —— | 19. Apply a tourniquet 3 to 4 inches above the venipuncture site to obstruct venous blood flow and distend the vein. Direct the ends of the tourniquet away from the entry site. Make sure the radial pulse is still present. | |
| —— | —— | —— | 20. Instruct the patient to hold the arm lower than the heart. | |

| Excellent | Satisfactory | Needs Practice | SKILL 15-1 **Initiating a Peripheral Venous Access IV Infusion** *(Continued)* | Comments |
|---|---|---|---|---|
| — | — | — | 21. Ask the patient to open and close the fist. Observe and palpate for a suitable vein. Try the following techniques if a vein cannot be felt: | |
| — | — | — | a. Massage the patient's arm from proximal to distal end and gently tap over intended vein. | |
| — | — | — | b. Remove tourniquet and place warm, moist compresses over intended vein for 10 to 15 minutes. | |
| — | — | — | 22. *Cleanse site with an antiseptic solution such as chlorhexidine or according to facility policy. Press applicator against the skin and apply chlorhexidine using a back and forth friction scrub for at least 30 seconds. Do not wipe or blot. Allow to dry completely.* | |
| — | — | — | 23. Use the nondominant hand, placed about 1 or 2 inches below the entry site, to hold the skin taut against the vein. *Avoid touching the prepared site.* Ask the patient to remain still while performing the venipuncture. | |
| — | — | — | 24. Enter the skin gently, holding the catheter by the hub in your dominant hand, bevel side up, at a 10- to 15-degree angle. Insert the catheter from directly over the vein or from the side of the vein. While following the course of the vein, advance the needle or catheter into the vein. A sensation of "give" can be felt when the needle enters the vein. | |
| — | — | — | 25. When blood returns through the lumen of the needle or the flashback chamber of the catheter, advance either device into the vein until the hub is at the venipuncture site. The exact technique depends on the type of device used. | |
| — | — | — | 26. Release the tourniquet. Quickly remove the protective cap from the extension tubing and attach it to the catheter or needle. Stabilize the catheter or needle with your nondominant hand. | |
| — | — | — | 27. Continue to stabilize the catheter or needle and flush gently with the saline, observing the site for infiltration and leaking. | |
| — | — | — | 28. Open the skin protectant wipe. Apply the skin protectant to the site, making sure to apply—at minimum—the area to be covered with the dressing. Place sterile transparent dressing or catheter securing/stabilization device over venipuncture site. Loop the tubing near the site of entry, and anchor with tape (nonallergenic) close to the site. | |
| — | — | — | 29. Label the IV dressing with the date, time, site, and type and size of catheter or needle used for the infusion. | |

# Initiating a Peripheral Venous Access IV Infusion *(Continued)*

| Excellent | Satisfactory | Needs Practice | | Comments |
|---|---|---|---|---|

| | | | |
|---|---|---|---|
| — — — | 30. | Using an antimicrobial swab, cleanse the access cap on the extension tubing. Remove the end cap from the administration set. Insert the end of the administration set into the end cap. Loop the administration set tubing near the site of entry, and anchor with tape (nonallergenic) close to the site. Remove gloves. | |
| — — — | 31. | Open the clamp on the administration set. Set the flow rate and begin the fluid infusion. Alternately, start the flow of solution by releasing the clamp on the tubing and counting the drops. Adjust until the correct drop rate is achieved. Assess the flow of the solution and function of the infusion device. Inspect the insertion site for signs of infiltration. | |
| — — — | 32. | Apply an IV securement/stabilization device if not already in place as part of dressing, as indicated, based on facility policy. Explain to patient the purpose of the device and the importance of safeguarding the site when using the extremity. | |
| — — — | 33. | Remove equipment and return the patient to a position of comfort. Lower bed, if not in lowest position. | |
| — — — | 34. | Remove additional PPE, if used. Perform hand hygiene. | |
| — — — | 35. | Return to check flow rate and observe IV site for infiltration 30 minutes after starting infusion, and at least hourly thereafter. Ask the patient if he or she is experiencing any pain or discomfort related to the IV infusion. | |

*Skill Checklists for Taylor's Clinical Nursing Skills:*
*A Nursing Process Approach, 3rd edition*

Name _____    Date _____

Unit _____    Position _____

Instructor/Evaluator: _____    Position _____

## SKILL 15-2

# Changing an IV Solution Container and Administration Set

**Goal:** The prescribed IV infusion continues without interruption and with infusion complications identified.

| Excellent | Satisfactory | Needs Practice | | Comments |
|---|---|---|---|---|
| —— | —— | —— | 1. Verify IV solution order on MAR/CMAR with the medical order. Clarify any inconsistencies. Check the patient's chart for allergies. Check for color, leaking, and expiration date. Know the purpose of the IV administration and medications if ordered. | |
| —— | —— | —— | 2. Gather all equipment and bring to bedside. | |
| —— | —— | —— | 3. Perform hand hygiene and put on PPE, if indicated. | |
| —— | —— | —— | 4. Identify the patient. | |
| —— | —— | —— | 5. Close curtains around bed and close the door to the room, if possible. Explain what you are going to do and why you are going to do it to the patient. Ask the patient about allergies to medications or tape, as appropriate. | |
| —— | —— | —— | 6. Compare IV container label with the MAR/CMAR. Remove IV bag from outer wrapper, if indicated. Check expiration dates. Scan bar code on container, if necessary. Compare patient identification band with the MAR/CMAR. Alternately, label solution container with the patient's name, solution type, additives, date, and time. Complete a time strip for the infusion and apply to IV container. | |
| —— | —— | —— | 7. Maintain aseptic technique when opening sterile packages and IV solution. Remove administration set from package. Apply label to tubing reflecting the day/date for next set change, per facility guidelines. | |

**To Change IV Solution Container**

| Excellent | Satisfactory | Needs Practice | | Comments |
|---|---|---|---|---|
| —— | —— | —— | 8. If using an electronic infusion device, pause the device or put on "hold." Close the slide clamp on the administration set closest to the drip chamber. If using gravity infusion, close the roller clamp on the administration set. | |
| —— | —— | —— | 9. Carefully remove the cap on the entry site of the new IV solution container and expose the entry site, taking care not to touch the exposed entry site. | |
| —— | —— | —— | 10. Lift empty container off IV pole and invert it. Quickly remove the spike from the old IV container, *being careful not to contaminate it.* Discard old IV container. | |

## SKILL 15-2

# Changing an IV Solution Container and Administration Set (Continued)

| Excellent | Satisfactory | Needs Practice | | Comments |
|---|---|---|---|---|

11. Using a twisting and pushing motion, insert the administration set spike into the entry site of the IV container. Alternately, follow the manufacturer's directions for insertion. Hang the container on the IV pole.

12. Alternately, hang the new IV fluid container on an open hook on the IV pole. Carefully remove the cap on the entry site of the new IV solution container and expose the entry site, taking care not to touch the exposed entry site. Lift empty container off the IV pole and invert it. Quickly remove the spike from the old IV container, *being careful not to contaminate it.* Discard old IV container. Using a twisting and pushing motion, insert the administration set spike into the entry port of the new IV container as it hangs on the IV pole.

13. If using an electronic infusion device, open the slide clamp, check the drip chamber of the administration set, verify the flow rate programmed in the infusion device, and turn the device to "run" or "infuse."

14. If using gravity infusion, slowly open the roller clamp on the administration set and count the drops. Adjust until the correct drop rate is achieved.

**To Change IV Solution Container and Administration Set**

15. Prepare the IV solution and administration set. Refer to Skill 15-1, Steps 7–11.

16. Hang the IV container on an open hook on the IV pole. Close the clamp on the existing IV administration set. Also, close the clamp on the short extension tubing connected to the IV catheter in the patient's arm.

17. If using an electronic infusion device, remove the current administration set from device. Following manufacturer's directions, insert a new administration set into infusion device.

18. Put on gloves. Remove the current infusion tubing from the access cap on the short extension IV tubing. Using an antimicrobial swab, cleanse access cap on extension tubing. Remove the end cap from the new administration set. Insert the end of the administration set into the access cap. Loop the administration set tubing near the entry site, and anchor with tape (nonallergenic) close to site.

19. Open the clamp on the extension tubing. Open the clamp on the administration set.

SKILL 15-2

# Changing an IV Solution Container and Administration Set *(Continued)*

| Excellent | Satisfactory | Needs Practice | | Comments |
|---|---|---|---|---|
| —— | —— | —— | 20. If using an electronic infusion device, open the slide clamp, check the drip chamber of the administration set, verify the flow rate programmed in the infusion device, and turn the device to "run" or "infuse." | |
| —— | —— | —— | 21. If using gravity infusion, slowly open the roller clamp on the administration set and count the drops. Adjust until the correct drop rate is achieved. | |
| —— | —— | —— | 22. Remove equipment. Ensure patient's comfort. Remove gloves. Lower bed, if not in lowest position. | |
| —— | —— | —— | 23. Remove additional PPE, if used. Perform hand hygiene. | |
| —— | —— | —— | 24. Return to check flow rate and observe IV site for infiltration 30 minutes after starting infusion, and at least hourly thereafter. Ask the patient if he or she is experiencing any pain or discomfort related to the IV infusion. | |

*Skill Checklists for Taylor's Clinical Nursing Skills:*
*A Nursing Process Approach, 3rd edition*

Name _____     Date _____

Unit _____     Position _____

Instructor/Evaluator: _____     Position _____

| Excellent | Satisfactory | Needs Practice | SKILL 15-3 **Monitoring an IV Site and Infusion** | Comments |
|---|---|---|---|---|
| | | | **Goal:** The patient remains free from complications and demonstrates signs and symptoms of fluid balance. | |
| ___ | ___ | ___ | 1. Verify IV solution order on the MAR/CMAR with the medical order. Clarify any inconsistencies. Check the patient's chart for allergies. Check for color, leaking, and expiration date. Know purpose of the IV administration and medications, if ordered. | |
| ___ | ___ | ___ | 2. *Monitor IV infusion every hour or per agency policy. More frequent checks may be necessary if medication is being infused.* | |
| ___ | ___ | ___ | 3. Perform hand hygiene and put on PPE, if indicated. | |
| ___ | ___ | ___ | 4. Identify the patient. | |
| ___ | ___ | ___ | 5. Close curtains around bed and close the door to the room, if possible. Explain what you are going to do to the patient. | |
| ___ | ___ | ___ | 6. If an electronic infusion device is being used, check settings, alarm, and indicator lights. Check set infusion rate. Note position of fluid in IV container in relation to time tape. Teach patient about the alarm features on the electronic infusion device. | |
| ___ | ___ | ___ | 7. If IV is infusing via gravity, check the drip chamber and time the drops. Refer to Box 15-1 to review calculation of IV flow rates for gravity infusion. | |
| ___ | ___ | ___ | 8. Check tubing for anything that might interfere with flow. Be sure clamps are in the open position. | |
| ___ | ___ | ___ | 9. Observe dressing for leakage of IV solution. | |
| ___ | ___ | ___ | 10. *Inspect the site for swelling, leakage at the site, coolness, or pallor, which may indicate infiltration. Ask if patient is experiencing any pain or discomfort. If any of these symptoms are present, the IV will need to be removed and restarted at another site. Check facility policy for treating infiltration.* See Fundamentals Review 15-3 and Box 15-2. | |
| ___ | ___ | ___ | 11. *Inspect site for redness, swelling, and heat. Palpate for induration. Ask if patient is experiencing pain. These findings may indicate phlebitis. Notify primary care provider if phlebitis is suspected. IV will need to be discontinued and restarted at another site. Check facility policy for treatment of phlebitis.* Refer to Fundamentals Review 15-3 and Box 15-3. | |

SKILL 15-3

# Monitoring an IV Site and Infusion *(Continued)*

| Excellent | Satisfactory | Needs Practice | | Comments |
|---|---|---|---|---|
| —— | —— | —— | 12. *Check for local manifestations (redness, pus, warmth, induration, and pain) that may indicate an infection is present at the site, or systemic manifestations (chills, fever, tachycardia, hypotension) that may accompany local infection at the site. If signs of infection are present, discontinue the IV and notify the primary care provider.* Be careful not to disconnect IV tubing when putting on patient's hospital gown or assisting the patient with movement. | |
| —— | —— | —— | 13. Be alert for additional complications of IV therapy. | |
| —— | —— | —— | a. *Fluid overload can result in signs of cardiac and/or respiratory failure. Monitor intake and output and vital signs. Assess for edema and auscultate lung sounds. Ask if patient is experiencing any shortness of breath.* | |
| —— | —— | —— | b. Check for bleeding at the site. | |
| —— | —— | —— | 14. If possible, instruct patient to call for assistance if any discomfort is noted at site, solution container is nearly empty, flow has changed in any way, or if the electronic pump alarm sounds. | |

*Skill Checklists for Taylor's Clinical Nursing Skills:*
*A Nursing Process Approach, 3rd edition*

Name _____     Date _____

Unit _____     Position _____

Instructor/Evaluator: _____     Position _____

SKILL 15-4

# Changing a Peripheral Venous Access Dressing

| Excellent | Satisfactory | Needs Practice | **Goal:** The patient exhibits an access site that is clean, dry, and without evidence of any signs and symptoms of infection, infiltration, or phlebitis. In addition, the dressing will be clean, dry, and intact and the patient will not experience injury. | Comments |
|---|---|---|---|---|
| ___ | ___ | ___ | 1. Determine the need for a dressing change. Check facility policy. Gather all equipment and bring to bedside. | |
| ___ | ___ | ___ | 2. Perform hand hygiene and put on PPE, if indicated. | |
| ___ | ___ | ___ | 3. Identify the patient. | |
| ___ | ___ | ___ | 4. Close curtains around bed and close the door to the room, if possible. Explain what you are going to do and why you are going to do it to the patient. Ask the patient about allergies to tape and skin antiseptics. | |
| ___ | ___ | ___ | 5. Put on mask and place a mask on patient, if indicated. Put on gloves. Place towel or disposable pad under the arm with the venous access. If solution is currently infusing, temporarily stop the infusion. Hold the catheter in place with your nondominant hand and *carefully remove old dressing and/or stabilization/securing device.* Use adhesive remover as necessary. Discard dressing. | |
| ___ | ___ | ___ | 6. *Inspect IV site for presence of phlebitis (inflammation), infection, or infiltration.* Discontinue and relocate IV, if noted. Refer to Fundamentals Review 15-3, Box 15-2, and Box 15-3. | |
| ___ | ___ | ___ | 7. *Cleanse site with an antiseptic solution such as chlorhexidine or according to facility policy. Press applicator against the skin and apply chlorhexidine using a back and forth friction scrub for at least 30 seconds. Do not wipe or blot. Allow to dry completely.* | |
| ___ | ___ | ___ | 8. Open the skin protectant wipe. Apply the skin protectant to the site, making sure to cover at minimum the area to be covered with the dressing. Allow to dry. Place sterile transparent dressing or catheter securing/stabilization device over venipuncture site. | |

| Excellent | Satisfactory | Needs Practice | SKILL 15-4<br>**Changing a Peripheral Venous<br>Access Dressing** *(Continued)* | |
|---|---|---|---|---|
| | | | | **Comments** |
| —— | —— | —— | 9. Label dressing with date, time of change, and initials. Loop the tubing near the entry site, and anchor with tape (nonallergenic) close to site. Resume fluid infusion, if indicated. Check that IV flow is accurate and system is patent. Refer to Skill 15-3. | |
| —— | —— | —— | 10. Remove equipment. Ensure patient's comfort. Remove gloves. Lower bed, if not in lowest position. | |
| —— | —— | —— | 11. Remove additional PPE, if used. Perform hand hygiene. | |

*Skill Checklists for Taylor's Clinical Nursing Skills:*
*A Nursing Process Approach, 3rd edition*

Name _____  Date _____

Unit _____  Position _____

Instructor/Evaluator: _____  Position _____

| Excellent | Satisfactory | Needs Practice | SKILL 15-5 |
|---|---|---|---|

### SKILL 15-5
## Capping for Intermittent Use and Flushing a Peripheral Venous Access Device

**Goal:** The patient remains free of injury and any signs and symptoms of IV complications.

**Comments**

| Excellent | Satisfactory | Needs Practice | | Comments |
|---|---|---|---|---|
| ___ | ___ | ___ | 1. Determine the need for conversion to an intermittent access. Verify medical order. Check facility policy. Gather all equipment and bring to bedside. | |
| ___ | ___ | ___ | 2. Perform hand hygiene and put on PPE, if indicated. | |
| ___ | ___ | ___ | 3. Identify the patient. | |
| ___ | ___ | ___ | 4. Close curtains around bed and close the door to the room, if possible. Explain what you are going to do and why you are going to do it to the patient. Ask the patient about allergies to tape and skin antiseptics. | |
| ___ | ___ | ___ | 5. Assess the IV site. Refer to Skill 15-3. | |
| ___ | ___ | ___ | 6. If using an electronic infusion device, stop the device. Close the roller clamp on the administration set. If using gravity infusion, close the roller clamp on the administration set. | |
| ___ | ___ | ___ | 7. Put on gloves. Close the clamp on the short extension tubing connected to the IV catheter in the patient's arm. | |
| ___ | ___ | ___ | 8. Remove the administration set tubing from the extension set. Cleanse the end cap with an antimicrobial swab. | |
| ___ | ___ | ___ | 9. Insert the saline flush syringe into the cap on the extension tubing. Pull back on the syringe to aspirate the catheter for positive blood return. If positive, instill the solution over 1 minute or flush the line according to facility policy. Remove syringe and reclamp the extension tubing. | |
| ___ | ___ | ___ | 10. If necessary, loop the extension tubing near the entry site and anchor it with tape (nonallergenic) close to site. | |
| ___ | ___ | ___ | 11. Remove equipment. Ensure patient's comfort. Remove gloves. Lower bed, if not in lowest position. | |
| ___ | ___ | ___ | 12. Remove additional PPE, if used. Perform hand hygiene. | |

Skill Checklists for Taylor's Clinical Nursing Skills:
A Nursing Process Approach, 3rd edition

Name _____  Date _____

Unit _____  Position _____

Instructor/Evaluator: _____  Position _____

SKILL 15-6

# Administering a Blood Transfusion

**Goal:** The patient receives the correct blood type and remains free of injury due to transfusion complications and/or reactions.

| Excellent | Satisfactory | Needs Practice | | Comments |
|---|---|---|---|---|
| —— | —— | —— | 1. Verify the medical order for transfusion of a blood product. Verify the completion of informed consent documentation in the medical record. Verify any medical order for pretransfusion medication. If ordered, administer medication at least 30 minutes before initiating transfusion. | |
| —— | —— | —— | 2. Gather all equipment and bring to bedside. | |
| —— | —— | —— | 3. Perform hand hygiene and put on PPE, if indicated. | |
| —— | —— | —— | 4. Identify the patient. | |
| —— | —— | —— | 5. Close curtains around bed and close the door to the room, if possible. Explain what you are going to do and why you are going to do it to the patient. Ask the patient about previous experience with transfusion and any reactions. Advise patient to report any chills, itching, rash, or unusual symptoms. | |
| —— | —— | —— | 6. Prime blood administration set with the normal saline IV fluid. Refer to Skill 15-2. | |
| —— | —— | —— | 7. Put on gloves. If patient does not have a venous access in place, initiate peripheral venous access. (Refer to Skill 15-1.) Connect the administration set to the venous access device via the extension tubing. (Refer to Skill 15-1.) Infuse the normal saline per facility policy. | |
| —— | —— | —— | 8. Obtain blood product from blood bank according to agency policy. Scan for bar codes on blood products if required. | |
| | | | 9. Two nurses compare and validate the following information with the medical record, patient identification band, and the label of the blood product: | |
| —— | —— | —— | • Medical order for transfusion of blood product | |
| —— | —— | —— | • Informed consent | |
| —— | —— | —— | • Patient identification number | |
| —— | —— | —— | • Patient name | |
| —— | —— | —— | • Blood group and type | |
| —— | —— | —— | • Expiration date | |
| —— | —— | —— | • Inspection of blood product for clots | |

## SKILL 15-6
# Administering a Blood Transfusion *(Continued)*

| Excellent | Satisfactory | Needs Practice | | Comments |
|---|---|---|---|---|

| Excellent | Satisfactory | Needs Practice | | Comments |
|---|---|---|---|---|
| —— | —— | —— | 10. *Obtain baseline set of vital signs before beginning transfusion.* | |
| —— | —— | —— | 11. Put on gloves. If using an electronic infusion device, put the device on "hold." Close the roller clamp closest to the drip chamber on the saline side of the administration set. Close the roller clamp on the administration set below the infusion device. Alternately, if using infusing via gravity, close the roller clamp on the administration set. | |
| —— | —— | —— | 12. Close the roller clamp closest to the drip chamber on the blood product side of the administration set. Remove the protective cap from the access port on the blood container. Remove the cap from the access spike on the administration set. Using a pushing and twisting motion, insert the spike into the access port on the blood container, taking care not to contaminate the spike. Hang blood container on the IV pole. Open the roller clamp on the blood side of the administration set. Squeeze drip chamber until the in-line filter is saturated. Remove gloves. | |
| —— | —— | —— | 13. *Start administration slowly (no more than 25 to 50 mL for the first 15 minutes). Stay with the patient for the first 5 to 15 minutes of transfusion.* Open the roller clamp on the administration set below the infusion device. Set the rate of flow and begin the transfusion. Alternately, start the flow of solution by releasing the clamp on the tubing and counting the drops. Adjust until the correct drop rate is achieved. Assess the flow of the blood and function of the infusion device. Inspect the insertion site for signs of infiltration. | |
| —— | —— | —— | 14. Observe patient for flushing, dyspnea, itching, hives or rash, or any unusual comments. | |
| —— | —— | —— | 15. After the observation period (5 to 15 minutes) increase the infusion rate to the calculated rate to complete the infusion within the prescribed time frame, no more than 4 hours. | |
| —— | —— | —— | 16. Reassess vital signs after 15 minutes. Obtain vital signs thereafter according to facility policy and nursing assessment. | |
| —— | —— | —— | 17. Maintain the prescribed flow rate as ordered or as deemed appropriate based on the patient's overall condition, keeping in mind the outer limits for safe administration. Ongoing monitoring is crucial throughout the entire duration of the blood transfusion for early identification of any adverse reactions. | |

SKILL 15-6

# Administering a Blood Transfusion *(Continued)*

| Excellent | Satisfactory | Needs Practice | | Comments |
|---|---|---|---|---|
| —— | —— | —— | 18. *During transfusion, assess frequently for transfusion reaction. Stop blood transfusion if you suspect a reaction. Quickly replace the blood tubing with a new administration set primed with normal saline for IV infusion. Initiate an infusion of normal saline for IV at an open rate, usually 40 mL/hour. Obtain vital signs. Notify physician and blood bank.* | |
| —— | —— | —— | 19. When transfusion is complete, close roller clamp on blood side of the administration set and open the roller clamp on the normal saline side of the administration set. Initiate infusion of normal saline. When all of blood has infused into the patient, clamp the administration set. Obtain vital signs. Put on gloves. Cap access site or resume previous IV infusion. (Refer to Skill 15-1 and Skill 15-5.) Dispose of blood-transfusion equipment or return to blood bank, according to facility policy. | |
| —— | —— | —— | 20. Remove equipment. Ensure patient's comfort. Remove gloves. Lower bed, if not in lowest position. | |
| —— | —— | —— | 21. Remove additional PPE, if used. Perform hand hygiene. | |

*Skill Checklists for Taylor's Clinical Nursing Skills:*
*A Nursing Process Approach, 3rd edition*

Name _____  Date _____

Unit _____  Position _____

Instructor/Evaluator: _____  Position _____

| Excellent | Satisfactory | Needs Practice | SKILL 15-7 **Changing the Dressing and Flushing Central Venous Access Devices** | Comments |
|---|---|---|---|---|
| | | | **Goal:** The dressing is changed and the CVAD flushed with the patient remaining free of signs of infection. | |
| ___ | ___ | ___ | 1. Verify the medical order and/or facility policy and procedure. Often, the procedure for CVAD flushing and dressing changes will be a standing protocol. Gather equipment and bring to bedside. | |
| ___ | ___ | ___ | 2. Perform hand hygiene and put on PPE, if indicated. | |
| ___ | ___ | ___ | 3. Identify the patient. | |
| ___ | ___ | ___ | 4. Close curtains around bed and close the door to the room, if possible. Explain what you are going to do and why you are going to do it to the patient. Ask the patient about allergies to tape and skin antiseptics. | |
| ___ | ___ | ___ | 5. Place a waste receptacle or bag at a convenient location for use during the procedure. | |
| ___ | ___ | ___ | 6. Adjust bed to comfortable working height, usually elbow height of the caregiver (VISN 8 Patient Safety Center, 2009). | |
| ___ | ___ | ___ | 7. Assist the patient to a comfortable position that provides easy access to the CVAD insertion site and dressing. If the patient has a PICC, position the patient with the arm extended from the body below heart level. Use the bath blanket to cover any exposed area other than the site. | |
| ___ | ___ | ___ | 8. Apply a mask. Ask patient to turn head away from access site. Alternately, have the patient put on a mask. Move the overbed table to a convenient location within easy reach. Set up a sterile field on the table. Open dressing supplies and add to sterile field. If IV solution is infusing via CVAD, interrupt and place on hold during dressing change. Apply slide clamp on each lumen of the CVAD. | |
| ___ | ___ | ___ | 9. Put on clean gloves. Assess CVAD insertion site (for inflammation, redness, and so forth) through old dressing. Note the status of any sutures that may be present. Remove old dressing by lifting it distally and then working proximally, making sure to stabilize the catheter. Discard dressing in trash receptacle. Remove gloves and discard. | |

| Excellent | Satisfactory | Needs Practice | SKILL 15-7<br><br>**Changing the Dressing and Flushing**<br>**Central Venous Access Devices** *(Continued)* |
|---|---|---|---|
| | | | **Comments** |
| —— | —— | —— | 10. Put on sterile gloves. Starting at insertion site and continuing in a circle, wipe off any old blood or drainage with a sterile antimicrobial wipe. Using the chlorhexidine swab, cleanse the site. Cleanse directly over the insertion site by pressing applicator against the skin. *Apply chlorhexidine using a back and forth friction scrub for at least 30 seconds.* Moving outward from the site, use a scrubbing motion to continue to clean, covering at least a 2- to 3-inch area. *Do not wipe or blot. Allow to dry completely.* Apply the skin protectant to the same area, avoiding direct application to insertion site and allow to dry. |
| —— | —— | —— | 11. Stabilize catheter hub by holding it in place with nondominant hand. Use an alcohol wipe to clean each lumen of the catheter, starting at the insertion site and move outward. |
| —— | —— | —— | 12. Apply transparent site dressing or securement/stabilization device, centering over insertion site. If patient has PICC in place, measure the length of the catheter that extends out from the insertion site. |
| —— | —— | —— | 13. Working with one lumen at a time, remove end cap. Cleanse the end of the lumen with an alcohol swab and apply new end cap. Repeat for each lumen. Secure catheter lumens and/or tubing that extend outside dressing with tape.<br><br>*If required, flush each lumen of the CVAD. Amount of saline and heparin flushes varies depending on specific CVAD and facility policy.* |
| —— | —— | —— | 14. Cleanse end cap with an antimicrobial swab. |
| —— | —— | —— | 15. Insert the saline flush syringe into the cap on the extension tubing. Pull back on the syringe to aspirate the catheter for positive blood return. If positive, instill the solution over 1 minute or flush the line according to facility policy. Remove syringe. Insert heparin syringe and instill the volume of solution designated by facility policy over 1 minute or according to facility policy. Remove syringe and reclamp the lumen. Remove gloves. |
| —— | —— | —— | 16. Label dressing with date, time of change, and initials. Resume fluid infusion, if indicated. Check that IV flow is accurate and system is patent. (Refer to Skill 15-3.) |
| —— | —— | —— | 17. Remove equipment. Ensure patient's comfort. Lower bed, if not in lowest position. |
| —— | —— | —— | 18. Remove additional PPE, if used. Perform hand hygiene. |

*Skill Checklists for Taylor's Clinical Nursing Skills:*
*A Nursing Process Approach, 3rd edition*

Name _____ Date _____

Unit _____ Position _____

Instructor/Evaluator: _____ Position _____

| Excellent | Satisfactory | Needs Practice | SKILL 15-8<br>**Accessing an Implanted Port** | Comments |
|---|---|---|---|---|
| | | | **Goal:** The port is accessed with minimal to no discomfort to the patient; the port site is free from trauma and infection; and the patient verbalizes an understanding of care associated with the port. | |
| ⎯ | ⎯ | ⎯ | 1. Verify medical order and/or facility policy and procedure. Often, the procedure for accessing an implanted port and dressing changes will be a standing protocol. Gather equipment and bring to bedside. | |
| ⎯ | ⎯ | ⎯ | 2. Perform hand hygiene and put on PPE, if indicated. | |
| ⎯ | ⎯ | ⎯ | 3. Identify the patient. | |
| ⎯ | ⎯ | ⎯ | 4. Close curtains around bed and close the door to the room, if possible. Explain what you are going to do, and why you are going to do it to the patient. Ask the patient about allergies to tape and skin antiseptics. | |
| ⎯ | ⎯ | ⎯ | 5. Place a waste receptacle or bag at a convenient location for use during the procedure. | |
| ⎯ | ⎯ | ⎯ | 6. Adjust bed to comfortable working height, usually elbow height of the caregiver (VISN 8 Patient Safety Center, 2009). | |
| ⎯ | ⎯ | ⎯ | 7. Assist the patient to a comfortable position that provides easy access to the port site. Use the bath blanket to cover any exposed area other than the site. | |
| ⎯ | ⎯ | ⎯ | 8. Put a mask on. Ask patient to turn head away from access site. Alternately, have the patient put on a mask. Move the overbed table to a convenient location within easy reach. Set up a sterile field on the table. Open dressing supplies and add to sterile field. | |
| ⎯ | ⎯ | ⎯ | 9. Put on clean gloves. Palpate the location of the port. Assess site. Note the status of any surgical incisions that may be present. Remove gloves and discard. | |
| ⎯ | ⎯ | ⎯ | 10. Put on sterile gloves. Connect the end cap to the extension tubing on the noncoring needle. Clean end cap with alcohol wipe. Insert syringe with normal saline into end cap. Fill extension tubing with normal saline and apply clamp. Place on sterile field. | |

| Excellent | Satisfactory | Needs Practice | | Comments |
|---|---|---|---|---|

**SKILL 15-8**

# Accessing an Implanted Port *(Continued)*

| | | | |
|---|---|---|---|
| —— —— —— | 11. Using the chlorhexidine swab, cleanse the port site. Press the applicator against the skin. *Apply chlorhexidine using a back and forth friction scrub for at least 30 seconds.* Moving outward from the site, use a circular, scrubbing motion to continue to clean, covering at least a 2- to 3-inch area. *Do not wipe or blot. Allow to dry completely.* | |
| —— —— —— | 12. Using the nondominant hand, locate the port. Hold the port stable, keeping the skin taut. | |
| —— —— —— | 13. Visualize the center of the port. Pick up the needle. Coil extension tubing into palm of hand. Holding needle at a 90-degree angle to the skin, insert *through the skin into the port septum until the needle hits the back of the port.* | |
| —— —— —— | 14. Cleanse the end cap on the extension tubing with an antimicrobial swab and insert the syringe with normal saline. *Open the clamp on extension tubing and flush with 3 to 5 mL of saline, while observing the site for fluid leak or infiltration. It should flush easily, without resistance.* | |
| —— —— —— | 15. Pull back on the syringe plunger to aspirate for blood return. Aspirate only a few milliliters of blood; do not allow blood to enter the syringe. If positive, instill the solution over 1 minute or flush the line according to facility policy. Remove syringe. Insert heparin syringe and instill the solution over 1 minute or according to facility policy. Remove syringe and clamp the extension tubing. Alternately, if IV fluid infusion is to be started, do not flush with heparin. | |
| —— —— —— | 16. If using a "Gripper" needle, remove the gripper portion from the needle by squeezing the sides together and lifting off the needle while holding the needle securely to the port with the other hand. | |
| —— —— —— | 17. Apply the skin protectant to the site, avoiding direct application to needle insertion site. Allow to dry. | |
| —— —— —— | 18. Apply tape or Steri-Strips in a star-like pattern over the needle to secure it. | |
| —— —— —— | 19. Apply transparent site dressing or securement/stabilization device, centering over insertion site. | |
| —— —— —— | 20. Label dressing with date, time of change, and initials. If IV fluid infusion is ordered, attach administration set to extension tubing and begin administration. Refer to Skill 15-1. | |
| —— —— —— | 21. Remove equipment. Ensure patient's comfort. Lower bed, if not in lowest position. | |
| —— —— —— | 22. Remove additional PPE, if used. Perform hand hygiene. | |

*Skill Checklists for Taylor's Clinical Nursing Skills:*
*A Nursing Process Approach, 3rd edition*

Name _____   Date _____

Unit _____   Position _____

Instructor/Evaluator: _____   Position _____

| Excellent | Satisfactory | Needs Practice | SKILL 15-9 **Deaccessing an Implanted Port** | Comments |
|---|---|---|---|---|
| | | | **Goal:** The needle is removed with minimal to no discomfort to the patient; the patient experiences no trauma or infection; and the patient verbalizes an understanding of port care. | |
| ___ | ___ | ___ | 1. Verify medical order and/or facility policy and procedure. Often, the procedure for accessing an implanted port and dressing changes will be a standing protocol. Gather equipment and bring to bedside. | |
| ___ | ___ | ___ | 2. Perform hand hygiene and put on PPE, if indicated. | |
| ___ | ___ | ___ | 3. Identify the patient. | |
| ___ | ___ | ___ | 4. Close curtains around bed and close the door to the room, if possible. Explain what you are going to do and why you are going to do it to the patient. | |
| ___ | ___ | ___ | 5. Adjust bed to comfortable working height, usually elbow height of the caregiver (VISN 8 Patient Safety Center, 2009). | |
| ___ | ___ | ___ | 6. Assist the patient to a comfortable position that provides easy access to the port site. Use the bath blanket to cover any exposed area other than the site. | |
| ___ | ___ | ___ | 7. Put on gloves. Stabilize port needle with nondominant hand. Gently pull back transparent dressing, beginning with edges and proceeding around the edge of the dressing. Carefully remove all the tape that is securing the needle in place. | |
| ___ | ___ | ___ | 8. Clean the end cap on the extension tubing and insert the saline-filled syringe. Unclamp the extension tubing and flush with a minimum of 10 mL of normal saline. | |
| ___ | ___ | ___ | 9. Remove the syringe and insert the heparin-filled syringe, flushing with 5 mL heparin (100 U/mL or per facility policy). Remove syringe and clamp the extension tubing. | |
| ___ | ___ | ___ | 10. Secure the port on either side with the fingers of your nondominant hand. Grasp the needle/wings with the fingers of dominant hand. Firmly and smoothly, pull the needle straight up at a 90-degree angle from the skin to remove it from the septum. Engage needle guard, if not automatic on removal. | |

SKILL 15-9

**Deaccessing an Implanted Port** *(Continued)*

| Excellent | Satisfactory | Needs Practice | | Comments |
|---|---|---|---|---|
| — | — | — | 11. Apply gentle pressure with the gauze to the insertion site. Apply a Band-Aid over the port if any oozing occurs. Otherwise, a dressing is not necessary. Remove gloves. | |
| — | — | — | 12. Ensure patient's comfort. Lower bed, if not in lowest position. Put on one glove to handle needle. Dispose of needle with extension tubing in sharps container. | |
| — | — | — | 13. Remove gloves and additional PPE, if used. Perform hand hygiene. | |

Copyright © 2011 by Wolters Kluwer Health | Lippincott Williams & Wilkins. *Skill Checklists for Taylor's Clinical Nursing Skills: A Nursing Process Approach,* 3rd edition, by Pamela Lynn and Marilee LeBon.

*Skill Checklists for Taylor's Clinical Nursing Skills:*
*A Nursing Process Approach, 3rd edition*

Name _____  Date _____

Unit _____  Position _____

Instructor/Evaluator: _____  Position _____

### SKILL 15-10

# Removing a Peripherally Inserted Central Catheter (PICC)

**Goal:** The PICC is removed with minimal to no discomfort to the patient and the patient experiences no trauma or infection.

| Excellent | Satisfactory | Needs Practice | | Comments |
|---|---|---|---|---|
| ___ | ___ | ___ | 1. Verify medical order for PICC removal and facility policy and procedure. Gather equipment and bring to bedside. | |
| ___ | ___ | ___ | 2. Perform hand hygiene and put on PPE, if indicated. | |
| ___ | ___ | ___ | 3. Identify the patient. | |
| ___ | ___ | ___ | 4. Close curtains around bed and close the door to the room, if possible. Explain what you are going to do and why you are going to do it to the patient. | |
| ___ | ___ | ___ | 5. Adjust bed to comfortable working height, usually elbow height of the caregiver (VISN 8 Patient Safety Center, 2009). | |
| ___ | ___ | ___ | 6. Assist the patient to a supine position with the arm straight and the catheter insertion site below heart level. Use the bath blanket to cover any exposed area other than the site. | |
| ___ | ___ | ___ | 7. Put on gloves. Stabilize catheter hub with your nondominant hand. Gently pull back transparent dressing, beginning with edges and proceeding around the edge of the dressing. Carefully remove all the tape that is securing the catheter in place. | |
| ___ | ___ | ___ | 8. Using dominant hand, remove the catheter slowly. Grasp the catheter close to the insertion site and slowly ease the catheter out, keeping it parallel to the skin. Continue removing in small increments, using a smooth and gentle motion (Best Practices, 2007). | |
| ___ | ___ | ___ | 9. After removal, apply pressure to the site with a sterile gauze until hemostasis is achieved (minimum 1 minute). Then apply a small sterile dressing to the site. | |
| ___ | ___ | ___ | 10. Measure the catheter and compare it with the length listed in the chart when it was inserted. Inspect the catheter for patency. Dispose of PICC according to facility policy. | |
| ___ | ___ | ___ | 11. Remove gloves. Ensure patient's comfort. Lower bed, if not in lowest position. | |
| ___ | ___ | ___ | 12. Remove additional PPE, if used. Perform hand hygiene. | |

*Skill Checklists for Taylor's Clinical Nursing Skills:*
*A Nursing Process Approach, 3rd edition*

Name _____  Date _____

Unit _____  Position _____

Instructor/Evaluator: _____  Position _____

## SKILL 16-1

# Obtaining an Electrocardiogram (ECG)

**Goal:** A cardiac electrical tracing is obtained without any complications.

| Excellent | Satisfactory | Needs Practice | | Comments |
|---|---|---|---|---|
| —— | —— | —— | 1. Verify the order for an ECG on the patient's medical record. | |
| —— | —— | —— | 2. Gather all equipment and bring to bedside. | |
| —— | —— | —— | 3. Perform hand hygiene and put on PPE, if indicated. | |
| —— | —— | —— | 4. Identify the patient. | |
| —— | —— | —— | 5. Close curtains around bed and close the door to the room, if possible. As you set up the machine to record a 12-lead ECG, explain the procedure to the patient. Tell the patient that the test records the heart's electrical activity, and it may be repeated at certain intervals. Emphasize that no electrical current will enter his or her body. Tell the patient the test typically takes about 5 minutes. Ask the patient about allergies to adhesive, as appropriate. | |
| —— | —— | —— | 6. Place the ECG machine close to the patient's bed, and plug the power cord into the wall outlet. | |
| —— | —— | —— | 7. If the bed is adjustable, raise it to a comfortable working height, usually elbow height of the caregiver (VISN 8 Patient Safety Center, 2009). | |
| —— | —— | —— | 8. Have the patient lie supine in the center of the bed with the arms at the sides. Raise the head of the bed if necessary to promote comfort. Expose the patient's arms and legs, and drape appropriately. Encourage the patient to relax the arms and legs. If the bed is too narrow, place the patient's hands under the buttocks to prevent muscle tension. Also use this technique if the patient is shivering or trembling. Make sure the feet do not touch the bed's footboard. | |
| —— | —— | —— | 9. Select flat, fleshy areas on which to place the electrodes. Avoid muscular and bony areas. If the patient has an amputated limb, choose a site on the stump. | |
| —— | —— | —— | 10. If an area is excessively hairy, clip the hair. *Do not shave hair.* Clean excess oil or other substances from the skin with soap and water and dry it completely. | |

# Obtaining an Electrocardiogram (ECG) *(Continued)*

| Excellent | Satisfactory | Needs Practice | | Comments |
|---|---|---|---|---|
| — | — | — | 11. Apply the limb lead electrodes. The tip of each lead wire is lettered and color coded for easy identification. The white or RA lead goes to the right arm; the green or RL lead to the right leg; the red or LL lead to the left leg; the black or LA lead to the left arm. Peel the contact paper off the self-sticking disposable electrode and apply directly to the prepared site, as recommended by the manufacturer. Position disposable electrodes on the legs with the lead connection pointing superiorly. | |
| — | — | — | 12. Connect the limb lead wires to the electrodes. Make sure the metal parts of the electrodes are clean and bright. | |
| | | | 13. Expose the patient's chest. Apply the precordial lead electrodes. The tip of each lead wire is lettered and color coded for easy identification. The brown or $V_1$ to $V_6$ leads are applied to the chest. Peel the contact paper off the self-sticking, disposable electrode and apply directly to the prepared site, as recommended by the manufacturer. | |
| — | — | — | Position chest electrodes as follows (Refer to Figure 1): | |
| — | — | — | • $V_1$: Fourth intercostal space at right sternal border | |
| — | — | — | • $V_2$: Fourth intercostal space at left sternal border | |
| — | — | — | • $V_3$: Halfway between $V_2$ and $V_4$ | |
| — | — | — | • $V_4$: Fifth intercostal space at the left midclavicular line | |
| — | — | — | • V5: Fifth intercostal space at anterior axillary line (halfway between $V_4$ and $V_6$) | |
| — | — | — | • $V_6$: Fifth intercostal space at midaxillary line, level with $V_4$ | |
| — | — | — | 14. Connect the precordial lead wires to the electrodes. Make sure the metal parts of the electrodes are clean and bright. | |
| — | — | — | 15. After the application of all the leads, make sure the paper-speed selector is set to the standard 25 m/second and that the machine is set to full voltage. | |
| — | — | — | 16. If necessary, enter the appropriate patient identification data into the machine. | |
| — | — | — | 17. Ask the patient to relax and breathe normally. ***Instruct the patient to lie still and not to talk while you record the ECG.*** | |

| Excellent | Satisfactory | Needs Practice | SKILL 16-1<br>**Obtaining an Electrocardiogram (ECG)** *(Continued)* | |
|---|---|---|---|---|
| | | | | **Comments** |
| —— | —— | —— | 18. Press the AUTO button. Observe the tracing quality. The machine will record all 12 leads automatically, recording 3 consecutive leads simultaneously. Some machines have a display screen so you can preview waveforms before the machine records them on paper. Adjust waveform, if necessary. If any part of the waveform extends beyond the paper when you record the ECG, adjust the normal standardization to half-standardization and repeat. Note this adjustment on the ECG strip, because this will need to be considered in interpreting the results. | |
| —— | —— | —— | 19. When the machine finishes recording the 12-lead ECG, remove the electrodes and clean the patient's skin, if necessary, with adhesive remover for sticky residue. | |
| —— | —— | —— | 20. After disconnecting the lead wires from the electrodes, dispose of the electrodes. Return the patient to a comfortable position. Lower bed height and adjust the head of bed to a comfortable position. | |
| —— | —— | —— | 21. Clean ECG machine per facility policy. If not done electronically from data entered into the machine, label the ECG with the patient's name, date of birth, location, date and time of recording, and other relevant information, such as symptoms that occurred during the recording (Jevon, 2007b). | |
| —— | —— | —— | 22. Remove additional PPE, if used. Perform hand hygiene. | |

*Skill Checklists for Taylor's Clinical Nursing Skills:*
*A Nursing Process Approach, 3rd edition*

Name _____     Date _____

Unit _____     Position _____

Instructor/Evaluator: _____     Position _____

| Excellent | Satisfactory | Needs Practice | SKILL 16-2 **Applying a Cardiac Monitor** | Comments |
|---|---|---|---|---|
| | | | **Goal:** A clear waveform, free from artifact, is displayed on the cardiac monitor. | |
| ___ | ___ | ___ | 1. Verify the order for cardiac monitoring on the patient's medical record. | |
| ___ | ___ | ___ | 2. Gather all equipment and bring to bedside. | |
| ___ | ___ | ___ | 3. Perform hand hygiene and put on PPE, if indicated. | |
| ___ | ___ | ___ | 4. Identify the patient. | |
| ___ | ___ | ___ | 5. Close curtains around bed and close the door to the room, if possible. Explain the procedure to the patient. Tell the patient that the monitoring records the heart's electrical activity. Emphasize that no electrical current will enter his or her body. Ask the patient about allergies to adhesive, as appropriate. | |
| ___ | ___ | ___ | 6. For hardwire monitoring, plug the cardiac monitor into an electrical outlet and turn it on to warm up the unit while preparing the equipment and the patient. For telemetry monitoring, insert a new battery into the transmitter. Match the poles on the battery with the polar markings on the transmitter case. Press the button at the top of the unit, test the battery's charge, and test the unit to ensure that the battery is operational. | |
| ___ | ___ | ___ | 7. Insert the cable into the appropriate socket in the monitor. | |
| ___ | ___ | ___ | 8. Connect the lead wires to the cable. In some systems, the lead wires are permanently secured to the cable. For telemetry, if the lead wires are not permanently affixed to the telemetry unit, attach them securely. If they must be attached individually, connect each one to the correct outlet. | |
| ___ | ___ | ___ | 9. Connect an electrode to each of the lead wires, carefully checking that each lead wire is in its correct outlet. | |
| ___ | ___ | ___ | 10. If the bed is adjustable, raise it to a comfortable working height, usually elbow height of the caregiver (VISN 8 Patient Safety Center, 2009). | |

| Excellent | Satisfactory | Needs Practice | |
|-----------|--------------|----------------|---|

## SKILL 16-2
# Applying a Cardiac Monitor *(Continued)*

**Comments**

— — — 11. Expose the patient's chest and determine electrode positions, based on which system and leads are being used. If necessary, clip the hair from an area about 10 cm in diameter around each electrode site. Clean the area with soap and water and dry it completely to remove skin secretions that may interfere with electrode function.

— — — 12. Remove the backing from the pregelled electrode. Check the gel for moistness. If the gel is dry, discard it and replace it with a fresh electrode. *Apply the electrode to the site and press firmly to ensure a tight seal.* Repeat with the remaining electrodes to complete the three-lead or five-lead system.

— — — 13. When all the electrodes are in place, connect the appropriate lead wire to each electrode. Check waveform for clarity, position, and size. *To verify that the monitor is detecting each beat, compare the digital heart rate display with an auscultated count of the patient's heart rate.* If necessary, use the gain control to adjust the size of the rhythm tracing, and use the position control to adjust the waveform position on the monitor.

— — — 14. Set the upper and lower limits of the heart rate alarm, based on the patient's condition or unit policy.

— — — 15. For telemetry, place the transmitter in the pouch in the hospital gown. If not available in gown, use a portable pouch. Tie the pouch strings around the patient's neck and waist, making sure that the pouch fits snugly without causing discomfort. If no pouch is available, place the transmitter in the patient's bathrobe pocket.

— — — 16. To obtain a rhythm strip, press the RECORD key either at the bedside for monitoring or at the central station for telemetry. Label the strip with the patient's name and room number, date, time, and rhythm identification. Analyze the strip, as appropriate. Place the rhythm strip in the appropriate location in the patient's chart.

— — — 17. Return the patient to a comfortable position. Lower bed height and adjust the head of bed to a comfortable position.

— — — 18. Remove additional PPE, if used. Perform hand hygiene.

*Skill Checklists for Taylor's Clinical Nursing Skills:*
*A Nursing Process Approach, 3rd edition*

Name _____   Date _____

Unit _____   Position _____

Instructor/Evaluator: _____   Position _____

| Excellent | Satisfactory | Needs Practice | SKILL 16-3<br>**Obtaining an Arterial Blood Sample From an Arterial Line–Stopcock System** | |
|---|---|---|---|---|
| | | | **Goal:** A specimen is obtained without compromise to the patency of the arterial line. | **Comments** |
| ___ | ___ | ___ | 1. Verify the order for laboratory testing on the patient's medical record. | |
| ___ | ___ | ___ | 2. Gather all equipment and bring to bedside. | |
| ___ | ___ | ___ | 3. Perform hand hygiene and put on PPE, if indicated. | |
| ___ | ___ | ___ | 4. Identify the patient. | |
| ___ | ___ | ___ | 5. Close curtains around bed and close the door to the room, if possible. Explain the procedure to the patient. | |
| ___ | ___ | ___ | 6. Compare specimen label with patient identification bracelet. Label should include patient's name and identification number, time specimen was collected, route of collection, identification of the person obtaining sample, and any other information required by agency policy. | |
| ___ | ___ | ___ | 7. Put on gloves and goggles or face shield. | |
| ___ | ___ | ___ | 8. Turn off or temporarily silence the arterial pressure alarms, depending on facility policy. | |
| ___ | ___ | ___ | 9. Locate the stopcock nearest the arterial line insertion site. Use the alcohol swab or chlorhexidine to scrub the sampling port on the stopcock. Allow to air dry. | |
| ___ | ___ | ___ | 10. Attach a 5-mL syringe into the sampling port on the stopcock to obtain the discard volume. Turn off the stopcock to the flush solution. Aspirate slowly until blood enters the syringe. Stop aspirating. Note the volume in the syringe, which is the dead-space volume. Continue to aspirate until the dead-space volume has been withdrawn a total of three times. For example, if the dead-space volume is 0.8 mL, aspirate 2.4 mL of blood. | |
| ___ | ___ | ___ | 11. Turn the stopcock to the halfway position between the flush solution and the sampling port to close the system in all directions. | |
| ___ | ___ | ___ | 12. Remove the discard syringe and dispose of appropriately. | |

# Obtaining an Arterial Blood Sample From an Arterial Line–Stopcock System (Continued)

| Excellent | Satisfactory | Needs Practice | | Comments |
|---|---|---|---|---|
| —— | —— | —— | 13. Place the syringe for the laboratory sample or the Vacutainer in the sampling port of the stopcock. Turn the stopcock off to the flush solution, and slowly withdraw the required amount of blood. For each additional sample required, repeat this procedure. If coagulation tests are included in the required tests, obtain blood for this from the final sample. | |
| —— | —— | —— | 14. Turn the stopcock to the halfway position between the flush solution and the sampling port to close the system in all directions. Remove the syringe or Vacutainer. Apply the rubber cap to the ABG syringe hub, if necessary. | |
| —— | —— | —— | 15. Insert a 5-mL syringe into the sampling port of the stopcock. Turn off the stopcock to the patient. Activate the in-line flushing device. *Flush through the sampling port into the syringe to clear the stopcock and sampling port of any residual blood.* | |
| —— | —— | —— | 16. Turn off the stopcock to the sampling port; remove the syringe. Remove sampling port cap and replace with new sterile one. *Intermittently flush the arterial catheter with the in-line flushing device until the tubing is clear of blood.* | |
| —— | —— | —— | 17. Remove gloves. Reactivate the monitor alarms. Record date and time the samples were obtained on the labels, as well as the required information to identify the person obtaining the samples. If ABG was collected, record oxygen flow rate (or room air) on label. Apply labels to the specimens, according to facility policy. Place in biohazard bags; place ABG sample in bag with ice. | |
| —— | —— | —— | 18. Check the monitor for return of the arterial waveform and pressure reading. | |
| —— | —— | —— | 19. Return the patient to a comfortable position. Lower bed height, if necessary, and adjust head of bed to a comfortable position. | |
| —— | —— | —— | 20. Remove goggles and additional PPE, if used. Perform hand hygiene. Send specimens to the laboratory immediately. | |

*Skill Checklists for Taylor's Clinical Nursing Skills:*
*A Nursing Process Approach, 3rd edition*

Name _____   Date _____

Unit _____   Position _____

Instructor/Evaluator: _____   Position _____

| Excellent | Satisfactory | Needs Practice | SKILL 16-4<br>**Removing Arterial and Femoral Lines** | |
|---|---|---|---|---|
| | | | **Goal:** The line is removed intact and without injury to the patient. | **Comments** |
| ___ | ___ | ___ | 1. Verify the order for removal of arterial or femoral line in the patient's medical record. | |
| ___ | ___ | ___ | 2. Gather all equipment and bring to bedside. | |
| ___ | ___ | ___ | 3. Perform hand hygiene and put on PPE, if indicated. | |
| ___ | ___ | ___ | 4. Identify the patient. | |
| ___ | ___ | ___ | 5. Close curtains around bed and close the door to the room, if possible. Explain the procedure to the patient. | |
| ___ | ___ | ___ | 6. Ask the patient to empty his or her bladder. Maintain an IV infusion of normal saline via another venous access during the procedure, as per medical orders or facility guidelines. | |
| ___ | ___ | ___ | 7. If the bed is adjustable, raise it to a comfortable working height, usually elbow height of the caregiver (VISN 8 Patient Safety Center, 2009). | |
| ___ | ___ | ___ | 8. Put on clean gloves, goggles, and gown. | |
| ___ | ___ | ___ | 9. If the line being removed is in a femoral site, use Doppler ultrasound to locate femoral artery 1 to 2 inches above the entrance site of the femoral line. Mark with 'X' using indelible pen. | |
| ___ | ___ | ___ | 10. Turn off the monitor alarms and then turn off the flow clamp to the flush solution. Carefully remove the dressing over the insertion site. Remove any sutures using the suture removal kit; make sure all sutures have been removed. | |
| ___ | ___ | ___ | 11. *Withdraw the catheter using a gentle, steady motion. Keep the catheter parallel to the blood vessel during withdrawal. Watch for hematoma formation during catheter removal by gently palpating surrounding tissue. If hematoma starts to form, reposition your hands until optimal pressure is obtained to prevent further leakage of blood.* | |
| ___ | ___ | ___ | 12. *Immediately after withdrawing the catheter, apply pressure 1 or 2 inches above the site at the previously marked spot with a sterile 4 × 4 gauze pad. Maintain pressure for at least 10 minutes, or per facility policy (longer if bleeding or oozing persists).* Apply additional pressure to a femoral site or if the patient has coagulopathy or is receiving anticoagulants. | |

SKILL 16-4

# Removing Arterial and Femoral Lines (Continued)

| Excellent | Satisfactory | Needs Practice | | Comments |
|---|---|---|---|---|
| — | — | — | 13. *Assess distal pulses every 3 to 5 minutes while pressure is being applied.* Note: dorsalis pedis and posterior tibial pulses should be markedly weaker from baseline if sufficient pressure is applied to the femoral artery. | |
| — | — | — | 14. Cover the site with an appropriate dressing and secure the dressing with tape. If stipulated by facility policy, make a pressure dressing for a femoral site by folding four sterile 4 × 4 gauze pads in half, and then applying the dressing. | |
| — | — | — | 15. Cover the dressing with a tight adhesive bandage, per policy, and then cover the femoral bandage with a sandbag. Remove gloves. Maintain the patient on bed rest, with the head of the bed elevated less than 30°, for 6 hours with the sandbag in place. Lower the bed height. Remind the patient not to lift his or her head while on bed rest. | |
| — | — | — | 16. Remove additional PPE. Perform hand hygiene. Send specimens to the laboratory immediately. | |
| — | — | — | 17. Observe the site for bleeding. Assess circulation in the extremity distal to the site by evaluating color, pulses, and sensation. Repeat this assessment every 15 minutes for the first 1 hour, every 30 minutes for the next 2 hours, hourly for the next 2 hours, then every 4 hours, or according to facility policy. Use log rolling to assist the patient in using the bedpan, if needed. | |

*Skill Checklists for Taylor's Clinical Nursing Skills:*
*A Nursing Process Approach, 3rd edition*

Name _____   Date _____

Unit _____   Position _____

Instructor/Evaluator: _____   Position _____

<table>
<thead>
<tr><th>Excellent</th><th>Satisfactory</th><th>Needs Practice</th><th>SKILL 16-5<br>**Performing Cardiopulmonary Resuscitation (CPR)**<br><br>**Goal:** CPR is performed effectively without adverse effect to the patient.</th><th>Comments</th></tr>
</thead>
<tbody>
<tr><td>——</td><td>——</td><td>——</td><td>1. Assess responsiveness. If the patient is not responsive, call for help, pull call bell, and call the facility emergency response number. Call for the automated external defibrillator (AED).</td><td></td></tr>
<tr><td>——</td><td>——</td><td>——</td><td>2. Put on gloves, if available. Position the patient supine on his or her back on a firm, flat surface, with arms alongside the body. If the patient is in bed, place a backboard or other rigid surface under the patient (often the footboard of the patient's bed).</td><td></td></tr>
<tr><td>——</td><td>——</td><td>——</td><td>3. Use the head tilt–chin lift maneuver to open the airway. Place one hand on the victim's forehead and apply firm, backward pressure with the palm to tilt the head back. Place the fingers of the other hand under the bony part of the lower jaw near the chin and lift the jaw upward to bring the chin forward and the teeth almost to occlusion. If trauma to the head or neck is present or suspected, use the jaw-thrust maneuver to open the airway. Place one hand on each side of the patient's head. Rest elbows on the flat surface under the patient, grasp the angle of the patient's lower jaw, and lift with both hands.</td><td></td></tr>
<tr><td>——</td><td>——</td><td>——</td><td>4. Look, listen, and feel for air exchange. Take at least 5 seconds and no more than 10 seconds (AHA, 2006).</td><td></td></tr>
<tr><td>——</td><td>——</td><td>——</td><td>5. If the patient resumes breathing or adequate respirations and signs of circulation are noted, place the patient in the recovery position.</td><td></td></tr>
<tr><td>——</td><td>——</td><td>——</td><td>6. If no spontaneous breathing is noted, seal the patient's mouth and nose with the face shield, one-way valve mask, or Ambu-bag (handheld resuscitation bag), if available. If not available, seal the patient's mouth with rescuer's mouth.</td><td></td></tr>
<tr><td>——</td><td>——</td><td>——</td><td>7. Instill two breaths, each lasting 1 second, making the chest rise.</td><td></td></tr>
</tbody>
</table>

| Excellent | Satisfactory | Needs Practice | | Comments |
|---|---|---|---|---|

## SKILL 16-5
# Performing Cardiopulmonary Resuscitation (CPR) *(Continued)*

____ ____ ____ 8. If you are unable to ventilate or the chest does not rise during ventilation, reposition the patient's head and reattempt to ventilate. If still unable to ventilate, begin CPR. Each subsequent time the airway is opened to administer breaths, look for an object. If an object is visible in the mouth, remove it. If no object is visible, continue with CPR.

____ ____ ____ 9. Check the carotid pulse, simultaneously evaluating for breathing, coughing, or movement. This assessment should take at least 5 seconds and no more than 10 seconds. Place the patient in the recovery position if breathing resumes.

____ ____ ____ 10. If patient has a pulse, but remains without spontaneous breathing, continue rescue breathing at a rate of one breath every 5 to 6 seconds, for a rate of 10 to 12 breaths per minute.

____ ____ ____ 11. If the patient is without signs of circulation, position the heel of one hand in the center of the chest between the nipples, directly over the lower half of the sternum. Place the other hand directly on top of the first hand. Extend or interlace fingers to keep fingers above the chest. Straighten arms and position shoulders directly over hands.

____ ____ ____ 12. Perform 30 chest compressions at a rate of 100 per minute, counting "one, two, etc." up to 30, keeping elbows locked, arms straight, and shoulders directly over the hands. Chest compressions should depress the sternum 1½ to 2 inches. Push straight down on the patient's sternum. Allow full chest recoil (re-expand) after each compression.

____ ____ ____ 13. Give two rescue breaths after each set of 30 compressions. Do five complete cycles of 30 compressions and two ventilations.

____ ____ ____ 14. ***Defibrillation should be provided at the earliest possible moment, as soon as AED becomes available.*** Refer to Skill 16-6: Automated External Defibrillation and Skill 16-7: Manual External Defibrillation.

____ ____ ____ 15. Continue CPR until advanced care providers take over, the patient starts to move, you are too exhausted to continue, or a physician discontinues CPR. Advanced care providers will indicate when a pulse check or other therapies are appropriate (AHA, 2006, p. 34).

____ ____ ____ 16. Remove gloves, if used. Perform hand hygiene.

*Skill Checklists for Taylor's Clinical Nursing Skills:*
*A Nursing Process Approach, 3rd edition*

Name _____  Date _____

Unit _____  Position _____

Instructor/Evaluator: _____  Position _____

| | | | SKILL 16-6 | |
|:---:|:---:|:---:|:---|:---:|
| | | | **Performing Emergency Automated External Defibrillation** | |
| Excellent | Satisfactory | Needs Practice | **Goal:** The defibrillation is performed correctly without adverse effect to the patient, and the patient regains signs of circulation, with organized electrical rhythm and pulse. | **Comments** |
| —— | —— | —— | 1. Assess responsiveness. If the patient is not responsive, call for help and pull call bell, and call the facility emergency response number. Call for the AED. Put on gloves, if available. Perform cardiopulmonary resuscitation (CPR) until the defibrillator and other emergency equipment arrive. | |
| —— | —— | —— | 2. Prepare the AED. Power on the AED. Push the power button. Some devices will turn on automatically when the lid or case is opened. | |
| —— | —— | —— | 3. Attach AED connecting cables to the AED (may be preconnected). Attach AED cables to the adhesive electrode pads (may be preconnected). | |
| —— | —— | —— | 4. Stop chest compressions. Peel away the covering from the electrode pads to expose the adhesive surface. Attach the electrode pads to the patient's chest. Place one pad on the upper right sternal border, directly below the clavicle. Place the second pad lateral to the left nipple, with the top margin of the pad a few inches below the axilla. | |
| —— | —— | —— | 5. Once the pads are in place and the device is turned on, follow the prompts given by the device. Clear the patient and analyze the rhythm. Ensure no one is touching the patient. Loudly state a "Clear the patient" message. Press 'Analyze' button to initiate analysis, if necessary. Some devices automatically begin analysis when the pads are attached. Avoid all movement affecting the patient during analysis. | |
| —— | —— | —— | 6. If ventricular tachycardia or ventricular fibrillation is present, the device will announce that a shock is indicated and begin charging. Once the AED is charged, a message will be delivered to shock the patient. | |
| —— | —— | —— | 7. Before pressing the 'Shock' button, loudly state a "Clear the patient" message. Visually check that no one is in contact with the patient. Press the 'Shock' button. If the AED is fully automatic, a shock will be delivered automatically. | |

| Excellent | Satisfactory | Needs Practice | SKILL 16-6<br>**Performing Emergency Automated**<br>**External Defibrillation** *(Continued)* | |
| --- | --- | --- | --- | --- |
| | | | | **Comments** |
| —— | —— | —— | 8. Immediately resume CPR, beginning with chest compressions. After five cycles (about 2 minutes), allow the AED to analyze the heart rhythm. If a shock is not advised, resume CPR, beginning with chest compressions. Do not recheck to see if there is a pulse. Follow the AED voice prompts. Continue until advanced care providers take over, the patient starts to move, you are too exhausted to continue, or a physician discontinues CPR. Advanced care providers will indicate when a pulse check or other therapies are appropriate (AHA, 2006, p. 34). | |
| —— | —— | —— | 9. Remove gloves, if used. Perform hand hygiene. | |

*Skill Checklists for Taylor's Clinical Nursing Skills:*
*A Nursing Process Approach, 3rd edition*

Name _____     Date _____

Unit _____     Position _____

Instructor/Evaluator: _____     Position _____

| Excellent | Satisfactory | Needs Practice | SKILL 16-7<br>**Performing Emergency Manual External Defibrillation (Asynchronous)** | |
|---|---|---|---|---|
| | | | **Goal:** The procedure is performed correctly without adverse effect to the patient; and the patient regains signs of circulation. | **Comments** |
| ___ | ___ | ___ | 1. Assess responsiveness. If the patient is not responsive, call for help and pull call bell, and call the facility emergency response number. Call for the AED. Put on gloves, if available. Perform cardiopulmonary resuscitation (CPR) until the defibrillator and other emergency equipment arrive. | |
| ___ | ___ | ___ | 2. Turn on the defibrillator. | |
| ___ | ___ | ___ | 3. If the defibrillator has "quick-look" capability, place the paddles on the patient's chest. Otherwise, connect the monitoring leads of the defibrillator to the patient and assess the cardiac rhythm. | |
| ___ | ___ | ___ | 4. Expose the patient's chest, and apply conductive pads at the paddle placement positions. For anterolateral placement, place one pad to the right of the upper sternum, just below the right clavicle, and the other over the fifth or sixth intercostal space at the left anterior axillary line. 'Hands-free' defibrillator pads can be used with the same placement positions, if available. For anteroposterior placement, place the anterior paddle directly over the heart at the precordium, to the left of the lower sternal border. Place the flat posterior paddle under the patient's body beneath the heart and immediately below the scapulae (but not on the vertebral column). | |
| ___ | ___ | ___ | 5. Set the energy level for 360 J (joules) for an adult patient when using a monophasic defibrillator. Use clinically appropriate energy levels for biphasic defibrillators, beginning with 150 to 200 J (AHA, 2005b). | |
| ___ | ___ | ___ | 6. Charge the paddles by pressing the charge buttons, which are located either on the machine or on the paddles themselves. | |
| ___ | ___ | ___ | 7. *Place the paddles over the conductive pads and press firmly against the patient's chest, using 25 pound (11 kg) of pressure. If using hands-off pads, do not touch the paddles.* | |
| ___ | ___ | ___ | 8. Reassess the cardiac rhythm. | |

# Performing Emergency Manual External Defibrillation (Asynchronous) *(Continued)*

| Excellent | Satisfactory | Needs Practice | | Comments |
|---|---|---|---|---|
| —— | —— | —— | 9. *If the patient remains in VF or pulseless VT, instruct all personnel to stand clear of the patient and the bed, including the operator.* | |
| —— | —— | —— | 10. Discharge the current by pressing both paddle charge buttons simultaneously. If using remote defibrillator pads, press the discharge or shock button on the machine. | |
| —— | —— | —— | 11. After the shock, immediately resume CPR, beginning with chest compressions. After five cycles (about 2 minutes), reassess the cardiac rhythm. Continue until advanced care providers take over, the patient starts to move, you are too exhausted to continue, or a physician discontinues CPR. Advanced care providers will indicate when a pulse check or other therapies are appropriate. | |
| —— | —— | —— | 12. If necessary, prepare to defibrillate a second time. Energy level on the monophasic defibrillator should remain at 360 J for subsequent shocks (AHA, 2005b). | |
| —— | —— | —— | 13. Announce that you are preparing to defibrillate and follow the procedure described above. | |
| —— | —— | —— | 14. If defibrillation restores a normal rhythm: | |
| —— | —— | —— |    a. Check for signs of circulation; check the central and peripheral pulses, and obtain a blood pressure reading, heart rate, and respiratory rate. | |
| —— | —— | —— |    b. If signs of circulation are present, check breathing. If breathing is inadequate, assist breathing. Start rescue breathing (one breath every 5 seconds). | |
| —— | —— | —— |    c. If breathing is adequate, place the patient in the recovery position. Continue to assess the patient. | |
| —— | —— | —— |    d. Assess the patient's level of consciousness, cardiac rhythm, breath sounds, and skin color and temperature. | |
| —— | —— | —— |    e. Obtain baseline ABG levels and a 12-lead ECG, if ordered. | |
| —— | —— | —— |    f. Provide supplemental oxygen, ventilation, and medications, as needed. | |
| —— | —— | —— | 15. Check the chest for electrical burns and treat them, as ordered, with corticosteroid- or lanolin-based creams. If using 'hands-free' pads, keep pads on in case of recurrent ventricular tachycardia or ventricular fibrillation. | |
| —— | —— | —— | 16. Remove gloves, if used. Perform hand hygiene. | |
| —— | —— | —— | 17. Prepare the defibrillator for immediate reuse. | |

*Skill Checklists for Taylor's Clinical Nursing Skills:*
*A Nursing Process Approach, 3rd edition*

Name _____  Date _____

Unit _____  Position _____

Instructor/Evaluator: _____  Position _____

## SKILL 16-8

# Using an External (Transcutaneous) Pacemaker

**Goal:** The equipment is applied correctly without adverse effect to the patient; and the patient regains signs of circulation, including the capture of at least the minimal set heart rate.

| Excellent | Satisfactory | Needs Practice | | Comments |
|---|---|---|---|---|
| ___ | ___ | ___ | 1. Bring necessary equipment to the bedside stand or overbed table. | |
| ___ | ___ | ___ | 2. Perform hand hygiene and put on PPE, if indicated. | |
| ___ | ___ | ___ | 3. Identify the patient. | |
| ___ | ___ | ___ | 4. If the patient is responsive, explain the procedure to the patient. Explain that it involves some discomfort and that you will administer medication to keep him or her comfortable and help him or her to relax. Administer analgesia and sedation, as ordered, if not an emergency situation. | |
| ___ | ___ | ___ | 5. Close curtains around bed and close the door to the room, if possible. | |
| ___ | ___ | ___ | 6. If necessary, clip the hair over the areas of electrode placement. ***Do not shave the area.*** | |
| ___ | ___ | ___ | 7. Attach cardiac monitoring electrodes to the patient in the lead I, II, and III positions. Do this even if the patient is already on telemetry monitoring. If you select the lead II position, adjust the LL (left leg) electrode placement to accommodate the anterior pacing electrode and the patient's anatomy. | |
| ___ | ___ | ___ | 8. Attach the patient monitoring electrodes to the ECG cable and into the ECG input connection on the front of the pacing generator. Set the selector switch to the 'Monitor on' position. | |
| ___ | ___ | ___ | 9. Note the ECG waveform on the monitor. Adjust the R-wave beeper volume to a suitable level and activate the alarm by pressing the 'Alarm on' button. Set the alarm for 10 to 20 beats lower and 20 to 30 beats higher than the intrinsic rate. | |
| ___ | ___ | ___ | 10. Press the 'Start/Stop' button for a printout of the waveform. | |
| ___ | ___ | ___ | 11. Apply the two pacing electrodes. Make sure the patient's skin is clean and dry to ensure good skin contact. Pull the protective strip from the posterior electrode (marked 'Back') and apply the electrode on the left side of the thoracic spinal column, just below the scapula. | |

| Excellent | Satisfactory | Needs Practice | SKILL 16-8<br>**Using an External (Transcutaneous)<br>Pacemaker** *(Continued)* | |
|---|---|---|---|---|
| | | | | **Comments** |
| —— | —— | —— | 12. Apply the anterior pacing electrode (marked 'Front'), which has two protective strips—one covering the gelled area and one covering the outer rim. Expose the gelled area and apply it to the skin in the anterior position, to the left side of the sternum in the usual $V_2$ to $V_5$ position, centered close to the point of maximal cardiac impulse. Move this electrode around to get the best waveform. Then expose the electrode's outer rim and firmly press it to the skin. | |
| —— | —— | —— | 13. Prepare to pace the heart. After making sure the energy output in milliamperes (mA) is on 0, connect the electrode cable to the monitor output cable. | |
| —— | —— | —— | 14. Check the waveform, looking for a tall QRS complex in lead II. | |
| —— | —— | —— | 15. Check the selector switch to 'Pacer on.' Select synchronous (demand) or asynchronous (fixed-rate or nondemand) mode, per medical orders. *Tell the patient he or she may feel a thumping or twitching sensation. Reassure the patient you will provide medication if the discomfort is intolerable.* | |
| —— | —— | —— | 16. Set the pacing rate dial to 10 to 20 beats higher than the intrinsic rhythm. Look for pacer artifact or spikes, which will appear as you increase the rate. If the patient does not have an intrinsic rhythm, set the rate at 80 beats/minute (Craig, 2005). | |
| —— | —— | —— | 17. Set the pacing current output (in milliamperes [mA]). For patients with bradycardia, start with the minimal setting and *slowly increase the amount of energy delivered to the heart by adjusting the 'Output' mA dial. Do this until electrical capture is achieved: you will see a pacer spike followed by a widened QRS complex and a tall broad T wave that resembles a premature ventricular contraction.* | |
| —— | —— | —— | 18. Increase output by 2 mA or 10%. *Do not go higher because of the increased risk of discomfort to the patient.* | |
| —— | —— | —— | 19. Assess for mechanical capture: Presence of a pulse and signs of improved cardiac output (increased blood pressure, improved level of consciousness, improved body temperature). | |
| —— | —— | —— | 20. For patients with asystole, start with the full output. If capture occurs, slowly decrease the output until capture is lost, then add 2 mA or 10% more. | |
| —— | —— | —— | 21. Secure the pacing leads and cable to the patient's body. | |

| Excellent | Satisfactory | Needs Practice | SKILL 16-8<br>**Using an External (Transcutaneous)<br>Pacemaker** *(Continued)* | |
|---|---|---|---|---|
| | | | | **Comments** |
| —— | —— | —— | 22. Monitor the patient's heart rate and rhythm to assess ventricular response to pacing. Assess the patient's vital signs, skin color, level of consciousness, and peripheral pulses. Take blood pressure in both arms. | |
| —— | —— | —— | 23. Assess the patient's pain and administer analgesia/sedation, as ordered, to ease the discomfort of chest wall muscle contractions (Craig, 2005). | |
| —— | —— | —— | 24. Perform a 12-lead ECG and additional ECG daily or with clinical changes. | |
| —— | —— | —— | 25. Continually monitor the ECG readings, noting capture, sensing, rate, intrinsic beats, and competition of paced and intrinsic rhythms. If the pacemaker is sensing correctly, the sense indicator on the pulse generator should flash with each beat. | |
| —— | —— | —— | 26. Remove PPE, if used. Perform hand hygiene. | |

*Skill Checklists for Taylor's Clinical Nursing Skills:*
*A Nursing Process Approach, 3rd edition*

Name _____  Date _____

Unit _____  Position _____

Instructor/Evaluator: _____  Position _____

## SKILL 17-1
## Logrolling a Patient

**Goal:** The patient's spine remains in proper alignment, thereby reducing the risk for injury.

| Excellent | Satisfactory | Needs Practice | | Comments |
|---|---|---|---|---|
| —— | —— | —— | 1. Review the medical record and nursing plan of care for activity orders and conditions that may influence the patient's ability to move or to be positioned. Assess for tubes, IV lines, incisions, or equipment that may alter the positioning procedure. Identify any movement limitations. | |
| —— | —— | —— | 2. Perform hand hygiene and put on PPE, if indicated. | |
| —— | —— | —— | 3. Identify the patient. | |
| —— | —— | —— | 4. Close curtains around bed and close the door to the room, if possible. Explain the purpose of the logrolling technique and what you are going to do, even if the patient is not conscious. Answer any questions. | |
| —— | —— | —— | 5. Place the bed at an appropriate and comfortable working height, usually elbow height of the caregiver (VISN 8 Patient Safety Center, 2009). | |
| —— | —— | —— | 6. Position at least one caregiver on one side of the bed and the two other caregivers on the opposite side of the bed. If a cervical collar is not in place, position one caregiver at the top of the bed, at the patient's head. Place the bed in flat position. Lower the side rails. Place a small pillow between the patient's knees. | |
| —— | —— | —— | 7. If a friction-reducing sheet is not in place under the patient, take the time to place one at this time, to facilitate future movement of the patient. | |
| —— | —— | —— | 8. If the patient can move the arms, ask the patient to cross the arms on the chest. Roll or fanfold the friction-reducing sheet close to the patient's sides and grasp it. In unison, gently slide the patient to the side of the bed opposite to that which the patient will be turned. | |
| —— | —— | —— | 9. Make sure the friction-reducing sheet under the patient is straight and wrinkle free. | |
| —— | —— | —— | 10. If necessary, reposition personnel to ensure two stand on the side of the bed to which the patient is turning. The third helper stands on the other side. *Grasp the friction-reducing sheet at hip and shoulder level.* | |

| Excellent | Satisfactory | Needs Practice | | Comments |
|---|---|---|---|---|

SKILL 17-1

# Logrolling a Patient *(Continued)*

|  |  |  |  |  |
|---|---|---|---|---|
| ___ | ___ | ___ | 11. Have everyone face the patient. On a predetermined signal, turn the patient by holding the friction-reducing sheet taut to support the body. The caregiver at the patient's head should firmly hold the patient's head on either side, directly above the ears. Turn the patient as a unit in one smooth motion toward the side of the bed with the two nurses. The patient's head, shoulders, spine, hips, and knees should turn simultaneously. | |
| ___ | ___ | ___ | 12. *Once the patient has been turned, use pillows to support the patient's neck, back, buttocks, and legs in straight alignment in a side-lying position.* Raise the side rails, as appropriate. | |
| ___ | ___ | ___ | 13. *Stand at the foot of the bed and assess the spinal column. It should be straight, without any twisting or bending.* Place the bed in the lowest position. Ensure that the call bell and telephone are within reach. Replace covers. Lower bed height. | |
| ___ | ___ | ___ | 14. Reassess the patient's neurologic status and comfort level. | |
| ___ | ___ | ___ | 15. Remove PPE, if used. Perform hand hygiene. | |

*Skill Checklists for Taylor's Clinical Nursing Skills:*
*A Nursing Process Approach, 3rd edition*

Name _____     Date _____

Unit _____     Position _____

Instructor/Evaluator: _____     Position _____

SKILL 17-2

# Applying a Two-Piece Cervical Collar

**Goal:** The patient's cervical spine is immobilized, preventing further injury to the spinal cord.

| Excellent | Satisfactory | Needs Practice | | Comments |
|---|---|---|---|---|
| —— | —— | —— | 1. Review the medical record and nursing plan of care to determine need for placement of a cervical collar. Identify any movement limitations. | |
| —— | —— | —— | 2. Gather the necessary supplies and bring to the bedside stand or overbed table. | |
| —— | —— | —— | 3. Perform hand hygiene and put on PPE, if indicated. | |
| —— | —— | —— | 4. Identify the patient. | |
| —— | —— | —— | 5. Close curtains around bed and close the door to the room, if possible. Explain what you are going to do and why you are going to do it to the patient. | |
| —— | —— | —— | 6. Assess patient for any changes in neurologic status. (See Chapter 2 for assessment details.) | |
| —— | —— | —— | 7. Place the bed at an appropriate and comfortable working height, usually elbow height of the caregiver (VISN 8 Patient Safety Center, 2009). Lower the side rails as necessary. | |
| —— | —— | —— | 8. Gently clean the face and neck with a mild soap and water. If the patient has experienced trauma, inspect the area for broken glass or other material that could cut the patient or the nurse. Pat the area dry. | |
| —— | —— | —— | 9. Have a second caregiver in position to hold the patient's head firmly on either side above the ears. Measure from the bottom of the chin to the top of the sternum, and measure around the neck. Match these height and circumference measurements to the manufacturer's recommended size chart. | |
| —— | —— | —— | 10. Slide the flattened back portion of the collar under the patient's head. *The center of the collar should line up with the center of the patient's neck. Do not allow the patient's head to move when passing the collar under the head.* | |
| —— | —— | —— | 11. Place the front of the collar centered over the chin, while ensuring that the chin area fits snugly in the recess. Be sure that the front half of the collar overlaps the back half. Secure Velcro straps on both sides. Check to see that at least one finger can be inserted between collar and patient's neck. | |

# Applying a Two-Piece Cervical Collar *(Continued)*

| Excellent | Satisfactory | Needs Practice | | Comments |
|---|---|---|---|---|
| —— | —— | —— | 12. Raise the side rails. Place the bed in lowest position. Make sure the call bell is in reach. | |
| —— | —— | —— | 13. Reassess the patient's neurologic status and comfort level. | |
| —— | —— | —— | 14. Remove PPE, if used. Perform hand hygiene. | |
| —— | —— | —— | 15. *Check the skin under the cervical collar at least every 4 hours for any signs of skin breakdown.* Remove the top half of the collar daily and cleanse the skin under the collar. *When the collar is removed, have a second person immobilize the cervical spine.* | |

*Skill Checklists for Taylor's Clinical Nursing Skills:*
*A Nursing Process Approach, 3rd edition*

Name _____  Date _____

Unit _____  Position _____

Instructor/Evaluator: _____  Position _____

| Excellent | Satisfactory | Needs Practice | SKILL 17-3<br>**Employing Seizure Precautions and Seizure Management** | Comments |
|---|---|---|---|---|
| | | | **Goal:** The patient remains free from injury related to seizure disorder. | |
| —— | —— | —— | 1. Review the medical record and nursing plan of care for conditions that would place the patient at risk for seizures. Review the medical orders and the nursing plan of care for orders for seizure precautions. | |
| | | | **Seizure Precautions** | |
| —— | —— | —— | 2. Gather the necessary supplies and bring to the bedside stand or overbed table. | |
| —— | —— | —— | 3. Perform hand hygiene and put on PPE, if indicated. | |
| —— | —— | —— | 4. Identify the patient. | |
| —— | —— | —— | 5. Close curtains around bed and close the door to the room, if possible. Explain what you are going to do and why you are going to do it to the patient. | |
| —— | —— | —— | 6. Place the bed in the lowest position with two to three side rails elevated. Apply padding to side rails. | |
| —— | —— | —— | 7. Attach oxygen apparatus to oxygen access in the wall at the head of the bed. Place nasal cannula or mask equipment in a location where it is easily reached if needed. | |
| —— | —— | —— | 8. Attach suction apparatus to vacuum access in the wall at the head of the bed. Place suction catheter, oral airway, and resuscitation bag in a location where they are easily reached if needed. | |
| —— | —— | —— | 9. Remove PPE, if used. Perform hand hygiene. | |
| | | | **Seizure Management** | |
| —— | —— | —— | 10. For patients with known seizures, be alert for the occurrence of an aura, if known. If the patient reports experiencing an aura, have the patient lie down. | |
| —— | —— | —— | 11. Once a seizure begins, close curtains around bed and close the door to the room, if possible. | |
| —— | —— | —— | 12. If the patient is seated, ease the patient to the floor. | |
| —— | —— | —— | 13. Remove patient's eyeglasses. Loosen any constricting clothing. Place something flat and soft, such as a folded blanket, under the head. Push aside furniture or other objects in area. | |

SKILL 17-3

# Employing Seizure Precautions and Seizure Management *(Continued)*

| Excellent | Satisfactory | Needs Practice | | Comments |
|---|---|---|---|---|
| —— | —— | —— | 14. If the patient is in bed, remove the pillow and raise side rails. | |
| —— | —— | —— | 15. Do not restrain patient. Guide movements, if necessary. Do not try to insert anything in the patient's mouth or open jaws. | |
| —— | —— | —— | 16. If possible, place patient on the side with the head flexed forward, head of bed elevated 30 degrees. Begin administration of oxygen, based on facility policy. Clear airway using suction, as appropriate. (Refer to Skill 14-9, Suctioning the nasopharyngeal and oropharyngeal airways, Chapter 14, Oxygenation.) | |
| —— | —— | —— | 17. Provide supervision throughout the seizure. | |
| —— | —— | —— | 18. Establish/maintain intravenous access, as necessary. Administer medications, as appropriate, based on medical order and facility policy. | |
| —— | —— | —— | 19. After the seizure, place the patient in a side-lying position. Clear airway using suction, as appropriate. | |
| —— | —— | —— | 20. Monitor vital signs, oxygen saturation, and capillary glucose as appropriate. | |
| —— | —— | —— | 21. Allow the patient to sleep after the seizure. On awakening, orient and reassure the patient. | |
| —— | —— | —— | 22. Remove PPE, if used. Perform hand hygiene. | |

*Skill Checklists for Taylor's Clinical Nursing Skills:*
*A Nursing Process Approach, 3rd edition*

Name _____    Date _____

Unit _____    Position _____

Instructor/Evaluator: _____    Position _____

SKILL 17-4

# Caring for a Patient in Halo Traction

**Goal:** The patient maintains cervical alignment.                    **Comments**

Columns: Excellent | Satisfactory | Needs Practice

| Excellent | Satisfactory | Needs Practice | |
|---|---|---|---|
| ―― | ―― | ―― | 1. Review the medical record and the nursing plan of care to determine the type of device being used and prescribed care. |
| ―― | ―― | ―― | 2. Gather the necessary supplies and bring to the bedside stand or overbed table. |
| ―― | ―― | ―― | 3. Perform hand hygiene and put on PPE, if indicated. |
| ―― | ―― | ―― | 4. Identify the patient. |
| ―― | ―― | ―― | 5. Close curtains around bed and close the door to the room, if possible. Explain what you are going to do and why you are going to do it to the patient. |
| ―― | ―― | ―― | 6. Assess the patient for possible need for nonpharmacologic, pain-reducing interventions or analgesic medication before beginning. Administer appropriate prescribed analgesic. Allow sufficient time for analgesic to achieve its effectiveness before beginning the procedure. |
| ―― | ―― | ―― | 7. Place a waste receptacle at a convenient location for use during the procedure. |
| ―― | ―― | ―― | 8. Adjust bed to comfortable working height, usually elbow height of the caregiver if the patient will remain in bed (VISN 8 Patient Safety Center, 2009). Alternatively, have the patient sit up, if appropriate. |
| ―― | ―― | ―― | 9. Assist the patient to a comfortable position that provides easy access to the head. Place a waterproof pad under the head if patient is lying down. |
| ―― | ―― | ―― | 10. Monitor vital signs and perform a neurologic assessment, including level of consciousness, motor function, and sensation, per facility policy. This is usually at least every 2 hours for 24 hours, or possibly every hour for 48 hours. |
| ―― | ―― | ―― | 11. Examine the halo vest unit every 8 hours for stability, secure connections, and positioning. Make sure the patient's head is centered in the halo without neck flexion or extension. Check each bolt for loosening. |
| ―― | ―― | ―― | 12. Check the fit of the vest. With the patient in a supine position, you should be able to insert one or two fingers under the jacket at the shoulder and chest. |

# Caring for a Patient in Halo Traction *(Continued)*

| Excellent | Satisfactory | Needs Practice | | Comments |
|:---:|:---:|:---:|---|---|
| —— | —— | —— | 13. Put on nonsterile gloves, if appropriate. Remove patient's shirt or gown. Wash the patient's chest and back daily. Loosen the bottom Velcro straps. | |
| —— | —— | —— | 14. Wring out a bath towel soaked in warm water. Pull the towel back and forth in a drying motion beneath the front. Do not use soap or lotion under the vest. | |
| —— | —— | —— | 15. Thoroughly dry the skin in the same manner with a dry towel. Inspect the skin for tender, reddened areas or pressure spots. Lightly dust the skin with a prescribed medicated powder or cornstarch. | |
| —— | —— | —— | 16. Turn the patient on his or her side, less than 45 degrees if lying supine, and repeat the process on the back. Close the Velcro straps. Assist the patient with putting on a new shirt, if desired. | |
| —— | —— | —— | 17. Perform a respiratory assessment. Check for respiratory impairment, such as absence of breath sounds, the presence of adventitious sounds, reduced inspiratory effort, or shortness of breath. | |
| —— | —— | —— | 18. Assess the pin sites for redness, tenting of the skin, prolonged or purulent drainage, swelling, and bowing, bending, or loosening of the pins. Monitor body temperature. | |
| —— | —— | —— | 19. Perform pin-site care. (See Skills 9-19 and 9-20.) | |
| —— | —— | —— | 20. Depending on physician order and facility policy, apply the antimicrobial ointment to pin sites and apply a dressing. | |
| —— | —— | —— | 21. Remove gloves and dispose of them appropriately. Raise rails, as appropriate, and place the bed in the lowest position. Assist patient to a comfortable position. | |
| —— | —— | —— | 22. Remove additional PPE, if used. Perform hand hygiene. | |

*Skill Checklists for Taylor's Clinical Nursing Skills:*
*A Nursing Process Approach, 3rd edition*

Name _____     Date _____

Unit _____     Position _____

Instructor/Evaluator: _____     Position _____

SKILL 17-5

# Caring for a Patient with an External Ventriculostomy (Intraventricular Catheter–Closed Fluid-Filled System)

**Goal:** The patient maintains intracranial pressure at less than 10 to 15 mm Hg, and cerebral perfusion pressure at 60 to 90 mm Hg.

| Excellent | Satisfactory | Needs Practice | | Comments |
|---|---|---|---|---|
| —— | —— | —— | 1. Review the medical orders for specific information about ventriculostomy parameters. | |
| —— | —— | —— | 2. Gather the necessary supplies and bring to the bedside stand or overbed table. | |
| —— | —— | —— | 3. Perform hand hygiene and put on PPE, if indicated. | |
| —— | —— | —— | 4. Identify the patient. | |
| —— | —— | —— | 5. Close curtains around bed and close the door to the room, if possible. Explain what you are going to do and why you are going to do it to the patient. | |
| —— | —— | —— | 6. Assess patient for any changes in neurologic status. (See Chapter 2, Health Assessment, for details of assessment.) | |
| —— | —— | —— | 7. *Assess the height of the ventriculostomy system to ensure that the stopcock is at the level of midpoint between the outer canthus of the patient's eye and the tragus of the patient's ear or external auditory canal (Littlejohns, 2005), using carpenter level, bubble-line level, or laser level, according to facility policy.* Adjust the height of the system if needed. *Move the drip chamber to the ordered height.* Assess the amount of CSF in the drip chamber if the ventriculostomy is draining. | |
| —— | —— | —— | 8. *Zero the transducer.* Turn stopcock off to the patient. Remove the cap from the transducer, being careful not to touch the end of the cap. Press and hold the calibration button on the monitor until the monitor beeps. Return the cap to the transducer. *Turn the stopcock off to the drip chamber to obtain an ICP reading. After obtaining a reading, turn the stopcock off to the transducer.* | |
| —— | —— | —— | 9. *Adjust the ventriculostomy height to prevent too much drainage, too little drainage, or inaccurate ICP readings.* | |

Excellent

Satisfactory

Needs Practice

## SKILL 17-5

# Caring for a Patient with an External Ventriculostomy (Intraventricular Catheter–Closed Fluid-Filled System) *(Continued)*

|  |  |  | | **Comments** |
| --- | --- | --- | --- | --- |
| Excellent | Satisfactory | Needs Practice | | |
| ___ | ___ | ___ | 10. Care for the insertion site according to the institution's policy. Assess the site for any signs of infection, such as purulent drainage, redness, or warmth. Ensure the catheter is secured at site per facility policy. | |
| ___ | ___ | ___ | 11. Calculate the CPP, if necessary. Calculate the difference between the systemic MAP and the ICP. | |
| ___ | ___ | ___ | 12. Remove PPE, if used. Perform hand hygiene. | |
| ___ | ___ | ___ | 13. Assess ICP, MAP, and CPP at least hourly. | |

Skill Checklists for Taylor's Clinical Nursing Skills:
A Nursing Process Approach, 3rd edition

Name _____  Date _____

Unit _____  Position _____

Instructor/Evaluator: _____  Position _____

## SKILL 17-6

# Caring for a Patient With a Fiber Optic Intracranial Catheter

**Goal:** The patient maintains ICP less than 10 to 15 mm Hg, and CPP 60 to 90 mm Hg.

| Excellent | Satisfactory | Needs Practice | | Comments |
|---|---|---|---|---|
| —— | —— | —— | 1. Review the medical orders for specific information about monitoring parameters. | |
| —— | —— | —— | 2. Gather the necessary supplies and bring to the bedside stand or overbed table. | |
| —— | —— | —— | 3. Perform hand hygiene and put on PPE, if indicated. | |
| —— | —— | —— | 4. Identify the patient. | |
| —— | —— | —— | 5. Close curtains around bed and close the door to the room, if possible. Explain what you are going to do and why you are going to do it to the patient. | |
| —— | —— | —— | 6. Assess patient for any changes in neurologic status. (See Chapter 2, Health Assessment, for details of assessment.) | |
| —— | —— | —— | 7. Assess ICP, MAP, and CPP at least hourly. Note ICP waveforms as shown on the monitor. *Notify the primary care provider if A or B waves are present.* | |
| —— | —— | —— | 8. Care for the insertion site according to the institution's policy. Assess the site for any signs of infection, such as drainage, redness, or warmth. Ensure the catheter is secured at site per facility policy. | |
| —— | —— | —— | 9. Calculate the CPP, if necessary. Calculate the difference between the systemic MAP and the ICP. | |
| —— | —— | —— | 10. Remove PPE, if used. Perform hand hygiene. | |

*Skill Checklists for Taylor's Clinical Nursing Skills:*
*A Nursing Process Approach, 3rd edition*

Name _____  Date _____

Unit _____  Position _____

Instructor/Evaluator: _____  Position _____

| Excellent | Satisfactory | Needs Practice | SKILL 18-1 **Testing Stool for Occult Blood** | Comments |
|---|---|---|---|---|
| | | | **Goal:** An uncontaminated stool sample is obtained, following collection guidelines, and then transported to the laboratory within the recommended time frame, without adverse effect. | |
| ___ | ___ | ___ | 1. Bring necessary equipment to the bedside stand or overbed table. | |
| ___ | ___ | ___ | 2. Perform hand hygiene and put on PPE, if indicated. | |
| ___ | ___ | ___ | 3. Identify the patient. Discuss with the patient the need for a stool sample. Explain to the patient the process by which the stool will be collected, either from a bedpan, commode, or plastic receptacle in the toilet. | |
| ___ | ___ | ___ | 4. If sending the specimen to the laboratory, check specimen label with patient identification bracelet. Label should include patient's name and identification number, time specimen was collected, route of collection, identification of the person obtaining the sample, and any other information required by agency policy. | |
| ___ | ___ | ___ | 5. Close curtains around bed or close the door to the room, if possible. | |
| ___ | ___ | ___ | 6. Place the plastic collection receptacle in the toilet, if applicable. Assist the patient to the bathroom or onto the bedside commode, or assist the patient onto the bedpan. Instruct the patient not to urinate or discard toilet paper with the stool. | |
| ___ | ___ | ___ | 7. After the patient defecates, assist the patient out of the bathroom, off the commode, or remove the bedpan. Perform hand hygiene and put on disposable gloves. | |
| ___ | ___ | ___ | 8. *With wooden applicator, apply a small amount of stool from the center of the bowel movement onto one window of the Hemoccult testing card. With opposite end of wooden applicator, obtain another sample of stool from another area and apply a small amount of stool onto second window of Hemoccult card.* | |
| ___ | ___ | ___ | 9. Close flap over stool samples. | |
| ___ | ___ | ___ | 10. If sending to the laboratory, label the specimen card per facility policy. Place in a sealable plastic biohazard bag and send to the laboratory immediately. | |

SKILL 18-1

## Testing Stool for Occult Blood *(Continued)*

| Excellent | Satisfactory | Needs Practice | | Comments |
|---|---|---|---|---|
| —— | —— | —— | 11. If testing at bedside, open flap on opposite side of card and *place two drops of developer over each window and wait the time stated in the manufacturer's instructions.* | |
| —— | —— | —— | 12. Observe card for any blue areas. | |
| —— | —— | —— | 13. Discard Hemoccult testing slide appropriately, according to facility policy. Remove gloves and any other PPE, if used. Perform hand hygiene. | |

*Skill Checklists for Taylor's Clinical Nursing Skills:*
*A Nursing Process Approach, 3rd edition*

Name _____    Date _____

Unit _____    Position _____

Instructor/Evaluator: _____    Position _____

| Excellent | Satisfactory | Needs Practice | SKILL 18-2 **Collecting a Stool Specimen for Culture** | Comments |
|---|---|---|---|---|
| | | | **Goal:** An uncontaminated specimen is obtained and sent to the laboratory promptly. | |
| —— | —— | —— | 1. Gather necessary equipment and bring to the bedside. | |
| —— | —— | —— | 2. Perform hand hygiene and put on PPE, if indicated. | |
| —— | —— | —— | 3. Identify the patient. Discuss with the patient the need for a stool sample. Explain to the patient the process by which the stool will be collected, either from a bedpan, commode, or plastic receptacle in the toilet to catch stool without urine. Instruct the patient to void first and not to discard toilet paper with stool. Tell the patient to call you as soon as a bowel movement is completed. | |
| —— | —— | —— | 4. Check specimen label with the patient's identification bracelet. Label should include patient's name and identification number, time specimen was collected, route of collection, identification of the person obtaining the sample, and any other information required by agency policy. | |
| —— | —— | —— | 5. After the patient has passed a stool, put on gloves. Use the tongue blades to obtain a sample, free of blood or urine, and place it in the designated clean container. | |
| —— | —— | —— | 6. Collect as much of the stool as possible to send to the laboratory. | |
| —— | —— | —— | 7. Place lid on container. Dispose of used equipment per facility policy. Remove gloves and perform hand hygiene. | |
| —— | —— | —— | 8. Place label on the container per facility policy. Place container in plastic, sealable biohazard bag. | |
| —— | —— | —— | 9. Remove other PPE, if used. Perform hand hygiene. | |
| —— | —— | —— | 10. Transport the specimen to the laboratory while stool is still warm. If immediate transport is impossible, check with laboratory personnel or policy manual whether refrigeration is contraindicated. | |

*Skill Checklists for Taylor's Clinical Nursing Skills:*
*A Nursing Process Approach, 3rd edition*

Name _____    Date _____

Unit _____    Position _____

Instructor/Evaluator: _____    Position _____

| Excellent | Satisfactory | Needs Practice | SKILL 18-3<br><br>**Obtaining a Capillary Blood Sample for Glucose Testing**<br><br>**Goal:** The blood glucose level is measured accurately without adverse effect. | Comments |
|---|---|---|---|---|
| ___ | ___ | ___ | 1. Check the patient's medical record or nursing plan of care for monitoring schedule. You may decide that additional testing is indicated based on nursing judgment and the patient's condition. | |
| ___ | ___ | ___ | 2. Gather equipment. | |
| ___ | ___ | ___ | 3. Perform hand hygiene and put on PPE, if indicated. | |
| ___ | ___ | ___ | 4. Identify the patient. Explain the procedure to the patient and instruct the patient about the need for monitoring blood glucose. | |
| ___ | ___ | ___ | 5. Close curtains around bed and close the door to the room, if possible. | |
| ___ | ___ | ___ | 6. Turn on the monitor. | |
| ___ | ___ | ___ | 7. Enter the patient's identification number, if required, according to facility policy. | |
| ___ | ___ | ___ | 8. Put on nonsterile gloves. | |
| ___ | ___ | ___ | 9. Prepare lancet using aseptic technique. | |
| ___ | ___ | ___ | 10. Remove test strip from the vial. *Recap container immediately.* Test strips also come individually wrapped. *Check that the code number for the strip matches code number on the monitor screen.* | |
| ___ | ___ | ___ | 11. Insert the strip into the meter according to directions for that specific device. | |
| ___ | ___ | ___ | 12. For adult, massage side of finger toward puncture site. | |
| ___ | ___ | ___ | 13. *Have the patient wash hands with soap and warm water and dry thoroughly. Alternately, cleanse the skin with an alcohol swab. Allow skin to dry completely.* | |
| ___ | ___ | ___ | 14. Hold lancet perpendicular to skin and pierce site with lancet. | |
| ___ | ___ | ___ | 15. Wipe away first drop of blood with gauze square or cotton ball if recommended by manufacturer of monitor. | |

# Obtaining a Capillary Blood Sample for Glucose Testing *(Continued)*

| Excellent | Satisfactory | Needs Practice | | Comments |
|---|---|---|---|---|
| —— | —— | —— | 16. Encourage bleeding by lowering the hand, making use of gravity. Lightly stroke the finger, if necessary, until sufficient amount of blood has formed to cover the sample area on the strip, based on monitor requirements (check instructions for monitor). Take care not to squeeze the finger, not to squeeze at puncture site, or not to touch puncture site or blood. | |
| —— | —— | —— | 17. Gently touch a drop of blood to pad to the test strip without smearing it. | |
| —— | —— | —— | 18. Press time button if directed by manufacturer. | |
| —— | —— | —— | 19. Apply pressure to puncture site with a cotton ball or dry gauze. *Do not use alcohol wipe.* | |
| —— | —— | —— | 20. Read blood glucose results and document appropriately at bedside. Inform patient of test result. | |
| —— | —— | —— | 21. Turn off meter, remove test strip, and dispose of supplies appropriately. Place lancet in sharps container. | |
| —— | —— | —— | 22. Remove gloves and any other PPE, if used. Perform hand hygiene. | |

*Skill Checklists for Taylor's Clinical Nursing Skills:*
*A Nursing Process Approach, 3rd edition*

Name _____   Date _____

Unit _____   Position _____

Instructor/Evaluator: _____   Position _____

SKILL 18-4

# Obtaining a Nasal Swab

**Goal:** An uncontaminated specimen is obtained without injury to the patient and sent to the laboratory promptly.

| Excellent | Satisfactory | Needs Practice | | Comments |
|---|---|---|---|---|
| —— | —— | —— | 1. Bring necessary equipment to the bedside stand or overbed table. Check the expiration date on the swab package. | |
| —— | —— | —— | 2. Perform hand hygiene and put on PPE, if indicated. | |
| —— | —— | —— | 3. Identify the patient. Discuss with the patient the need for a nasal swab. Explain to the patient the process by which the specimen will be collected. | |
| —— | —— | —— | 4. Check specimen label with patient identification bracelet. Label should include patient's name and identification number, time specimen was collected, route of collection, identification of the person obtaining the sample, and any other information required by agency policy. | |
| —— | —— | —— | 5. Close curtains around bed or close the door to the room, if possible. | |
| —— | —— | —— | 6. Put on nonsterile gloves. | |
| —— | —— | —— | 7. Ask the patient to tip his or her head back. Assist as necessary. | |
| —— | —— | —— | 8. Peel open the swab packaging to expose the swab and collection tube. Remove the white plug from the collection tube and discard. Remove the swab from packaging by grasping the exposed end. Take care not to contaminate the swab by touching it to any other surface. Moisten with sterile water, depending on facility policy. | |
| —— | —— | —— | 9. Insert swab 2 cm into one **naris** and rotate against the anterior nasal mucosa for 3 seconds or five rotations, depending on facility policy. | |
| —— | —— | —— | 10. Remove the swab and repeat in the second naris, using the same swab. | |
| —— | —— | —— | 11. Insert the swab fully into the collection tube, taking care not to touch any other surface. The handle end of the swab should fit snugly into the collection tube. | |
| —— | —— | —— | 12. Dispose of used equipment per facility policy. Remove gloves. Perform hand hygiene. | |

SKILL 18-4

# Obtaining a Nasal Swab *(Continued)*

| Excellent | Satisfactory | Needs Practice | | Comments |
|---|---|---|---|---|
| —— | —— | —— | 13. Place label on the collection tube per facility policy. Place container in plastic, sealable biohazard bag. | |
| —— | —— | —— | 14. Remove other PPE, if used. Perform hand hygiene. | |
| —— | —— | —— | 15. Transport specimen to the laboratory immediately. If immediate transport is not possible, check with laboratory personnel or policy manual whether refrigeration is contraindicated. | |

*Skill Checklists for Taylor's Clinical Nursing Skills:*
*A Nursing Process Approach, 3rd edition*

Name _____   Date _____

Unit _____   Position _____

Instructor/Evaluator: _____   Position _____

| Excellent | Satisfactory | Needs Practice | SKILL 18-5<br>**Obtaining a Nasopharyngeal Swab**<br><br>**Goal:** An uncontaminated specimen is obtained without injury to the patient and sent to the laboratory promptly. | Comments |
|---|---|---|---|---|
| ___ | ___ | ___ | 1. Bring necessary equipment to the bedside stand or overbed table. Check the expiration date on the swab package. | |
| ___ | ___ | ___ | 2. Perform hand hygiene and put on PPE, if indicated. | |
| ___ | ___ | ___ | 3. Identify the patient. Discuss with patient the need for a nasal swab. Explain to patient the process by which the specimen will be collected. | |
| ___ | ___ | ___ | 4. Check the specimen label with the patient's identification bracelet. Label should include patient's name and identification number, time specimen was collected, route of collection, identification of person obtaining the sample, and any other information required by agency policy. | |
| ___ | ___ | ___ | 5. Close curtains around bed or close the door to the room, if possible. | |
| ___ | ___ | ___ | 6. Put on nonsterile gloves. | |
| ___ | ___ | ___ | 7. Ask the patient to cough and then to tip his or her head back. Assist, as necessary. | |
| ___ | ___ | ___ | 8. Peel open the swab packaging to expose the swab and collection tube. Remove the cap from the collection tube and discard. Remove the swab from packaging by grasping the exposed end. Take care not to contaminate the swab by touching it to any other surface. | |
| ___ | ___ | ___ | 9. Ask the patient to open the mouth. Inspect the back of the patient's throat using the tongue depressor. | |
| ___ | ___ | ___ | 10. Continue to observe the nasopharynx and insert the swab approximately 6 inches (adult) through one naris to the nasopharynx. Rotate the swab. Leave the swab in the nasopharynx for 15 to 30 seconds and remove. Take care not to touch the swab to the patient's tongue or sides of the nostrils. | |
| ___ | ___ | ___ | 11. Insert the swab into the collection tube, taking care not to touch any other surface. | |
| ___ | ___ | ___ | 12. Dispose of used equipment per facility policy. Remove gloves. Perform hand hygiene. | |

SKILL 18-5

# Obtaining a Nasopharyngeal Swab (Continued)

| Excellent | Satisfactory | Needs Practice | | Comments |
|---|---|---|---|---|
| ___ | ___ | ___ | 13. Place label on the collection tube per facility policy. Place container in plastic, sealable biohazard bag. | |
| ___ | ___ | ___ | 14. Remove other PPE, if used. Perform hand hygiene. | |
| ___ | ___ | ___ | 15. Transport the specimen to the laboratory immediately. If immediate transport is not possible, check with laboratory personnel or policy manual whether refrigeration is contraindicated. | |

*Skill Checklists for Taylor's Clinical Nursing Skills:*
*A Nursing Process Approach, 3rd edition*

Name _____    Date _____

Unit _____    Position _____

Instructor/Evaluator: _____    Position _____

SKILL 18-6

# Collecting a Sputum Specimen for Culture

**Goal:** The patient produces an adequate sample from the lungs.

| Excellent | Satisfactory | Needs Practice | | Comments |
|---|---|---|---|---|
| —— | —— | —— | 1. Bring necessary equipment to the bedside stand or overbed table. | |
| —— | —— | —— | 2. Perform hand hygiene and put on PPE, if indicated. | |
| —— | —— | —— | 3. Identify the patient. Explain the procedure to the patient. If the patient might have pain with coughing, administer pain medication, if ordered. If the patient can perform the task without assistance after instruction, leave the container at bedside with instructions to call the nurse as soon as specimen is produced. | |
| —— | —— | —— | 4. Check specimen label with the patient's identification bracelet. Label should include patient's name and identification number, time specimen was collected, route of collection, identification of the person obtaining the sample, and any other information required by agency policy. | |
| —— | —— | —— | 5. Close curtains around bed and close the door to the room, if possible. | |
| —— | —— | —— | 6. Put on disposable gloves and goggles. | |
| —— | —— | —— | 7. Adjust the bed to a comfortable working height, usually elbow height of the caregiver (VISN 8 Patient Safety Center, 2009). Lower side rail closest to you. Place patient in semi-Fowler's position. *Have patient clear nose and throat and rinse mouth with water before beginning procedure.* | |
| —— | —— | —— | 8. *Instruct the patient to inhale deeply two or three times and cough with exhalation.* If the patient has had abdominal surgery, assist the patient to splint abdomen. | |
| —— | —— | —— | 9. If the patient produces sputum, open the lid to the container and have the patient **expectorate** the specimen into container. | |
| —— | —— | —— | 10. If patient believes he or she can produce more of the specimen, have the patient repeat the procedure. | |
| —— | —— | —— | 11. Close lid to container. Offer oral hygiene to the patient. | |
| —— | —— | —— | 12. Remove equipment and return the patient to a position of comfort. Raise side rail and lower bed. | |
| —— | —— | —— | 13. Remove goggles and gloves. Perform hand hygiene. | |

# Collecting a Sputum Specimen for Culture *(Continued)*

| Excellent | Satisfactory | Needs Practice | | Comments |
|---|---|---|---|---|
| —— | —— | —— | 14. Place label on the container per facility policy. Place container in plastic, sealable biohazard bag. | |
| —— | —— | —— | 15. Remove other PPE, if used. Perform hand hygiene. | |
| —— | —— | —— | 16. Transport the specimen to the laboratory immediately. If immediate transport is not possible, check with laboratory personnel or policy manual whether refrigeration is contraindicated. | |

*Skill Checklists for Taylor's Clinical Nursing Skills:*
*A Nursing Process Approach, 3rd edition*

Name _____     Date _____

Unit _____     Position _____

Instructor/Evaluator: _____     Position _____

| Excellent | Satisfactory | Needs Practice | SKILL 18-7<br><br>**Collecting a Urine Specimen (Clean Catch, Midstream) for Urinalysis and Culture**<br><br>**Goal:** An adequate amount of urine is obtained from the patient without contamination. | Comments |
|---|---|---|---|---|
| ___ | ___ | ___ | 1. Bring necessary equipment to the bedside stand or overbed table. | |
| ___ | ___ | ___ | 2. Perform hand hygiene and put on PPE, if indicated. | |
| ___ | ___ | ___ | 3. Identify the patient. Explain the procedure to the patient. If the patient can perform the task without assistance after instruction, leave the container at bedside with instructions to call the nurse as soon as a specimen is produced. | |
| ___ | ___ | ___ | 4. Have the patient perform hand hygiene, if performing self-collection. | |
| ___ | ___ | ___ | 5. Check the specimen label with the patient's identification bracelet. Label should include patient's name and identification number, time specimen was collected, route of collection, identification of the person obtaining sample, and any other information required by agency policy. | |
| ___ | ___ | ___ | 6. Close curtains around bed and close the door to the room, if possible. | |
| ___ | ___ | ___ | 7. Put on unsterile gloves. Assist the patient to the bathroom, or onto the bedside commode or bedpan. Instruct the patient not to defecate or discard toilet paper into the urine. | |
| ___ | ___ | ___ | 8. Instruct the female patient to separate the labia for cleaning of the area and during collection of urine. Female patients should use the towelettes or wet washcloth to clean each side of the urinary meatus, then the center over the meatus, from front to back, using a new wipe or a clean area of the washcloth for each stroke. Male patients should use a towelette to clean the tip of the penis, wiping in a circular motion away from the urethra. Instruct the uncircumcised male patient to retract the foreskin before cleaning and during collection. | |
| ___ | ___ | ___ | 9. *Have patient void a small amount of urine into the toilet, bedpan, or commode. The patient should then stop urinating briefly, then void into collection container. Collect specimen (10 to 20 mL is sufficient), and then finish voiding. Do not touch the inside of the container or the lid.* | |

SKILL 18-7

# Collecting a Urine Specimen (Clean Catch, Midstream) for Urinalysis and Culture *(Continued)*

| Excellent | Satisfactory | Needs Practice | | Comments |
|---|---|---|---|---|
| —— | —— | —— | 10. Place lid on container. If necessary, transfer the specimen to appropriate containers for ordered test, according to facility policy. | |
| —— | —— | —— | 11. Assist the patient from the bathroom, off the commode, or off the bedpan. Provide perineal care, if necessary. | |
| —— | —— | —— | 12. Remove gloves and perform hand hygiene. | |
| —— | —— | —— | 13. Place label on the container per facility policy. Place container in plastic, sealable biohazard bag. | |
| —— | —— | —— | 14. Remove other PPE, if used. Perform hand hygiene. | |
| —— | —— | —— | 15. Transport the specimen to the laboratory as soon as possible. If unable to take the specimen to the laboratory immediately, refrigerate it. | |

*Skill Checklists for Taylor's Clinical Nursing Skills:*
*A Nursing Process Approach, 3rd edition*

Name _____  Date _____

Unit _____  Position _____

Instructor/Evaluator: _____  Position _____

## SKILL 18-8

# Obtaining a Urine Specimen From an Indwelling Urinary Catheter

**Goal:** An adequate amount of urine is obtained from the patient without contamination or adverse effect; the patient experiences minimal anxiety during the collection process; and the patient demonstrates an understanding of the reason for the specimen.

| Excellent | Satisfactory | Needs Practice | | Comments |
|---|---|---|---|---|
| ____ | ____ | ____ | 1. Bring necessary equipment to the bedside stand or overbed table. | |
| ____ | ____ | ____ | 2. Perform hand hygiene and put on PPE, if indicated. | |
| ____ | ____ | ____ | 3. Identify the patient. Explain the procedure to the patient. | |
| ____ | ____ | ____ | 4. Check the specimen label with the patient's identification bracelet. Label should include patient's name and identification number, time specimen was collected, route of collection, identification of person obtaining the sample, and any other information required by agency policy. | |
| ____ | ____ | ____ | 5. Close curtains around bed and close the door to the room, if possible. | |
| ____ | ____ | ____ | 6. Put on unsterile gloves. | |
| ____ | ____ | ____ | 7. Clamp the catheter drainage tubing or bend it back on itself distal to the port. If an insufficient amount of urine is present in the tubing, allow the tubing to remain clamped up to 30 minutes, to collect a sufficient amount of urine, unless contraindicated (Fischbach & Dunning, 2006). Remove lid from specimen container, keeping the inside of the container and lid free from contamination. | |
| ____ | ____ | ____ | 8. *Cleanse aspiration port with alcohol wipe and allow port to air dry.* | |
| ____ | ____ | ____ | 9. Insert the needle or blunt-tipped cannula into the port, or attach the syringe to the needleless port. Slowly aspirate enough urine for specimen (usually 10 mL is adequate; check facility requirements). Remove the needle, blunt-tipped cannula, or syringe from the port. Engage the needle guard. *Unclamp the drainage tubing.* | |
| ____ | ____ | ____ | 10. *If a needle or blunt-tipped cannula was used on the syringe, remove from the syringe before emptying the urine from the syringe into the specimen cup. Place the needle into sharps collection container. Slowly inject urine into specimen container. Replace lid on container. Dispose of syringe appropriately.* | |

SKILL 18-8

# Obtaining a Urine Specimen From an Indwelling Urinary Catheter *(Continued)*

| Excellent | Satisfactory | Needs Practice | | Comments |
|---|---|---|---|---|
| —— | —— | —— | 11. Remove gloves and perform hand hygiene. | |
| —— | —— | —— | 12. Place label on the container per facility policy. Place container in plastic sealable biohazard bag. | |
| —— | —— | —— | 13. Remove other PPE, if used. Perform hand hygiene. | |
| —— | —— | —— | 14. Transport the specimen to the laboratory as soon as possible. If unable to take the specimen to laboratory immediately, refrigerate it. | |

*Skill Checklists for Taylor's Clinical Nursing Skills:*
*A Nursing Process Approach, 3rd edition*

Name _____   Date _____

Unit _____   Position _____

Instructor/Evaluator: _____   Position _____

SKILL 18-9

# Using Venipuncture to Collect a Venous Blood Sample for Routine Testing

**Goal:** An uncontaminated specimen is obtained without causing anxiety, injury, or infection to the patient

| Excellent | Satisfactory | Needs Practice | | Comments |
|---|---|---|---|---|
| ___ | ___ | ___ | 1. Gather the necessary supplies. Check product expiration dates. Identify ordered tests and select the appropriate blood-collection tubes. | |
| ___ | ___ | ___ | 2. Bring necessary equipment to the bedside stand or overbed table. | |
| ___ | ___ | ___ | 3. Perform hand hygiene and put on PPE, if indicated. | |
| ___ | ___ | ___ | 4. Identify the patient. Explain the procedure. Allow the patient time to ask questions and verbalize concerns about the venipuncture procedure. | |
| ___ | ___ | ___ | 5. Close curtains around bed and close the door to the room, if possible. | |
| ___ | ___ | ___ | 6. Check the specimen label with the patient's identification bracelet. Label should include the patient's name and identification number, time specimen was collected, route of collection, identification of the person obtaining the sample, and any other information required by agency policy. | |
| ___ | ___ | ___ | 7. Provide for good light. Artificial light is recommended. Place a trash receptacle within easy reach. | |
| ___ | ___ | ___ | 8. Assist the patient to a comfortable position, either sitting or lying. If the patient is lying in bed, raise the bed to a comfortable working height, usually elbow height of the caregiver (VISN 8 Patient Safety Center, 2009). | |
| ___ | ___ | ___ | 9. Determine the patient's preferred site for the procedure based on his or her previous experience. Expose the arm, supporting it in an extended position on a firm surface, such as a tabletop. Position self on the same side of the patient as the site selected. Apply a tourniquet to the upper arm on the chosen side approximately 3 to 4 inches above the potential puncture site. Apply sufficient pressure to impede venous circulation but not arterial blood flow. | |
| ___ | ___ | ___ | 10. Put on gloves. Assess the veins using inspection and palpation to determine the best puncture site. Refer to the Assessment information above. | |
| ___ | ___ | ___ | 11. ***Release the tourniquet. Check that the vein has decompressed (Lavery & Ingram, 2005).*** | |

# Using Venipuncture to Collect a Venous Blood Sample for Routine Testing *(Continued)*

| Excellent | Satisfactory | Needs Practice | | Comments |
|---|---|---|---|---|
| —— | —— | —— | 12. Attach the needle to the Vacutainer device. Place first blood-collection tube into the Vacutainer, but not engaged in the puncture device in the Vacutainer. | |
| —— | —— | —— | 13. Clean the patient's skin at the selected puncture site with the antimicrobial swab. If using chlorhexidine, use a back-and-forth motion, applying friction for 30 seconds to the site, or use the procedure recommended by the manufacturer. If using alcohol, wipe in a circular motion spiraling outward. Allow the skin to dry before performing the venipuncture. Alternately, the skin can be dried with a sterile gauze (Fischbach & Dunning, 2009). Check facility policy. | |
| —— | —— | —— | 14. Reapply the tourniquet approximately 3 to 4 inches above the identified puncture site. *Apply sufficient pressure to impede venous circulation but not arterial blood flow.* | |
| —— | —— | —— | 15. Hold the patient's arm in a downward position with your nondominant hand. Align the needle and Vacutainer device with the chosen vein, holding the Vacutainer and needle in your dominant hand. Use the thumb or first finger of your nondominant hand to apply pressure and traction to the skin just below the identified puncture site. | |
| —— | —— | —— | 16. *Inform the patient that he or she is going to feel a pinch.* With the bevel of the needle up, insert the needle into the vein at a 15-degree angle to the skin (Fischbach & Dunning, 2009). | |
| —— | —— | —— | 17. Grasp the Vacutainer securely to stabilize it in the vein with your nondominant hand, and push the first collection tube into the puncture device in the Vacutainer, until the rubber stopper on the collection tube is punctured. You will feel the tube push into place on the puncture device. Blood will flow into the tube automatically. | |
| —— | —— | —— | 18. *Remove the tourniquet as soon as blood flows adequately into the tube.* | |
| —— | —— | —— | 19. Continue to hold Vacutainer in place in the vein and continue to fill the required tubes, removing one and inserting another. Gently rotate each tube as you remove it. | |
| —— | —— | —— | 20. After you have drawn all required blood samples, remove the last collection tube from the Vacutainer. *Place a gauze pad over the puncture site and slowly and gently remove the needle from the vein. Engage needle guard. Do not apply pressure to site until the needle has been fully removed.* | |
| —— | —— | —— | 21. Apply gentle pressure to the puncture site for 2 to 3 minutes or until bleeding stops. | |

## SKILL 18-9
# Using Venipuncture to Collect a Venous Blood Sample for Routine Testing *(Continued)*

| Excellent | Satisfactory | Needs Practice | | Comments |
|---|---|---|---|---|
| —— | —— | —— | 22. After bleeding stops, apply an adhesive bandage. | |
| —— | —— | —— | 23. Remove equipment and return the patient to a position of comfort. Raise side rail and lower bed. | |
| —— | —— | —— | 24. Discard Vacutainer and needle in sharps container. | |
| —— | —— | —— | 25. Remove gloves and perform hand hygiene. | |
| —— | —— | —— | 26. Place label on the container per facility policy. Place container in plastic, sealable biohazard bag. | |
| —— | —— | —— | 27. Check the venipuncture site to see if a hematoma has developed. | |
| —— | —— | —— | 28. Remove other PPE, if used. Perform hand hygiene. | |
| —— | —— | —— | 29. Transport the specimen to the laboratory immediately. If immediate transport is not possible, check with laboratory personnel or policy manual whether refrigeration is contraindicated. | |

*Skill Checklists for Taylor's Clinical Nursing Skills:*
*A Nursing Process Approach, 3rd edition*

Name _____   Date _____

Unit _____   Position _____

Instructor/Evaluator: _____   Position _____

| Excellent | Satisfactory | Needs Practice | SKILL 18-10 **Obtaining a Venous Blood Specimen for Culture and Sensitivity** **Goal:** An uncontaminated specimen is obtained without causing anxiety, injury, or infection to the patient. | Comments |
|---|---|---|---|---|
| ___ | ___ | ___ | 1. Gather the necessary supplies. Check product expiration dates. Identify ordered number of blood culture sets and select the appropriate blood-collection bottles (at least one anaerobic and one aerobic bottle). If tests are ordered in addition to the blood cultures, collect the blood-culture specimens before other specimens. | |
| ___ | ___ | ___ | 2. Bring necessary equipment to the bedside stand or overbed table. | |
| ___ | ___ | ___ | 3. Perform hand hygiene and put on PPE, if indicated. | |
| ___ | ___ | ___ | 4. Identify the patient. Explain the procedure. Allow the patient time to ask questions and verbalize concerns about the venipuncture procedure. | |
| ___ | ___ | ___ | 5. Close curtains around bed and close the door to the room, if possible. | |
| ___ | ___ | ___ | 6. Check specimen label with the patient's identification bracelet. Label should include patient's name and identification number, time specimen was collected, route of collection, identification of person obtaining the sample, and any other information required by agency policy. | |
| ___ | ___ | ___ | 7. Provide for good light. Artificial light is recommended. Place a trash receptacle within easy reach. | |
| ___ | ___ | ___ | 8. Assist the patient to a comfortable position, either sitting or lying. If the patient is lying in bed, raise the bed to a comfortable working height, usually elbow height of the caregiver (VISN 8 Patient Safety Center, 2009). | |
| ___ | ___ | ___ | 9. Determine the patient's preferred site for the procedure based on his or her previous experience. Expose the arm, supporting it in an extended position on a firm surface, such as a tabletop. Position self on the same side of the patient as the site selected. Apply a tourniquet to the upper arm on the chosen side approximately 3 to 4 inches above the potential puncture site. Apply sufficient pressure to impede venous circulation, but not arterial blood flow. | |
| ___ | ___ | ___ | 10. Put on unsterile gloves. Assess the veins using inspection and palpation to determine the best puncture site. | |

## SKILL 18-10

# Obtaining a Venous Blood Specimen for
# Culture and Sensitivity *(Continued)*

| Excellent | Satisfactory | Needs Practice | | Comments |
|---|---|---|---|---|

| | | | | |
|---|---|---|---|---|
| —— | —— | —— | 11. *Release the tourniquet. Check that the vein has decompressed (Lavery & Ingram, 2005).* | |
| —— | —— | —— | 12. Attach the butterfly needle extension tubing to the Vacutainer device. | |
| —— | —— | —— | 13. Move collection bottles to a location close to arm, with bottles sitting upright on tabletop. | |
| —— | —— | —— | 14. Clean the patient's skin at the selected puncture site with the antimicrobial swab, according to facility policy. If using chlorhexidine, use a back-and-forth motion, applying friction for 30 seconds to the site, or use the procedure recommended by the manufacturer. Allow the site to dry. | |
| —— | —— | —— | 15. Using a new antimicrobial swab, clean the stoppers of the culture bottles with the appropriate antimicrobial, per facility policy. Cover bottle top with sterile gauze square, based on facility policy. | |
| —— | —— | —— | 16. Reapply the tourniquet approximately 3 to 4 inches above the identified puncture site. Apply sufficient pressure to impede venous circulation, but not arterial blood flow. *After disinfection, do not palpate the venipuncture site unless sterile gloves are worn.* | |
| —— | —— | —— | 17. Hold the patient's arm in a downward position with your nondominant hand. Align the butterfly needle with the chosen vein, holding the needle in your dominant hand. Use the thumb or first finger of your nondominant hand to apply pressure and traction to the skin just below the identified puncture site. *Do not touch the insertion site.* | |
| —— | —— | —— | 18. *Inform the patient that he or she is going to feel a pinch.* With the bevel of the needle up, insert the needle into the vein at a 15-degree angle to the skin (Fischbach & Dunning, 2006). You should see a flash of blood in the extension tubing close to the needle when the vein is entered. | |
| —— | —— | —— | 19. Grasp the butterfly needle securely to stabilize it in the vein with your nondominant hand, and push the Vacutainer onto the first collection bottle (anaerobic bottle), until the rubber stopper on the collection bottle is punctured. You will feel the bottle push into place on the puncture device. Blood will flow into the bottle automatically. | |
| —— | —— | —— | 20. *Remove the tourniquet as soon as blood flows adequately into the bottle.* | |

# Obtaining a Venous Blood Specimen for Culture and Sensitivity *(Continued)*

| Excellent | Satisfactory | Needs Practice | | Comments |
|---|---|---|---|---|
| —— | —— | —— | 21. Continue to hold the butterfly needle in place in the vein. Once first bottle is filled, remove it from the Vacutainer and insert the second bottle. After the blood culture specimens are obtained, continue to fill any additional required tubes, removing one and inserting another. Gently rotate each bottle and tube as you remove it. | |
| —— | —— | —— | 22. *After you have drawn all required blood samples, remove the last collection tube from the Vacutainer. Place a gauze pad over the puncture site and slowly and gently remove the needle from the vein. Engage needle guard.* Do not apply pressure to the site until the needle has been fully removed. | |
| —— | —— | —— | 23. Apply gentle pressure to the puncture site for 2 to 3 minutes or until bleeding stops. | |
| —— | —— | —— | 24. After bleeding stops, apply an adhesive bandage. | |
| —— | —— | —— | 25. Remove equipment and return patient to a position of comfort. Raise side rail and lower bed. | |
| —— | —— | —— | 26. Discard Vacutainer and butterfly needle in sharps container. | |
| —— | —— | —— | 27. Remove gloves and perform hand hygiene. | |
| —— | —— | —— | 28. Place label on the container, per facility policy. Place containers in plastic, sealable biohazard bag. Refer to facility policy regarding the need for separate biohazard bags for blood culture specimens and other blood specimens. | |
| —— | —— | —— | 29. Check the venipuncture site to see if a hematoma has developed. | |
| —— | —— | —— | 30. Remove other PPE, if used. Perform hand hygiene. | |
| —— | —— | —— | 31. Transport the specimen to the laboratory immediately. If immediate transport is not possible, check with laboratory personnel or policy manual as to appropriate handling. | |

*Skill Checklists for Taylor's Clinical Nursing Skills:*
*A Nursing Process Approach, 3rd edition*

Name _____     Date _____

Unit _____     Position _____

Instructor/Evaluator: _____     Position _____

---

SKILL 18-11

# Obtaining an Arterial Blood Specimen for Blood Gas Analysis

**Goal:** The blood sample is obtained from the artery without damage to the artery.

| Excellent | Satisfactory | Needs Practice | | Comments |
|---|---|---|---|---|
| ___ | ___ | ___ | 1. Gather the necessary supplies. Check product expiration dates. Identify ordered arterial blood gas analysis. Check the chart to make sure the patient has not been suctioned within the past 15 minutes. Check facility policy and/or procedure for guidelines on administering local anesthesia for arterial punctures. Administer anesthetic and allow sufficient time for full effect before beginning procedure (American Association of Critical Care Nurses [AACN], 2005; Hudson, et al., 2006). | |
| ___ | ___ | ___ | 2. Bring necessary equipment to the bedside stand or overbed table. | |
| ___ | ___ | ___ | 3. Perform hand hygiene and put on PPE, if indicated. | |
| ___ | ___ | ___ | 4. Check the patient's identification and confirm the patient's identity. Tell the patient you need to collect an arterial blood sample, and explain the procedure. Tell the patient that the needlestick will cause some discomfort but that he or she must remain still during the procedure. | |
| ___ | ___ | ___ | 5. Close curtains around bed and close the door to the room, if possible. | |
| ___ | ___ | ___ | 6. Check specimen label with the patient's identification bracelet. Label should include patient's name and identification number, time specimen was collected, route of collection, identification of person obtaining the sample, amount of oxygen the patient is receiving, and any other information required by agency policy. | |
| ___ | ___ | ___ | 7. Provide for good light. Artificial light is recommended. Place a trash receptacle within easy reach. | |
| ___ | ___ | ___ | 8. If the patient is on bed rest, ask him or her to lie in a supine position, with the head slightly elevated and the arms at the sides. Ask the ambulatory patient to sit in a chair and support the arm securely on an armrest or a table. Place a waterproof pad under the site and a rolled towel under the wrist. | |

# Obtaining an Arterial Blood Specimen for Blood Gas Analysis (Continued)

| Excellent | Satisfactory | Needs Practice | | Comments |
|---|---|---|---|---|
| —— | —— | —— | 9. *Perform Allen's test before obtaining a specimen from the radial artery:* | |
| —— | —— | —— | a. Have the patient clench the wrist to minimize blood flow into the hand. | |
| —— | —— | —— | b. Using your index and middle fingers, press on the radial and ulnar arteries. Hold this position for a few seconds. | |
| —— | —— | —— | c. Without removing your fingers from the arteries, ask the patient to unclench the fist and hold the hand in a relaxed position. The palm will be blanched because pressure from your fingers has impaired the normal blood flow. | |
| —— | —— | —— | d. Release pressure on the ulnar artery. If the hand becomes flushed, which indicates that blood is filling the vessels, it is safe to proceed with the radial artery puncture. This is considered a positive test. If the hand does not flush, perform the test on the other arm. | |
| —— | —— | —— | 10. Put on unsterile gloves. Locate the radial artery and lightly palpate it for a strong pulse. | |
| —— | —— | —— | 11. Clean the site with the antimicrobial swab. If using chlorhexidine, use a back-and-forth motion, applying friction for 30 seconds to the site, or use the procedure recommended by the manufacturer. Allow the site to dry. *After disinfection, do not palpate the site unless sterile gloves are worn.* | |
| —— | —— | —— | 12. Stabilize the hand with the wrist extended over the rolled towel, palm up. Palpate the artery above the puncture site with the index and middle fingers of your nondominant hand while holding the syringe over the puncture site with your dominant hand. *Do not directly touch the area to be punctured.* | |
| —— | —— | —— | 13. Hold the needle bevel up at a 45-degree angle at the site of maximal pulse impulse, with the shaft parallel to the path of the artery. (When puncturing the brachial artery, hold the needle at a 60-degree angle.) | |
| —— | —— | —— | 14. Puncture the skin and arterial wall in one motion. Watch for blood backflow in the syringe. The pulsating blood will flow into the syringe. Do not pull back on the plunger. Fill the syringe to the 5-mL mark. | |

**Excellent**

**Satisfactory**

**Needs Practice**

SKILL 18-11

# Obtaining an Arterial Blood Specimen for
# Blood Gas Analysis *(Continued)*

**Comments**

——  ——  ——  15. After collecting the sample, withdraw the syringe while your nondominant hand is beginning to place pressure proximal to the insertion site with the 2 × 2 gauze. Press a gauze pad firmly over the puncture site until the bleeding stops—at least 5 minutes. *If the patient is receiving anticoagulant therapy or has a blood dyscrasia, apply pressure for 10 to 15 minutes; if necessary, ask a coworker to hold the gauze pad in place while you prepare the sample for transport to the laboratory, but do not ask the patient to hold the pad.*

——  ——  ——  16. When the bleeding stops and the appropriate time has lapsed, apply a small adhesive bandage or small pressure dressing (fold a 2 × 2 gauze into fourths and firmly apply tape, stretching the skin tight).

——  ——  ——  17. Once the sample is obtained, check the syringe for air bubbles. If any appear, remove them by holding the syringe upright and slowly ejecting some of the blood onto a 2 × 2 gauze pad.

——  ——  ——  18. Engage the needle guard and remove the needle. Place the airtight cap on the syringe. Gently rotate the syringe to ensure that heparin is well distributed. Do not shake. Insert the syringe into a cup or bag of ice.

——  ——  ——  19. Place label on the syringe per facility policy. Place iced syringe in plastic, sealable biohazard bag.

——  ——  ——  20. Discard the needle in sharps container. Remove gloves and perform hand hygiene.

——  ——  ——  21. Remove other PPE, if used. Perform hand hygiene.

——  ——  ——  22. Transport the specimen to the laboratory immediately.